Rhinosinusitis

Editor

SANDRA Y. LIN

IMMUNOLOGY AND ALLERGY CLINICS OF NORTH AMERICA

www.immunology.theclinics.com

Consulting Editor
LINDA S. COX

May 2020 • Volume 40 • Number 2

ELSEVIER

1600 John F. Kennedy Boulevard • Suite 1800 • Philadelphia, Pennsylvania, 19103-2899

http://www.theclinics.com

IMMUNOLOGY AND ALLERGY CLINICS OF NORTH AMERICA Volume 40, Number 2

May 2020 ISSN 0889-8561, ISBN-13: 978-0-323-75814-7

Editor: Katerina Heidhausen

Developmental Editor: Kristen Helm

Immunology and Allergy Clinics of North America (ISSN 0889–8561) is published quarterly by Elsevier Inc., 360 Park Avenue South, New York, NY 10010-1710. Months of issue are February, May, August, and November. Periodicals postage paid at New York, NY and additional mailing offices. Subscription prices are $344.00 per year for US individuals, $623.00 per year for US institutions, $100.00 per year for US students and residents, $423.00 per year for Canadian individuals, $100.00 per year for Canadian students, $791.00 per year for Canadian institutions, $447.00 per year for international individuals, $791.00 per year for international institutions, $220.00 per year for international students. To receive student/resident rate, orders must be accompanied by name of affiliated institution, date of term, and the *signature* of program/residency coordinator on institution letterhead. Orders will be billed at individual rate until proof of status is received. Foreign air speed delivery is included in all *Clinics* subscription prices. All prices are subject to change without notice. **POSTMASTER**: Send address changes to *Immunology and Allergy Clinics of North America*, Elsevier Health Sciences Division, Subscription Customer Service, 3251 Riverport Lane, Maryland Heights, MO 63043. **Customer Service: 1-800-654-2452 (U.S. and Canada); 314-447-8871 (outside U.S. and Canada). Fax: 314-447-8029. E-mail: journalscustomerservice-usa@elsevier.com (for print support); journalsonlinesupport-usa@elsevier.com (for online support).**

Reprints. For copies of 100 or more, of articles in this publication, please contact the Commercial Reprints Department, Elsevier Inc., 360 Park Avenue South, New York, New York 10010-1710. Tel. 212-633-3874, Fax: 212-633-3820, E-mail: reprints@elsevier.com.

Immunology and Allergy Clinics of North America is covered in MEDLINE/PubMed (Index Medicus), Current Contents/Life Sciences, Science Citation Index, ISI/BIOMED, Chemical Abstracts, and EMBASE/Excerpta Medica.

Contributors

CONSULTING EDITOR

LINDA S. COX, MD, FACP, AAAAI
Department of Medicine and Dermatology, Nova Southeastern University, Casper, Wyoming

EDITOR

SANDRA Y. LIN, MD
Professor and Vice Director, Johns Hopkins Department of Otolaryngology–Head and Neck Surgery, Johns Hopkins School of Medicine, Baltimore, Maryland

AUTHORS

OMAR G. AHMED, MD
Rhinology Fellow, Department of Otolaryngology–Head and Neck Surgery, The Johns Hopkins Hospital, Baltimore, Maryland

JEREMIAH A. ALT, MD, PhD
Associate Professor, Division of Otolaryngology–Head and Neck Surgery, University of Utah, Salt Lake City, Utah

EMILY BARROW, MD
Department of Otolaryngology, Emory University, Medical Office Tower (MOT), Atlanta, Georgia

ASHLEY M. BAUER, MD
Instructor, Department of Otolaryngology–Head and Neck Surgery, Vanderbilt University Medical Center, Nashville, Tennessee

DANIEL M. BESWICK, MD
Department of Otolaryngology–Head and Neck Surgery, University of Colorado, Aurora, Colorado

DO-YEON CHO, MD
Department of Otolaryngology–Head and Neck Surgery, Gregory Fleming James Cystic Fibrosis Research Center, The University of Alabama at Birmingham, Birmingham, Alabama

NAWEED CHOWDHURY, MD
Department of Otolaryngology–Head and Neck Surgery, Vanderbilt University Medical Center, Vanderbilt University, Nashville, Tennessee

JOHN M. DELGAUDIO, MD
Department of Otolaryngology, Emory University, Medical Office Tower (MOT), Atlanta, Georgia

THOMAS EDWARDS, MD
Department of Otolaryngology, Emory University, Medical Office Tower (MOT), Atlanta, Georgia

CHRISTINE B. FRANZESE, MD
Professor of Clinical Otolaryngology, Director of Allergy, Department of Otolaryngology–Head and Neck Surgery, University of Missouri, Columbia, Missouri

ASHLEIGH A. HALDERMAN, MD
Assistant Professor, Department of Otolaryngology–Head and Neck Surgery, The University of Texas Southwestern Medical Center, Dallas, Texas

SAMUEL N. HELMAN, MD
Department of Otolaryngology, Emory University, Medical Office Tower (MOT), Atlanta, Georgia

RYAN C. HUNTER, PhD
Department of Microbiology and Immunology, University of Minnesota, Minneapolis, Minnesota

CAMILLE HUWYLER, MD
Department of Head and Neck Surgery, Kaiser Permanente Oakland Medical Center, Oakland, California

KATHLEEN M. KELLY, MD
Department of Otolaryngology–Head and Neck Surgery, The University of Texas Southwestern Medical Center, Dallas, Texas

STELLA E. LEE, MD
University of Pittsburgh School of Medicine, Department of Otolaryngology–Head and Neck Surgery, University of Pittsburgh Medical Center, Pittsburgh, Pennsylvania

VICTORIA S. LEE, MD
Department of Otolaryngology–Head and Neck Surgery, The University of Illinois at Chicago, Chicago, Illinois

KATHERINE A. LEES, MD
Instructor, Division of Otolaryngology–Head and Neck Surgery, University of Utah, Salt Lake City, Utah

JOSHUA M. LEVY, MD, MPH
Department of Otolaryngology, Emory University, Medical Office Tower (MOT), Atlanta, Georgia

JONATHAN LIANG, MD
Department of Head and Neck Surgery, Kaiser Permanente Oakland Medical Center, Rhinology and Endoscopic Skull Base Surgery, Oakland, California

SANDRA Y. LIN, MD
Professor and Vice Director, Johns Hopkins Department of Otolaryngology–Head and Neck Surgery, Johns Hopkins School of Medicine, Baltimore, Maryland

AMBER U. LUONG, MD, PhD
Associate Professor, Department of Otorhinolaryngology–Head and Neck Surgery, McGovern Medical School, The University of Texas Health Science Center at Houston,

Texas Sinus Institute, Center for Immunology and Autoimmune Diseases, Institute of Molecular Medicine, Houston, Texas

KATHLEEN LUSKIN, MD
Fellow, Allergy-Immunology, Scripps Health, Scripps Clinic Carmel Valley, San Diego, California

LEILA J. MADY, MD, PhD, MPH
Department of Otolaryngology–Head and Neck Surgery, University of Pittsburgh Medical Center, Pittsburgh, Pennsylvania

HILLARY A. NEWSOME, MD
Rhinology and Skull Base Division, Department of Otolaryngology and Communication Sciences, Medical College of Wisconsin, Zablocki VAMC, Milwaukee, Wisconsin

GRETCHEN OAKLEY, MD
Assistant Professor, Division of Otolaryngology–Head and Neck Surgery, University of Utah, Salt Lake City, Utah

SOMTOCHI OKAFOR, BA
Department of Otolaryngology–Head and Neck Surgery, The University of Texas Southwestern Medical Center, Dallas, Texas

RICHARD R. ORLANDI, MD
Professor, Division of Otolaryngology–Head and Neck Surgery, University of Utah, Salt Lake City, Utah

DAVID M. POETKER, MD
Professor and Chief, Rhinology and Skull Base Division, Department of Otolaryngology and Communication Sciences, Medical College of Wisconsin, Zablocki VAMC, Milwaukee, Wisconsin

VIJAY R. RAMAKRISHNAN, MD
Department of Otolaryngology–Head and Neck Surgery, University of Colorado, Aurora, Colorado

NICHOLAS R. ROWAN, MD
Assistant Professor, Department of Otolaryngology–Head and Neck Surgery, The Johns Hopkins Hospital, Baltimore, Maryland

HANNAH L. SCHWARZBACH, BA
University of Pittsburgh School of Medicine, Pittsburgh, Pennsylvania

TIMOTHY L. SMITH, MD, MPH
Department of Otolaryngology–Head and Neck Surgery, Oregon Health & Science University, Portland, Oregon

HIRAL THAKRAR, MD
Fellow, Allergy-Immunology, Scripps Health, Scripps Clinic Carmel Valley, San Diego, California

JUSTIN H. TURNER, MD, PhD
Associate Professor, Department of Otolaryngology–Head and Neck Surgery, Vanderbilt University Medical Center, Nashville, Tennessee

MATTHEW A. TYLER, MD
Assistant Professor, Department of Otolaryngology–Head and Neck Surgery, University of Minnesota Medical School, Minneapolis, Minnesota

ANDREW WHITE, MD
Faculty, Allergy-Immunology, Scripps Health, Scripps Clinic Carmel Valley, San Diego, California

SARAH K. WISE, MD, MSCR
Department of Otolaryngology, Emory University, Medical Office Tower (MOT), Atlanta, Georgia

Contents

Foreword: Rhinosinusitis Diagnosis and Management: The Hoops and Hurdles xiii

Linda S. Cox

Preface: Chronic Rhinosinusitis: An Evolution of Knowledge xvii

Sandra Y. Lin

The Role of Allergic Rhinitis in Chronic Rhinosinusitis 201

Samuel N. Helman, Emily Barrow, Thomas Edwards, John M. DelGaudio, Joshua M. Levy, and Sarah K. Wise

> This literature review collates and summarizes recent literature to explore the relationship between chronic rhinosinusitis (CRS) and allergy. The relationship between CRS and allergy is not fully understood. However, current evidence suggests a relationship between allergy and specific endotypes of CRS with nasal polyposis, including allergic fungal rhinosinusitis and central compartment atopic disease. Specific endotypes of CRS with nasal polyps seem to have an association with allergy. More evidence is necessary to better characterize this relationship. Level of evidence: 5.

What is the Role of Air Pollution in Chronic Rhinosinusitis? 215

Hannah L. Schwarzbach, Leila J. Mady, and Stella E. Lee

> Chronic rhinosinusitis (CRS) is a heterogeneous inflammatory disorder, and several environmental factors may be contributing to disease pathophysiology, including air pollutants. Tobacco smoke and occupational exposures also have been associated with CRS, and environmental exposures may contribute to the variability seen in disease endotype. Animal models that investigate the potential of air pollutants to induce chronic inflammation provide further insight into plausible triggers and modifiers of disease, including contributions to barrier disruption, alterations in the microbiome, and immune dysfunction. Additional studies are needed to further elucidate the role of environmental exposures on CRS pathophysiology and patient outcomes.

Olfactory Dysfunction and Chronic Rhinosinusitis 223

Omar G. Ahmed and Nicholas R. Rowan

> Olfactory dysfunction (OD) is one of the cardinal symptoms of chronic rhinosinusitis (CRS), and its prevalence ranges from 60% to 80% in patients with CRS. It is much more common in CRS with nasal polyposis patients compared to CRS without nasal polyposis. Decreased olfactory function is associated with significant decreases in patient-reported quality of life (QOL), and notably, depression and the enjoyment of food. Objective measures can help detail the degree of OD, whereas subjective measures can help to determine in the impact on patient. There is variable treatment response to OD with both medical and surgical therapies.

Primary Immunodeficiency and Rhinosinusitis   233

Camille Huwyler, Sandra Y. Lin, and Jonathan Liang

Refractory rhinosinusitis can be related to comorbid medical conditions, including primary immunodeficiency. Given the prevalence of immunodeficiency, clinicians should have a low threshold to consider these diagnoses. This article reviews primary immunodeficiencies contributing to chronic rhinosinusitis, including a proposed diagnostic work-up and the evidence for treatment in this unique population.

The Microbiome and Chronic Rhinosinusitis   251

Do-Yeon Cho, Ryan C. Hunter, and Vijay R. Ramakrishnan

Chronic rhinosinusitis (CRS) is persistent inflammation and/or infection of the nasal cavity and paranasal sinuses. Recent advancements in culture-independent molecular techniques have enhanced understanding of interactions between sinus microbiota and upper airway microenvironment. The dysbiosis hypothesis—alteration of microbiota associated with perturbation of the local ecological landscape—is suggested as a mechanism involved in CRS pathogenesis. This review discusses the complex role of the microbiota in health and in CRS and considerations in sinus microbiome investigation, dysbiosis of sinus microbiota in CRS, microbial interactions in CRS, and development of preclinical models. The authors conclude with future directions for CRS-associated microbiome research.

Measuring Success in the Treatment of Patients with Chronic Rhinosinusitis   265

Naweed Chowdhury, Timothy L. Smith, and Daniel M. Beswick

Chronic rhinosinusitis (CRS) has a substantial impact on patients' quality of life (QOL). Among the many metrics available for measuring treatment success in CRS, patient-reported outcome measures that quantify changes in QOL are the most widely used methods. In addition, objective data from imaging, endoscopy, and olfactory testing are useful adjunct measures to diagnose and prevent progression of disease, although these metrics have mixed correlations with symptoms and QOL. In the future, molecular biology, and multiomics techniques may change how successful CRS treatment is defined.

**Personalized Medicine in Chronic Rhinosinusitis: Phenotypes, Endotypes, and
Biomarkers**   281

Ashley M. Bauer and Justin H. Turner

Chronic rhinosinusitis (CRS) is a heterogeneous disease process with a complex underlying cause. Improved understanding of CRS pathophysiology has facilitated new approaches to management of the patient with CRS that rely on targeting patient-specific characteristics and individual inflammatory pathways. A more personalized approach to care will ultimately incorporate a combination of phenotypic and endotypic classification systems to guide treatment. This review summarizes current evidence with respect to CRS phenotypes and endotypes, as well as the identification of potential biomarkers with potential to guide current and future treatment algorithms.

The Role of Biologics in the Treatment of Nasal Polyps 295

Christine B. Franzese

Chronic rhinosinusitis with nasal polyps (CRSwNP) is a heteromorphic disease with both medical and surgical aspects to its treatment. CRSwNP is a chronic inflammatory condition with exacerbations that can be controlled through surgical and/or medical interventions, including biological agents. The role of biological agents in the treatment of CRSwNP as well as the patient characteristics that make suitable candidates for biologics are discussed.

The Role of Macrolides and Doxycycline in Chronic Rhinosinusitis 303

Katherine A. Lees, Richard R. Orlandi, Gretchen Oakley, and Jeremiah A. Alt

Antibiotic therapy has become an important adjunct in the management of recalcitrant chronic rhinosinusitis (CRS) because of some antibiotics' immunomodulatory properties even at subtherapeutic antimicrobial levels. Macrolide antibiotics, such as clarithromycin and azithromycin, decrease production of proinflammatory cytokines, impair neutrophil recruitment, inhibit bacterial biofilm formation, and improve mucus quality. Doxycycline, a tetracycline antibiotic, inhibits the activity of matrix metalloproteinases in CRS with nasal polyposis. This article reviews the clinical applications for macrolide and doxycycline use in CRS, considerations for dosing and duration of treatment, and important side effects and drug interactions associated with these medications.

Topical Irrigations for Chronic Rhinosinusitis 317

Victoria S. Lee

As the understanding of the primary cause of chronic rhinosinusitis has shifted away from infection toward inflammation, topical corticosteroid sprays and saline irrigations have become mainstays of treatment. Topical corticosteroid irrigations are recommended particularly in the postoperative setting, but further research on their effect and possible hypothalamic-pituitary-adrenal axis suppression is needed. The popularity of topical antibiotics has subsequently waned with their use reserved for recalcitrant cases. Further research is needed on the effect of topical antifungals in allergic fungal rhinosinusitis. Topical alternative therapies that target biofilms have gained increasing recognition, and investigations on topical probiotics are on the horizon.

Nasal Polyposis and Aspirin-Exacerbated Respiratory Disease 329

Kathleen Luskin, Hiral Thakrar, and Andrew White

Aspirin-exacerbated respiratory disease (AERD) is characterized by eosinophilic chronic rhinosinusitis with nasal polyps, asthma, and upper-/lower-respiratory tract reactions to nonsteroidal antiinflammatory drugs. Persistent, severe disease, anosmia, and alcohol sensitivity is typical. AERD is mediated by multiple pathways, including aberrant arachidonic acid metabolism leading to elevated leukotriene E4 and decreased prostaglandin E2. Mast cell mediators (prostaglandin D2) and unique properties of eosinophils and type 2 innate lymphoid cells, along with receptor-mediated signaling, also contribute to AERD pathogenesis. Pharmacologic therapies are a cornerstone of AERD treatment and include leukotriene modifiers, corticosteroids, biologics, and aspirin.

Current Concepts in the Management of Allergic Fungal Rhinosinusitis   345

Matthew A. Tyler and Amber U. Luong

Allergic fungal rhinosinusitis (AFRS) represents a subtype of chronic rhinosinusitis with nasal polyposis that exhibits a unique, often striking clinical presentation. Since its initial description more than a quarter century ago, a more sophisticated understanding of the pathophysiology of AFRS has been achieved and significant advancements in improving clinical outcomes made. This review focuses on the latest developments involving the pathophysiology and clinical management of this fascinating disease.

Odontogenic Sinusitis: Current Concepts in Diagnosis and Treatment   361

Hillary A. Newsome and David M. Poetker

Odontogenic sinusitis is a unique cause of sinus disease that deserves special consideration. An astute clinician can elicit historical findings such as recent dental work, and symptoms such as unilateral facial pain and foul drainage, despite a relatively benign oral cavity examination. Otolaryngologists and dental professionals who care for these patients must be able to interpret imaging studies for dental disorder such as periapical abscesses and periodontal disease. Treatment is frequently some combination of antibiotic therapy, dental procedures, and endoscopic sinus surgery. More prospective studies are needed to determine the best approach to caring for this patient population.

Management of Sinusitis in the Cystic Fibrosis Patient   371

Somtochi Okafor, Kathleen M. Kelly, and Ashleigh A. Halderman

Chronic rhinosinusitis (CRS) is present in up to 100% of patients with cystic fibrosis (CF). CF-associated CRS is particularly recalcitrant, and sinus disease can have important implications in the health of the lower airways and overall quality of life in these patients. Both medical and surgical management play important roles in treating CF-associated CRS, but guidelines are lacking. This review summarizes the current literature on both medical and surgical management of this disease to provide an up-to-date analysis and recommendations on the treatment of CF-associated CRS.

IMMUNOLOGY AND ALLERGY CLINICS OF NORTH AMERICA

FORTHCOMING ISSUES

August 2020
Immunodeficiencies
Mark Ballow and Elena Perez, *Editors*

November 2020
Biologics for the Treatments of Allergic Conditions
Lanny J. Rosenwasser, *Editor*

February 2021
Climate Change and Allergy
Jae Won Oh, *Editor*

RECENT ISSUES

February 2020
Update on Immunotherapy for Aeroallergens, Foods, and Venoms
Linda S. Cox and Anna Nowak-Wegrzyn, *Editors*

November 2019
Pediatric Allergy
David R. Stukus, *Editor*

August 2019
Infections and Asthma
Mitchell H. Grayson, *Editor*

SERIES OF RELATED INTEREST

Otolaryngologic Clinics of North America
Available at: https://www.oto.theclinics.com/

THE CLINICS ARE AVAILABLE ONLINE!
Access your subscription at:
www.theclinics.com

Foreword

Rhinosinusitis Diagnosis and Management: The Hoops and Hurdles

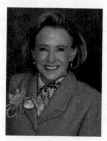

Linda S. Cox, MD, FACP, AAAAI
Consulting Editor

In my nearly 3 decades of clinical practice as an allergist/immunologist, I can think of no other condition more difficult and frustrating than chronic rhinosinusitis (CRS). Most of my CRS patients were refractory to treatment. At times, in frustration, I would "throw the kitchen sink at them" (ie, oral corticosteroids, topical and oral antibiotics, topical antifungal agents) to try to improve their quality of life. There are several reasons CRS diagnosis and management are so challenging. CRS is a complex, heterogeneous disease with several subgroups (also known as endotypes), which are defined by biomarkers that reflect their biological mechanism. As CRS endotypes may vary in their response to a specific agent, proper classification is important for determining optimal treatment. This foreword reviews the "hoops and hurdles" that a clinician must navigate to properly diagnose and effectively treat CRS.

The term rhinosinusitis infers an inflammatory process involving the sinus and passageways. It is a relatively recent term that was introduced because the majority of persons with chronic sinusitis had concurrent nasal disease. There is no billable *International Classification of Diseases, Tenth Revision (ICD-10)* code for acute or chronic rhinosinusitis. Several *ICD-10* codes are generally used to bill for CRS services. This may be partly because there is no uniform definition of CRS. The Rhinosinusitis and Nasal Polyps expert committee position paper proposed the following definition for CRS: "rhinosinusitis is defined as inflammation of the nose and the paranasal sinuses characterized by 2 or more symptoms, one of which should be either nasal blockage/obstruction or nasal discharge (anterior/posterior nasal drip)" for 12 weeks or longer.[1] The US practice guidelines on rhinosinusitis offered a less specific definition: "rhinosinusitis, defined as inflammation of at least 1 paranasal sinus, is characterized as acute when lasting shorter than 12 weeks and chronic when lasting at

Immunol Allergy Clin N Am 40 (2020) xiii–xv
https://doi.org/10.1016/j.iac.2020.02.002
0889-8561/20/© 2020 Published by Elsevier Inc.

least 12 weeks."[2] The problem with these definitions is that they are based largely on patient symptoms. CRS is a complex disease with several variants, which can be classified according to clinical features (phenotype) or biomarkers (endotype).[1] The presence or absence of nasal polyps (NP) defines the 2 most common CRS phenotypes in "primary" CRS (see Ashley M. Bauer and Justin H. Turner's article, "Personalized Medicine in Chronic Rhinosinusitis: Phenotypes, Endotypes, and Biomarkers," in this issue). Phenotype classification system does not account for the various biological mechanisms that have been identified in different CRS subgroups. Endotype classification is based on biomarkers that reflect biological mechanisms, such as eosinophilia, neutrophilic mediators, cytokine production, T-cell markers, and interferon-gamma. Endotype-based CRS management should result in a more personalized approach to CRS management and aid in treatment-related decisions, such as who is the best candidate for surgery, corticosteroids, antibiotics, or biologics. CRS endotype classification is a relatively new phenomenon. More research is needed to establish the predictive utility of CRS biomarkers in terms of optimal treatment and disease progression. The diagnosis of "primary" CRS requires consideration of other medical conditions or factors that impact nasal/sinus mucosal defense mechanisms (eg, immune deficiencies, autoimmune, vasculitis, immotile-cilia syndrome, sinus surgery, and cystic fibrosis; see Huwyler C, Lin SY, Liang J: Primary Immunodeficiency and Rhinosinusitis, and Okafor S, Kelly KM, Halderman AA: Management of Sinusitis in the Cystic Fibrosis Patient, in this issue).

Confirmation of CRS diagnosis can be challenging for several reasons. There are no pathognomonic signs or symptoms that definitively confirm or exclude the diagnosis,[2] nor are there any diagnostic tests that definitely confirm a specific CRS endotype. Sinus CT imaging can confirm the presence of sinus inflammation, but it generally cannot distinguish between a chronic or an acute process. Although Air-fluid levels may suggest an acute process, this finding can be seen after nasal irrigation, In addition, the resolution of infection-related inflammation on CT imaging may lag significantly after clinical resolution. Allergy testing only confirms the presence of allergen-specific immunoglobulin E. The clinician must determine the relevance of the positive allergy tests in terms of the patient's CRS. Some tests may only be available at specialized centers (eg, nasal secretion analysis for cytokines, cellularity, mediators, and nasal mucosa biopsy for cilia function or local production of immunoglobulin E). The lack of test availability poses a significant barrier to making the correct CRS endotype diagnosis.

In my opinion, the greatest challenge in CRS management is determining the best treatment approach for each patient. Ideally, the treatment plan should be evidence based and "personalized" per the patient's endotype. To warrant a "high-grade" or strong recommendation in a practice guideline, a treatment must have demonstrated efficacy in a systematic review, randomized, controlled clinical trial. Large randomized, controlled clinical trials are expensive and time consuming but a requirement for regulatory authority approval. Unfortunately, few CRS treatment interventions have not been this extensively studied. Thus, the evidence supporting many CRS interventions is largely empiric. For example, there is little evidence supporting the efficacy of topical corticosteroids, nasal saline irrigation, or oral or topical antibiotics in CRS management, but many clinicians prescribe them, likely because they recognize that the lack of evidence does not necessarily prove lack of efficacy. It may be due to lack of published studies. My primary frustration with CRS treatment is not the paucity of published evidence, but the limited effectiveness of the available treatments. The good news is there has been a breakthrough in CRS treatment with the Food and Drug Administration approval of the biologic, dupilumab, for NP. Several other biologics have completed phase 3 trials, and more biologics for CRS treatment may soon be available (see Franzese CB: The Role of Biologics in the Treatment of Nasal Polyps, in this issue).

Once a clinician has successfully navigated the "hoops and hurdles" of CRS diagnosis and management, there remains one last "hurdle": how should treatment success be measured and monitored (see Chowdhury N, Smith TL, Beswick DM: Measuring Success in the Treatment of Patients with Chronic Rhinosinusitis, in this issue)? This "hurdle" poses several questions. Is there a single test or tool that best reflects treatment success or failure? Should treatment success be based on the following:

- Composite or a single outcome(s) or
- Objective (eg, CT scan, nasal endoscopy) versus subjective (SNOT-22 and other quality of life questionnaires)?

This issue of *Immunology and Allergy Clinics of North America*, masterfully orchestrated by Sandra Lin, provides more in-depth and up-to-date information about the topics discussed in this foreword. In addition, this issue reviews the role of the microbiome and role of air pollution in CRS, the role of doxycycline and macrolides, and nasal irrigations in the treatment of CRS. Other topics reviewed in this issue are primary immunodeficiency, allergic fungal sinusitis, nasal polyposis and aspirin-exacerbated respiratory disease, olfactory dysfunction, odontogenic sinusitis, and cystic fibrosis. Each article has key points and a synopsis, which nicely summarize the article's important points and findings. This issue should be read cover to cover as it provides valuable information for clinicians navigating the "hoops and hurdles" of proper diagnosis and management of CRS.

Linda S. Cox, MD, FACP, AAAAI
Department of Medicine and Dermatology
1108 South Wolcott Street
Casper, WY 82601, USA

E-mail address:
lindaswolfcox@msn.com

REFERENCES

1. Akdis CA, Bachert C, Cingi C, et al. Endotypes and phenotypes of chronic rhinosinusitis: a PRACTALL document of the European Academy of Allergy and Clinical Immunology and the American Academy of Allergy, Asthma and Immunology. J Allergy Clin Immunol 2013;131(6):1479–90.
2. Peters AT, Spector S, Hsu J, et al. Diagnosis and management of rhinosinusitis: a practice parameter update. Ann Allergy Asthma Immunol 2014;113(4):347–85.

Preface
Chronic Rhinosinusitis: An Evolution of Knowledge

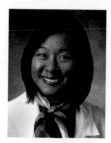

Sandra Y. Lin, MD
Editor

Chronic rhinosinusitis (CRS) is a common medical problem, frequently seen by those in primary care, allergy, and otolaryngology. Our understanding of chronic sinusitis is continuously evolving, with some recent substantial advancements in the knowledge of the pathophysiology of CRS and new treatment options. For example, there is a greater understanding of how the environment, through allergic rhinitis, air pollution, and the patient's own microbiome, may play a role in the development of CRS. The recognition of CRS as an inflammatory disease state has been further refined, but trying to define the disease in terms of phenotype, endotype, and biomarkers (a better understanding particularly of endotypes and biomarkers) will, it is hoped, allow for future refinement of treatment into a personalized approach for each patient. One of the newest breakthroughs in CRS treatment is the recent Food and Drug Administration approval of a biologic agent specifically indicated for the treatment of nasal polyps (dupilumab), but questions remain about what roles biologics should play in the treatment algorithm and which are the ideal patients to be treated with a biologic for nasal polyps. The understanding of different types of CRS inflammation has led to the recognition that certain patients with non-steroid-responsive inflammation may benefit from the anti-inflammatory effects of macrolides or doxycycline as a treatment regimen. There is continued interest in how to deliver treatment for CRS topically, with topical steroid irrigations becoming a mainstay of treatment prescribed by many physicians. There are also several subsets of chronic sinusitis patients that present unique diagnostic and treatment challenges that are discussed in this issue. Patients with nasal polyps and aspirin-exacerbated respiratory disease frequently have difficult-to-control asthma and nasal polyps that often recur quickly after surgery, a frustrating situation for both the patient and the physician. Similarly, patients with allergic fungal sinusitis may present with massive polyposis and must be correctly diagnosed and managed to optimize the chance for resolution of the disease. The authors of the articles in

Immunol Allergy Clin N Am 40 (2020) xvii–xviii
https://doi.org/10.1016/j.iac.2020.02.001
0889-8561/20/© 2020 Published by Elsevier Inc.

immunology.theclinics.com

this issue present the most up-to-date concepts on the above topics (and more!), touching on recent interesting topics and developments in our understanding of CRS.

Sandra Y. Lin, MD
Johns Hopkins Department of Otolaryngology–
Head & Neck Surgery
Johns Hopkins Outpatient Center
601 North Caroline Street, #6223
Baltimore, MD 21287, USA

E-mail address:
Slin30@jhmi.edu

The Role of Allergic Rhinitis in Chronic Rhinosinusitis

Samuel N. Helman, MD, Emily Barrow, MD, Thomas Edwards, MD, John M. DelGaudio, MD, Joshua M. Levy, MD, MPH, Sarah K. Wise, MD, MSCR*

KEYWORDS

- Allergy • Atopy • Allergic rhinitis • Chronic rhinosinusitis • Nasal polyposis
- Sinusitis

KEY POINTS

- There is limited evidence linking allergic rhinitis (AR) and chronic rhinosinusitis in general; however, certain endotypes of chronic rhinosinusitis with nasal polyps (CRSwNP) may be better linked.
- The hypersensitivity reactions of AR and the cytokine pathways of some CRSwNP subtypes are both subserved by a type 2 inflammatory response involving eosinophils and interleukins 4, 5, and 13, among others.
- Intranasal allergens may not penetrate the paranasal sinuses, but instead exert their effects indirectly by means of downstream, systemic factors that then feedback to the sinuses.
- Allergic fungal rhinosinusitis and the newly characterized central compartment atopic disease have immunologic differences from other types of CRS, and may be most related to AR.

INTRODUCTION

Allergic rhinitis (AR) is an inflammatory condition mediated by IgE pathways. It is a disease characterized by nasal obstruction, nasal itching, nasal discharge, and sneezing. Although AR may exist in isolation, rhinitis theoretically may worsen chronic rhinosinusitis (CRS) by adding more fuel to the inflammatory milieu. CRS has been defined as lasting 12 weeks or more and is characterized by nasal discharge, nasal obstruction, hyposmia, or anosmia, and facial pressure. CRS is diagnosed with the support of computed tomography (CT) or endoscopic findings of inflammation, polyps, or active infection.[1,2]

CRS, such as AR, is an inflammatory process with an indolent course. Chronic rhinosinusitis is frequently parsed into 2 phenotypic groups, namely CRS with nasal polyps

Department of Otolaryngology, Emory University, Medical Office Tower (MOT), 11th Floor, 550 Peachtree Street Northeast, Atlanta, GA 30308, USA
* Corresponding author. Department of Otolaryngology-Head and Neck Surgery, Emory University, MOT, 11th Floor, 550 Peachtree Street, Atlanta, GA 30308.
E-mail address: skmille@emory.edu

Immunol Allergy Clin N Am 40 (2020) 201–214
https://doi.org/10.1016/j.iac.2019.12.010
0889-8561/20/© 2019 Elsevier Inc. All rights reserved.
immunology.theclinics.com

(CRSwNP) and CRS without nasal polyps (CRSsNP). The mechanism behind CRS is multifactorial, and increasing evidence has mounted to suggest inflammation as a common manifestation of this disease process. Generally speaking, local tissue aberrations, such as epithelial tissue hypersensitivity, disruptions of innate immunity, the presence of bacterial colonization and biofilm, and genetic and environmental factors may all play a role in disease pathogenesis. CRSwNP and CRSsNP paint the disease process in broad strokes, however, and recent data suggest that there are discrete endotypes within these categories that better refine treatment and management strategies.[3] Nonetheless, inflammation serves as a common denominator for these seemingly disparate causes of sinusitis. Therefore, it is reasonable that allergy may produce or exacerbate CRS. However, data are conflicting when analyzing this relationship, particularly when patients are placed into broad phenotypic categories, such as CRSsNP and CWRwNP.[4]

Better evidence exists when looking at the relationship between AR and specific CRS subtypes, such as allergic fungal rhinosinusitis (AFRS) and the newly characterized central compartment atopic disease (CCAD). This article focuses on the confluence of these entities, with attention to the symptoms that characterize this phenomenon, the mechanism by which they synergize, and suggestions for the management of these patients. Special attention will be placed on CCAD, which lends itself well to characterize the synergistic relationship of allergy and CRS.

EPIDEMIOLOGY AND RISK FACTORS
Epidemiology

Allergic rhinitis is a common pathologic condition, with an estimated prevalence of 10% to 40% of adults worldwide, and 5% to 22% in the United States.[5,6] The prevalence of AR peaks in childhood and adolescence, and troughs in the elderly. Allergic rhinitis is most frequently triggered by trees, grasses, or weeds for seasonal AR and by dust mites or mold for perennial AR.[6] CRS is a common and costly disease process, affecting 5% of the United States populace, or approximately 31 million patients, and costs an estimated $8.6 billion per annum.[7,8] Allergic rhinitis is also costly, with estimates of $5.9 to $7.9 billion for direct patient care and upward of $3.4 billion in indirect costs (work/school absenteeism) in the treatment of this disease.[6,9]

PATHOPHYSIOLOGY

Allergy is a hypersensitivity to an antigen that yields reproducible symptoms at a dose that is otherwise tolerated by nonallergic individuals. In the case of AR, nasal allergy is the result of an allergen-specific IgE. Chronic rhinosinusitis *without* nasal polyposis and CRSwNP can be broadly differentiated based on the different cytokine pathways involved in inflammation. CRS *without* nasal polyposis is generally characterized by type 1 inflammation, with neutrophils serving as the common cell type and releasing cytokines, such as interferon-gamma. CRS *with* nasal polyposis is most often mediated by a type 2 inflammatory response involving eosinophils and cytokines, such as interleukin (IL-4), IL-5, and IL-13. Atopic and allergic responses, such as AR, also involve type 2 inflammation. In the AR patient, inhaled allergen activates nasal dendritic cells or other antigen presenting cells. Eosinophils, macrophages, B lymphocytes, and mast cells involved in this process activate downstream T-helper lymphocytes.[10–12]

Putative Mechanism Supporting a Relationship Between Allergic Rhinitis and Chronic Rhinosinusitis

Several studies have implicated allergens and cytokine mediators of allergy in CRS. A putative mechanism is that inhaled allergens are processed by nasal immune cells, which in turn activate T-helper lymphocytes that then migrate to the bone marrow, leading to the release of type 2 inflammatory mediators, such as IL-4, IL-5, and IL-13. This in turn yields the production of eosinophils, mast cells, and basophils, which precipitates nasal eosinophilia. Moreover, nasal and paranasal mucosal cells express cell surface molecules that attract inflammatory mediators and also release inflammatory cytokines leading to a feedback loop.[12,13] In patients with CRS, these cell surface adhesion molecules (such as vascular cell adhesion molecule-1 or VCAM-1) and chemotactic molecules are expressed in abundance and have been postulated to underlie the mechanism by which AR mediates CRS.[10–12] Changes in cellular transcription may serve to further link AR and CRS. As an example, eotaxin, an eosinophil-specific chemokine that directly recruits eosinophils to target tissues, is upregulated in both allergic and nonallergic sinusitis, and is correlated to eosinophil cell infiltrate commonly observed in CRS. Eotaxin mRNA is also upregulated following aeroallergen exposure in patients with AR.[13]

The above mechanism is supported in part by several animal models and human studies. Klemens and colleagues[14] demonstrated a hyper-responsiveness to histamine in a murine model of acute bacterial sinusitis, and Blair and colleagues[15] described an enhanced sinusitis disease state in mice exposed to aeroallergens. Several studies have demonstrated an increased rate (60%–63.2%) of positive skin prick testing in patients with CRSwNP when compared with a control cohort.[16–18] However, systemic allergy symptoms or testing is neither necessary nor solely sufficient for detecting intranasal IgE. Indeed, there are instances in which patients test negative for systemic allergy, but nonetheless demonstrate local sinonasal IgE. In this scenario, called local AR or "entopy," there is a confined IgE-mediated nasal inflammatory response.[19,20] This phenomenon could also explain why some patients who test negative for systemic allergen could still have a local inflammatory response that could worsen CRS.

Kennedy and Borish[12] suggest that aeroallergens may have limited access to the sinuses as a result of physical barriers, inability for allergen particles to diffuse adequately into adjacent sinus cavities, and mucociliary flow. The authors suggest that a systemic inflammatory process is more likely the cause of sinusitis. In their estimation, a nasally triggered allergen response leads to nasal eosinophilia by several downstream effector mechanisms. Newly created eosinophils are also nonspecifically recruited by tissues displaying addressins and chemotactic factors, as can occur in patients with sinusitis. The authors also posit that *Staphylococcus* species residing in the nose and paranasal sinuses can create a biofilm and serve as a source of superantigen, suggesting an active inflammatory role for these bacteria and their enterotoxins, despite being in an indolent, biofilm-associated state. The superantigens trigger IL-4, IL-13, and T_H2 cytokines further leading to IgE in the sinus tissues and further promoting the inflammatory response.[12,21]

Conflicting Data Regarding the Relationship Between Allergic Rhinitis and Chronic Rhinosinusitis

Although the pathways described above seem convincing, this relationship is controversial as several studies do not correlate allergy and atopy with CRS, and indeed only 0.5% of patients with atopy develop nasal polyposis.[22] Adkins and colleagues[23] used radiolabeled allergen to demonstrate that inhaled allergen is unable to permeate the adjoining sinuses and remained sequestered in the nasal cavity and oropharynx, suggesting that there is a natural physical limitation to allergy exacerbating disease of the sinuses. There is additional evidence that demonstrates no relationship between allergies and CRSwNP, including the extent of nasal polyposis, sinonasal symptom severity, or CRS disease recurrence.[24,25] Li and colleagues,[26] characterized the relationship of atopy, or the state of being sensitized to an allergen but not being symptomatic, to clinical severity and disease recurrence in CRSwNP patients. Their data showed no correlation between atopy test results (total IgE, eosinophil cationic protein levels, or Phadiatop testing) and disease severity score as measured by visual analog scoring, Lund-Kennedy endoscopy, or Lund-Mackay CT scoring. In a recent systematic review of CRSwNP, 7 of 18 studies showed no relationship between allergy and CRSwNP, 10 studies demonstrated a relationship between allergy and CRSwNP, and 1 study was equivocal.[4]

Less intuitive is the relationship between allergy and CRS without nasal polyposis. Indeed there is a dearth of literature addressing this question. Some studies suggest that inflammation on imaging seems worse in CRSsNP patients with allergy.[27,28] However, of 9 reviewed studies, only 4 demonstrated a relationship between CRSsNP and allergy.[4] Gelincik and colleagues[29] demonstrated no difference in the rates of CRS in allergic and nonallergic rhinitis patients. In a recent consensus statement, the evidence linking allergy to CRSsNP is quite low (level D).[1] What is more likely is the association between allergy and CRSwNP, or to be more specific, with select subtypes of CRSwNP, such as AFRS and CCAD.[30]

The missing link: AR is better associated with discrete endotypes of CRSwNP—Allergic Fungal Rhinosinusitis and Central Compartment Atopic Disease.

AFRS and CCAD are subtypes of CRSwNP that seem to be linked to allergen-mediated inflammation. AFRS is a known CRSwNP entity with strong geographic associations. Bent and Kuhn established 5 criteria for AFRS, among which is a type 1 hypersensitivity reaction to aeroallergens as confirmed by history, serologic testing, or skin prick testing.[31] Hutcheson and colleagues[32] demonstrated a heightened fungal responsiveness (including increased total serum IgE and IgG anti-alternaria antibodies) in AFRS compared with CRS, thus distinguishing AFRS as having a clear immunologic difference from other forms of CRS and tying the disease process closely with allergy.

In 2014, White and colleagues[33] demonstrated a correlation between isolated middle turbinate polypoid edema and polyps and positive skin or in-vitro testing to inhalant allergy. Hamizan and colleagues,[34] in a large retrospective study, showed that increasing degrees of middle turbinate polypoid edema on nasal endoscopy were associated with significant likelihood of AR. Brunner and colleagues[35] compared groups of patients with isolated middle turbinate polyps or with diffuse sinonasal polyposis, and found that these were 2 distinct entities, with the isolated middle turbinate polyp group having a significantly higher incidence of allergy (83% versus 34%), significantly lower incidence of sinusitis (10% versus 100%), and significantly lower Lund McKay scores (2.8 versus 14.9).

DelGaudio and colleagues[36] in 2017 first coined the term "central compartment atopic disease" in patients demonstrating polyps or polypoid changes of the superior nasal septum, along with the middle and superior turbinates, with a strong association to inhalant allergy. In the original paper on CCAD, 15 of 15 patients in the series suffered from AR symptoms and had positive allergy testing.

The central compartment structures include the superior nasal septum, the middle turbinate, and superior turbinate. These structures are involved because they are in the path of normal nasal airflow. Nasal airflow arcs over the head of the inferior turbinate to enter the area between the nasal septum and middle and superior turbinates, then descends over the posterior tail of the inferior turbinate to enter the nasopharynx. In a more recent publication, DelGaudio and colleagues[37] reported that 80.6% of patients with aspirin-exacerbated respiratory disease (AERD) have endoscopic evidence of central compartment disease, and over 80% have clinical AR. Among patients with AERD with central compartment involvement and with available allergy data, 100% had clinical AR and 93.8% had positive allergy testing.

CLINICAL FEATURES

CRS *without* nasal polyposis is defined as at least 12 consecutive weeks of 2 or more symptoms of nasal drainage, congestion, attenuated smell or loss of smell, sinus pressure, and evidence of inflammation on CT scan or on nasal endoscopy. Chronic rhinosinusitis *with* nasal polyposis mirrors that of CRSsNP, except with the presence of sinonasal polyposis.[2] Diagnosis of AR hinges of the presence of atopy, or the characteristic of becoming triggered to an allergen and mounting an IgE response.[4] The presence of atopy can be supported by skin prick or serum testing. To further complicate the diagnosis, there may be discord between the systemic response to an allergen and the intranasal release of IgE in response to an allergen, a response termed local AR. This discordance has been well characterized, and indeed in 1 study, using a nasal allergen provocation test, 26.5% of previously determined nonatopic individuals had an intranasal IgE response to an allergen.[34,38] Diagnosing AR concomitant with CRS is, therefore, complex, and requires thoughtful evaluation.

History and Physical Examination

A thorough history and physical examination can identify features of both CRS and AR occurring in unison. From the patient's history, the presence of seasonal or perennial allergy symptoms, rhinitis associated with specific triggers, itchy eyes and nose, responsiveness to anti-allergy medications, and comorbid asthma can help tease out atopic individuals.

Determining the time course and type of allergen exposure is also helpful. Indeed, CRS seems to be more associated with perennial rather than seasonal allergies.[39] It follows that chronic exposure to perennial allergens, such as cockroaches, dust mites, pets, and house mold, can yield a chronic inflammatory environment that reinforces CRS. In patients undergoing functional endoscopic sinus surgery for medically refractory CRSwNP, 56.4% of patients had a perennial allergy, a value that exceeds that of the general population, which is estimated between 5% and 22%.[40] In 1 study, among 225 patients undergoing surgery for CRS, 59.6% demonstrated sensitivity to 1 or more antigens, and among these patients 61.2% had perennial and seasonal allergies, 33.6% had perennial allergies only, and 5.2% had seasonal allergies only.[40]

AFRS can present with varying clinical severity ranging from nasal obstruction, taste and smell disturbance, to facial deformity, proptosis, and vision changes.[2] Questioning should ascertain a history of airway reactivity. In conjunction with the aforementioned history, the physical examination finding of nasal polyposis or polypoid edema is important for a diagnosis of AFRS or CCAD. Patients with endoscopic findings of central compartment polyposis, with involvement of structures, such as the superior nasal septum, and the middle and/or superior turbinate, in conjunction with allergic symptoms speaks to the disease entity of CCAD.[33,36,41] This finding in conjunction with positive allergy testing should lead the clinician to suspect CCAD (**Figs. 1** and **2**).

Allergy Testing

Allergy testing is the initial step in determining allergen sensitivity to correlate with clinical symptoms. There are several mechanisms to test for inhalant allergen sensitivity, including skin prick testing, intradermal testing, and serum allergen-specific IgE

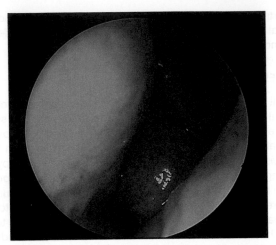

Fig. 1. Left-sided endoscopy image of central compartment atopic disease.

testing (described below). Testing for local AR Involves nasal provocation, quantification of allergen-specific IgE in nasal secretions/tissues, and/or basophil activation testing. These methods to detect local AR are most commonly used in research protocols at the present time.

Systemic allergy testing

A combination of serum and skin prick testing is considered most accurate to correctly identify offending allergens. Some allergic sensitivities may be missed if only 1 type of testing modality is performed.[42] Although clinically this may not always be practical, there is potential variance between the 2 techniques; with controversy regarding which technique is superior.[16,18] A thorough discussion of the benefits, downsides, and specific techniques for skin and in-vitro allergy testing is beyond the scope of this article.

DelGaudio and colleagues demonstrated that, in patients with CCAD, 100% of this cohort had a clinical history of AR and had positive allergy testing. Conversely, there

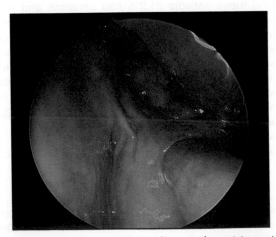

Fig. 2. Left-sided CCAD; suction demonstrates polyp attachment to septum.

are data to suggest a lack of association between allergy and CRSwNP as a broad phenotype, with no association between positive skin prick testing and polyposis, sinus imaging opacification, sinusitis symptoms, or likelihood for recurrent disease.[24,25,43] Although these 2 statements may seem to be contradictory at first, we now understand that CRSwNP describes a general phenotype of CRS that should be further broken down into subtypes (ie, AFRS, CCAD, AERD, nonatopic CRSwNP). Association of allergy with specific CRSwNP subtypes (namely CCAD, AFRS, and AERD with CCAD features) has been demonstrated. Attempting to associate AR and CRSwNP broadly is problematic because of the various disease processes and causes contributing to CRSwNP as a whole. Future studies and approaches may reduce the issues that have been present in the past.

Intranasal provocation with allergens and its relationship to sinonasal inflammation
Although geographic and regional differences exist, up to 85% of nasal polyps have a high concentration of IL-5.[26,44] Interestingly, nasal polyps can also express Th17- and Th1-associated cytokines, such as IL-17 and interferon-gamma, and in CRSsNP, tissues can express profiles associated with Th1, Th2, and Th17 signatures, suggesting a veritable cross-pollination of cytokine profiles.[44] Nonetheless, in CRSwNP, in response to a unilateral intranasal allergen challenge, there is a robust eosinophilic response that occurs in bilateral sinonasal cavities and renders a high tissue concentration of eosinophil cationic protein, IL-5, and tissue IgE.[45–47] Baroody and colleagues[45] observed an increased eosinophil count after cannulating the maxillary sinuses of seasonal allergy patients treated with an allergen challenge. The authors postulate that increased albumin, eosinophil cationic protein, histamine, and eosinophilia are not directly from allergen entering the sinus cleft but rather the result of a downstream reaction to a localized allergen challenge. Although these methodologies of intranasal testing provide excellent pathophysiologic information, commercial testing for intranasal cytokines and inflammatory cell types is not currently used in everyday clinical practice.

Imaging Studies

Kirtsreesakul and Ruttanaphol[27] and Berrettini and colleagues[28] demonstrated the presence of increased sinonasal inflammation in allergic patients on plain film radiographs and CT, respectively, when compared with nonallergic patients (67.5% compared with 33.4% in the CT cohort). Patients sensitized to cypress pollens undergoing a nasal provocation test have demonstrable radiologic changes in their osteomeatal complexes and ethmoid sinuses.[48] CT studies are used to identify paranasal sinus disease and can serve as an adjunct in diagnosing different disease subtypes. For example, in the presence of endoscopic findings of polyposis and allergic mucin, CT of the paranasal sinuses can identify heterogeneous intrasinus densities with possible bone thinning and expansion of the sinuses that is characteristic of AFRS (**Figs. 3** and **4**). On MRI, a signal void may be present in regions of fungal involvement with allergic mucin on T2-rendered images.[49] CCAD has characteristic endoscopic and imaging correlates. On endoscopy and CT imaging these patients demonstrate central compartment soft tissue thickening and/or frank polyposis. Patients with the radiologic finding of central opacification with peripheral clearing have a high association with allergy, and predicts atopy with a 90.82% specificity, and a 73.53% positive predictive value.[50] In isolated CCAD, as this is primarily a nasal inflammatory process, the sinuses are only affected late in the disease process, when the central compartment polyps obstruct the sinuses by lateralization and/or extensive polypoid changes of the middle turbinates, and cause a secondary obstructive sinusitis (**Figs. 5** and **6**).[36]

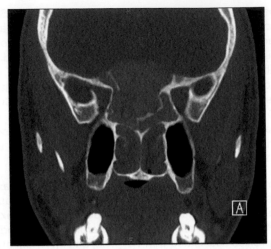

Fig. 3. Coronal computed tomography image of allergic fungal sinusitis with marked thinning of the skull base from local expansion of fungal mucin.

DIFFERENTIAL DIAGNOSIS

A patient with allergies and nasal polyposis may have various causes for their sinonasal disease that should be elucidated. As stated above, AFRS and CCAD should be strongly considered if the characteristics of history, nasal endoscopy, and imaging fit these entities. Other CRSwNP entities should be taken into account—AERD, cystic

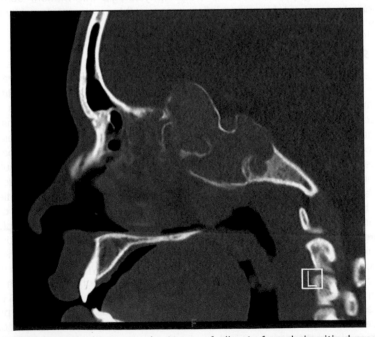

Fig. 4. Sagittal computed tomography image of allergic fungal sinusitis demonstrating expansion of allergic mucin above the sella.

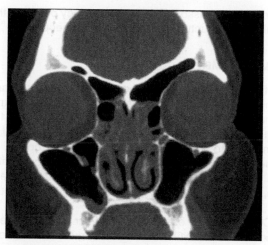

Fig. 5. Coronal computed tomography image demonstrating mild central compartment atopic disease with sparing of lateral sinuses.

fibrosis, or CRSwNP not otherwise specified, depending on the individual patient evaluation. Inverted papilloma should be considered for unilateral polyposis or bilateral polyposis in the setting of a communicating nasal septal perforation. Respiratory epithelial adenomatoid hamartoma is a rare process that is, frequently identified in the upper nasal septum as a primary process or concomitant with mucosal inflammatory disease, such as CRSwNP. It can be unilateral or bilateral.[51,52] It is further important to establish allergy as the underlying cause of rhinitis, since rhinitis may have nonallergic or mixed causes as well. Indeed, a careful history, physical examination, and allergy testing can be used to differentiate between infectious rhinitis, rhinitis medicamentosa, nonallergic vasomotor rhinitis, nonallergic inflammatory rhinitis with

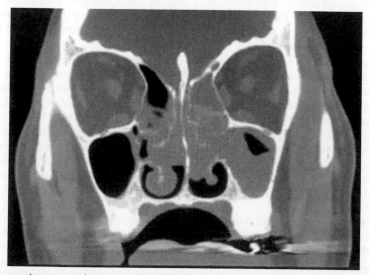

Fig. 6. Coronal computed tomography image demonstrating severe central compartment atopic disease with postobstructive involvement of lateral sinuses.

eosinophilia, hormonal rhinitis associated with pregnancy or a hypothyroid state, and finally reactive rhinitis from structural considerations or neoplasm.[1,6]

TREATMENT AND MANAGEMENT

The management for AR is multifactorial, and treatment is particularly nuanced as it relates to AR compounding CRS. Chronic aerosolized allergen exposure may lead to chronic inflammation, and indeed in patients with CRSwNP, 56.4% have a sensitivity to a perennial allergen compared with 5% of the general populace.[40] Therefore, reducing hypersensitivity to exacerbating allergens is an option, and the role of allergen immunotherapy has been well characterized in patients with AR.[1] Although immunotherapy is effective in AR, it is difficult to fully extrapolate this success to CRS. Nonetheless, immunotherapy may serve as an adjunct, particularly in the postoperative setting.

In the case of CCAD, allergen exposures and their sequelae are best addressed following surgical intervention. DelGaudio and colleagues[36] describes a cohort of patients with CCAD pretreated with intranasal corticosteroids, antihistamines, oral corticosteroids, antibiotics, and/or immunotherapy. Antibiotics were given for indication of endoscopic or CT imaging findings demonstrating purulence or air-fluid levels. Despite this pretreatment, medical management did not yield complete resolution of symptoms, and CT images obtained after treatment showed persisting thickening of the central nasal cavity and pathologic involvement of adjacent sinuses or sinuses whose outflow tracks were disturbed by middle turbinate lateralization by central compartment polyps. Therefore, surgical therapy was undertaken to remove obstructive sinonasal pathologic material with the goal of sculpting the polypoid central compartment. In some instances, and particularly in revision CCAD surgical cases, performing a Draf 2b or Draf 3 procedure is a helpful adjunct to clear frontal sinus disease, central compartment polyp and scar, and to resect the polyp-bearing upper nasal septum to provide better access for topical therapy to this portion of the central compartment. Postoperatively, these patients are treated with topical steroids and allergen immunotherapy. Maintenance of topical therapies and immunotherapy is essential, as opening the affected sinuses could in theory expose previously allergen-naive mucosa to a greater burden of environmental allergens and lead to new or recurrent disease.[23,36]

Surgery also has an essential role in the management of AFRS. Surgical relief of entrapped allergic mucin serves to halt progressive sinonasal symptoms as well as local tissue response to inflammatory mucin. Creating capacious and evacuated sinus cavities allows for irrigations to continuously remove debris and allergen and distributes topical anti-inflammatory medications to the mucosa. Just as in CCAD, patients with AFRS should undergo a regimen of preoperative systemic steroids and topical nasal steroid (preferably in rinse form), with allergen immunotherapy as an option postoperatively. Despite an underlying type I hypersensitivity reaction to fungal elements, allergen-specific immunotherapy has not undergone rigorous clinical trials in AFRS and currently carries a relatively low level of evidence in the treatment of this disease.[2,53]

The role of targeted anti-IgE and anti-cytokine therapy deserves mention. In particular, the Food and Drug Administration approval of omalizumab in the treatment of refractory allergen-exacerbated asthma and chronic urticaria has led to the study of this agent in CRSwNP.[54] Bachert and colleagues[46] demonstrated a reduction in total nasal endoscopic polyp scores in the omalizumab cohort, suggesting the role of IgE levels in the pathophysiology of CRSwNP. In a subgroup analysis, allergic patients had

Table 1
Comparisons between allergic fungal rhinosinusitis and central compartment atopic disease

	Allergic Fungal Rhinosinusitis	Central Compartment Atopic Disease
Presentation	Nasal obstruction, hyposmia/anosmia, facial pain/pressure Thick rhinorrhea, proptosis or telecanthus (in later stages)	Clear rhinorrhea, itchy nose, sneezing
Endoscopy	Large, diffuse nasal polyps with thick, yellow/brown, "allergic" or "eosinophilic" mucin	Mucosal edema or polypoid change of the middle turbinate, posterior-superior nasal septum, and/or superior turbinate
Imaging	Unilateral or asymmetric disease, bony remodeling, heterogenous signal in sinuses	Central nasal opacification with peripheral clearing of the sinuses, lateralization of the middle turbinates
Treatment	• Endoscopic sinus surgery to remove polyps and allergic mucin and widely open sinuses for postoperative irrigation • Topical corticosteroid irrigations • Allergen immunotherapy may be used but it is not well supported	• Endoscopic sinus surgery to sculpt the polypoid areas of the central sinonasal compartment and relieve obstructive sinusitis • Topical corticosteroid irrigations • Allergen immunotherapy is suggested but the role is currently unstudied

significant improvements in Lund-Mackay score compared with nonallergic patients (**Table 1**).

SUMMARY

This article highlights the pathophysiology, diagnosis, and management for AR associated with CRS. There are several putative links between AR and CRS. Although there are no definitive studies that prove this association, there are key features of the 2 disease processes that share common ground. Chronic inflammation may be a mechanism by which AR triggers or exacerbates CRS. Examples of this are the recently identified phenomenon of CCAD, as well as AFRS. Additional study of the relationship between AR and specific CRS subtypes will further our understanding of the interplay between these 2 entities in the future.

FINANCIAL DISCLOSURES AND POTENTIAL CONFLICTS OF INTEREST

None (S.N. Helman, E. Barrow, and T. Edwards). Medtronic (consultant); IntersectENT (stockholder) (J.M. DelGaudio). Research support by the Triological Society and National Center for Advancing Translational Sciences of the National Institutes of Health under award numbers UL1TR002378 and KL2TR002381. The content is solely the responsibility of the authors and does not necessarily represent the official views of the NIH (J.M. Levy). OptiNose (scientific advisory board); SinopSys Surgical (scientific advisory board); ALK-Abello (scientific advisory board; Stryker (consultant); NeurENT (consultant) (S.K. Wise).

REFERENCES

1. Wise SK, Lin SY, Toskala E, et al. International consensus statement on allergy and rhinology: allergic rhinitis. Int Forum Allergy Rhinol 2018;8(2):108–352.

2. Orlandi RR, Kingdom TT, Hwang PH, et al. International consensus statement on allergy and rhinology: rhinosinusitis. Int Forum Allergy Rhinol 2016;6:S22–209.
3. Gurrola J 2nd, Borish L. Chronic rhinosinusitis: endotypes, biomarkers, and treatment response. J Allergy Clin Immunol 2017;140:1499–508.
4. Wilson KF, McMains C, Orlandi RF. The association between allergy and chronic rhinosinusitis with and without nasal polyposis: an evidence-based review with recommendations. Int Forum Allergy Rhinol 2014;4:93–103.
5. Brozek JL, Bousquet J, Agache I, et al. Allergic rhinitis and its impact on asthma (ARIA) guidelines—2016 revision. J Allergy Clin Immunol 2017;140:950–8.
6. Bellanti JA, Wallerstedt DB. Allergic rhinitis update: epidemiology and natural history. Allergy Asthma Proc 2000;21:367–70.
7. Bhattacharyya N. Incremental health care utilization and expenditures for chronic rhinosinusitis in the United States. Ann Otol Rhinol Laryngol 2011;120:423–7.
8. Meltzer EO, Hamilos DL, Hadley JA, et al. Rhinosinusitis: establishing definitions for clinical research and patient care. Otolaryngol Head Neck Surg 2004; 131(suppl 6):S1–62.
9. Emanuel IA, Parker MJ, Traub O. Undertreatment of allergy: exploring the utility of sublingual immunotherapy. Otolaryngol Head Neck Surg 2009;140(5):615–21.
10. Jahnsen FL, Haraldsen G, Aanesen JP, et al. Eosinophil infiltration is related to increased expression of vascular cell adhesion molecule-1 in nasal polyps. Am J Respir Cell Mol Biol 1995;12:624–32.
11. Inman MD, Ellis R, Wattie J, et al. Allergen-induced increase in airway responsiveness, airway eosinophilia, and bone-marrow eosinophil progenitors in mice. Am J Respir Cell Mol Biol 1999;21:473–9.
12. Kennedy JL, Borish L. Chronic sinusitis pathophysiology: the role of allergy. Am J Rhinol 2013;27:367–71.
13. Minshall EM, Cameron L, Lavigne F, et al. Eotaxin mRNA and protein expression in chronic sinusitis and allergen-induced nasal responses in seasonal allergic rhinitis. Am J Respir Cell Mol Biol 1997;17:683–90.
14. Klemens JJ, Kirtsreesakul V, Luxameechanporn T, et al. Acute bacterial rhinosinusitis causes hyperresponsiveness to histamine challenge in mice. Arch Otolaryngol Head Neck Surg 2005;131:905–10.
15. Blair C, Nelson M, Thompson K, et al. Allergic inflammation enhances bacterial sinusitis in mice. J Allergy Clin Immunol 2001;108:424–9.
16. Munoz del Castillo F, Jurado-Ramos A, Fernandez-Conde BL, et al. Allergenic profile of nasal polyposis. J Investig Allergol Clin Immunol 2009;19:110–6.
17. Pumhirun P, Limitlaohapanth C, Wasuwat P. Role of allergy in nasal polyps of Thai patients. Asian Pac J Allergy Immunol 1999;17:13–5.
18. Tan BK, Zirkle W, Chandra R, et al. Atopic profile of patients failing medical therapy for chronic rhinosinusitis. Int Forum Allergy Rhinol 2011;1:88–94.
19. Smurthwaite L, Durham SR. Local IgE synthesis in allergic rhinitis and asthma. Curr Allergy Asthma Rep 2002;2:231–8.
20. Wise SK, Ahn CN, Schlosser RJ. Localized immunoglobulin E expression in allergic rhinitis and nasal polyposis. Curr Opin Otolaryngol Head Neck Surg 2009;17:216–22.
21. Zhang N, Holtappels G, Gevaert P, et al. Mucosal tissue polyclonal IgE is functional in response to allergen and SEB. Allergy 2011;66:141–8.
22. Caplin I, Haynes TJ, Spahn J. Are nasal polyps an allergic phenomenon? Ann Allergy 1971;29:631–4.
23. Adkins TN, Goodgold HM, Hendershott L, et al. Does inhaled pollen enter the sinus cavities? Ann Allergy Asthma Immunol 1998;81:181–4.

24. Erbek SS, Erbek S, Topal O, et al. The role of allergy in the severity of nasal polyposis. Am J Rhinol 2007;21:686–90.
25. Bonfils P, Avan P, Malinvaud D. Influence of allergy on the symptoms and treatment of nasal polyposis. Acta Otolaryngol 2006;126:839–44.
26. Li QC, Cheng KJ, Wang F, et al. Role of atopy in chronic rhinosinusitis with nasal polyps: does an atopic condition affect the severity and recurrence of disease? J Laryngol Otol 2016;130:640–4.
27. Kirtsreesakul V, Ruttanaphol S. The relationship between allergy and rhinosinusitis. Rhinology 2008;46:204–8.
28. Berrettini S, Carabelli A, Sellari-Franceschini S, et al. Perennial allergic rhinitis and chronic sinusitis: correlation with rhinologic risk factors. Allergy 1999;54:242–8.
29. Gelincik A, Buyukozturk S, Aslan I, et al. Allergic vs nonallergic rhinitis: which is more predisposing to chronic rhinosinusitis? Ann Allergy Asthma Immunol 2008; 101:18–22.
30. Marcus S, Roland LT, DelGaudio JM, et al. The relationship between allergy and chronic rhinosinusitis. Laryngoscope Investig Otolaryngol 2018;4(1):13–7.
31. Bent JP, Kuhn FA. Diagnosis of allergic fungal sinusitis. Otolaryngol Head Neck Surg 1994;111(5):580–8.
32. Hutcheson PS, Schubert MS, Slavin RG. Distinctions between allergic fungal rhinosinusitis and chronic rhinosinusitis. Am J Rhinol Allergy 2010;24:405–40.
33. White LJ, Rotella MR, DelGaudio JM. Polypoid changes of the middle turbinate as an indicator of atopic disease. Int Forum Allergy Rhinol 2014;4:376–80.
34. Hamizan AW, Rimmer J, Alvarado R, et al. Positive allergen reaction in allergic and nonallergic rhinitis: a systematic review. Int Forum Allergy Rhinol 2017;7: 868–77.
35. Brunner JP, Jawad BA, McCoul ED. Polypoid change of the middle turbinate and paranasal sinus polyposis are distinct entities. Otolaryngol Head Neck Surg 2017;157(3):519–23.
36. DelGaudio JM, Loftus PA, Hamizan AW, et al. Central compartment atopic disease. Am J Rhinol Allergy 2017;31(4):228–34.
37. DelGaudio JM, Levy JM, Wise SK. Central compartment involvement in aspirin-associated respiratory disease: the roll of allergy and previous sinus surgery. Int Forum Allergy Rhinol 2019;9(9):1017–22.
38. Settipane RA, Borish L, Peters AT. Chapter 16: determining the role of allergy in sinonasal disease. Am J Rhinol Allergy 2013;27:S56–8.
39. Gutman M, Torres A, Keen KJ, et al. Prevalence of allergy in patients with chronic rhinosinusitis. Otolaryngol Head Neck Surg 2004;130:545–52.
40. Houser SM, Keen KJ. The role of allergy and smoking in chronic rhinosinusitis and polyposis. Laryngoscope 2008;118:1521–7.
41. Hamizan AW, Christensen JW, Ebenzer J, et al. Middle turbinate edema as a diagnostic marker of inhalant allergy. Int Forum Allergy Rhinol 2016;7:37–42.
42. de Vos G. Skin testing versus serum-specific IgE testing: which is better for diagnosing aeroallergen sensitization and predicting clinical allergy? Curr Allergy Asthma Rep 2014;14:430.
43. Gorgulu O, Ozdemir S, Canbolat EP, et al. Analysis of the roles of smoking and allergy in nasal polyposis. Ann Otol Rhinol Laryngol 2012;121:615–9.
44. Wang X, Zhang N, Bo M, et al. Diversity of TH cytokine profiles in patients with chronic rhinosinusitis: a multicenter study in Europe, Asia, and Oceania. J Allergy Clin Immunol 2016;138:1344–53.
45. Baroody FM, Mucha SM, Detineo M, et al. Nasal challenge with allergen leads to maxillary sinus inflammation. J Allergy Clin Immunol 2008;121:1126–32.

46. Bachert C, Gevaert P, Holtappels G, et al. Total and specific IgE in nasal polyps is related to local eosinophilic inflammation. J Allergy Clin Immunol 2001;107: 607–14.

47. Mygind N, Dahl R, Bachert C. Nasal polyposis, eosinophil dominated inflammation, and allergy. Thorax 2000;55(suppl 2):S79–83.

48. Piette V, Bousquet C, Kvedariene V, et al. Sinus CT scans and mediator release in nasal secretions after nasal challenge with cypress pollens. Allergy 2004;59: 863–8.

49. Manning SC, Merkel M, Kriesel K, et al. Computed tomography and magnetic resonance diagnosis of allergic fungal sinusitis. Laryngoscope 1997;107:170–6.

50. Hamizan AW, Loftus PA, Alvarado R, et al. Allergic phenotype of chronic rhinosinusitis based on radiologic pattern of disease. Laryngoscope 2018;128:2015–21.

51. Mortuaire G, Pasquesoone X, Leroy X, et al. Respiratory epithelial adenomatoid hamartomas of the sinonasal tract. Eur Arch Otorhinolaryngol 2007;264(4):451–3.

52. Nguyen DT, Jankowski R, Bey A, et al. Respiratory epithelial adenomatoid hamartoma is frequent in olfactory cleft after nasalization. Laryngoscope 2019. https://doi.org/10.1002/lary.28298.

53. Gan EC, Thamboo A, Rudmik L, et al. Medical management of allergic fungal rhinosinusitis following endoscopic sinus surgery: an evidence-based review and recommendations. Int Forum Allergy Rhinol 2014;4:702–15.

54. Gevaert P, Calus L, Van Zele T, et al. Omalizumab is effective in allergic and nonallergic patients with nasal polyps and asthma. J Allergy Clin Immunol 2013;131:110–6.e1.

What is the Role of Air Pollution in Chronic Rhinosinusitis?

Hannah L. Schwarzbach, BA[a],[1], Leila J. Mady, MD, PhD, MPH[b],[2],
Stella E. Lee, MD[a],[b],*

KEYWORDS

- Air pollutants • Environmental exposure • Occupational exposure
- Particulate matter • Rhinitis • Allergic • Sinusitis • Nasal polyps

KEY POINTS

- The negative health effects of air pollution have been recognized in the lower airway, for example, chronic obstructive pulmonary disease, and asthma, but more recent studies demonstrate interactions between pollutant exposure and chronic rhinosinusitis (CRS) as well as nonallergic rhinitis.
- Pollutant exposure may be associated with CRS pathophysiology, and, among CRS patients without nasal polyps, exposure is associated with disease severity and decreased quality of life.
- Mechanisms of pollutant exposure in disease may be due to several factors, including disruption in the integrity of the sinonasal barrier, induction of chronic inflammation, and alteration of the nasal microbiome, among other causes not yet investigated.

GLOBAL AND LOCAL HEALTH EFFECTS OF ENVIRONMENTAL POLLUTANTS

Air pollution poses significant and pressing risks to the environment and human health worldwide. Although generally agreed that both environmental and host factors play a role in chronic rhinosinusitis (CRS), the effects of exposures encountered daily, such as pollutants in the air and occupational exposures, is unclear.[1] The US Environmental Protection Agency has identified 6 criteria pollutants that are common in the United States and pose a threat to the environment and human health. These pollutants include

[a] University of Pittsburgh School of Medicine, Pittsburgh, PA, USA; [b] Department of Otolaryngology–Head and Neck Surgery, University of Pittsburgh Medical Center, Pittsburgh, PA, USA
[1] Present address: University of Pittsburgh School of Medicine, 3550 Terrace Street - S594, Scaife Hall, Pittsburgh, PA 15261.
[2] Present address: University of Pittsburgh Department of Otolaryngology, 203 Lothrop Street - Suite 500, Pittsburgh, Pennsylvania 15213.
* Corresponding author. UPMC Mercy, 1400 Locust Street – Suite 2100, Pittsburgh, PA 15219.
E-mail address: lee6@upmc.edu

Immunol Allergy Clin N Am 40 (2020) 215–222
https://doi.org/10.1016/j.iac.2019.12.011
0889-8561/20/© 2020 Elsevier Inc. All rights reserved.
immunology.theclinics.com

lead, carbon monoxide, sulfur dioxide, ozone, nitrogen dioxide, and particulate matter (PM) 2.5 ($PM_{2.5}$) and PM 10 (PM_{10}), and although National Ambient Air Quality Standards attempt to regulate ambient pollutant levels, many parts of the United States are in nonattainment.[2] In regard to $PM_{2.5}$, 3 Pennsylvania counties, 1 county in Idaho, and 14 in California are in nonattainment as of August 2019. There are nonattainment regions for ozone in Arizona, California, Colorado, Connecticut, District of Columbia, Georgia, Illinois, Kentucky, Maryland, Michigan, Nevada, New Jersey, New Mexico, New York, Ohio, Pennsylvania, Texas, Utah, Virginia, and Wisconsin.[3] Studies have shown significant associations of poor air quality with chronic obstructive pulmonary disease (COPD) and asthma as well as other conditions, such as rheumatoid arthritis, anxiety and depression, cognitive impairment, and cardiovascular disease.[4–8] In COPD, pollutant exposure is associated with increased rescue inhaler use, more frequent emergency room visits, hospitalizations, and decreased pulmonary function.[9,10] Among a unique tobacco-naïve population of COPD patients, the most important risk factor was exposure to biomass smoke, which is a major source of airborne particulates and gaseous pollutants that originate from burning organic matter.[11] Comparable findings have been described in asthma, and a study on the effectiveness of air pollutant emission reduction policies found that hospital visits decreased by up to 16% in the first 10 years after these environmental policies were enforced.[12]

AIR POLLUTION AND EFFECTS ON CLINICAL OUTCOMES IN CHRONIC RHINOSINUSITIS AND ALLERGIC RHINITIS

Earlier studies investigating the role of air pollution in sinonasal disease examined the effects of exposure to sulfur dioxide, nitrogen dioxide, ozone, carbon monoxide, and PM. There was a significant association between PM_{10} exposure and the risk of CRS, with risk increasing by 1.22% with each 1 $\mu g/m^3$ increase in PM_{10}, but there was no association between ear, nose, and throat pathology and the other 4 pollutants.[13] This same study found no association between pollutant exposure and the prevalence of allergic rhinitis (AR). A similar study on traffic-related air pollution (TRAP) measured near patients' homes and schools reported no association between exposure and AR or asthma.[14] These findings conflict with 2 studies that did report an association between pollutant exposure and AR, but it is important to note that most of these studies were specifically measuring TRAP exposure.[15,16] TRAP typically consists of carbon monoxide, carbon dioxide, nitrogen oxides, hydrocarbons, and PM, but the amount and relative concentrations of each component vary significantly based on factors, including vehicle type, age, condition, and fuel. Study participants also likely encountered a heterogeneous mixture of TRAP components, depending on distance from the road, meteorologic conditions, and pollutant characteristics, so it is difficult to classify exposure specifics in each study.[17]

The authors' group studied the relationship between $PM_{2.5}$ and black carbon exposure and disease severity in CRS using spatial modeling data from regional pollutant monitoring sites. The authors analyzed CRS with nasal polyps (CRSwNP) and CRS without nasal polyps (CRSsNP) and found that among CRSsNP patients, increased $PM_{2.5}$ exposure was associated with increased risk of proceeding to functional endoscopic sinus surgery (FESS). When specifically looking at 6 patients who were exposed to $PM_{2.5}$ levels greater than 12.0 $\mu g/m^3$, which is the exposure limit proposed by the Environmental Protection Agency to protect public health, 4 patients (66.7%) required FESS compared with 38 patients (42.2%) with significantly less $PM_{2.5}$ exposure. Levels of exposure seem directly related because ordinal logistic regression found a 1.89-fold increase in the proportion of CRSsNP patients requiring surgery for each unit increase in $PM_{2.5}$ exposure ($P = .015$). Black carbon exposure had a significant impact on subjective symptom severity among CRSsNP patients, with higher levels associated with increased Sino-Nasal Outcome Test (SNOT)-22 scores. There were no significant associations between $PM_{2.5}$ or black carbon exposure and CRSwNP outcomes in the authors' cohort.[18]

The authors also investigated how air pollutant exposure relates to AR in CRS patients. Reports of AR prevalence among CRS patients range from 50% to 80% compared with 10% to 20% of the general population.[19,20] The authors' study showed that both $PM_{2.5}$ and black carbon exposure were significantly higher, however, among CRS patients with negative allergy testing compared with atopic CRS patients. These findings show that pollutant exposure may contribute to nonallergic rhinitis (NAR) in the CRS population.[1] The role of NAR in CRS is poorly understood and has not been studied extensively, but the authors' findings align with another study that examined AR and NAR in CRS. In a study of 115 patients, NAR patients had higher average global symptom scores than their allergic counterparts.[21] In the authors' study, among patients who tested negative for allergies, CRSsNP patients had significantly higher SNOT-22 scores than CRSwNP patients, suggesting that air pollutants could be driving the increased symptomatology seen in CRS patients without atopy.[1]

OCCUPATIONAL EXPOSURES, TOBACCO, AND CHRONIC RHINOSINUSITIS PATHOPHYSIOLOGY

Although the relationship between air pollution and CRS has not been studied as extensively as its role in lower respiratory conditions, there is a growing body of literature on the relationship between other environmental exposures and sinonasal disease. A 2015 systematic review on occupational and environmental risk factors for CRS identified 41 studies on occupational risk and environmental risk but determined that no strong conclusions could be drawn, because the definition of CRS used in these studies did not fit accepted diagnostic guidelines, and many exposure assessments relied on patient-reported exposures.[22] A more recent study that used participant interviews to study occupational and environmental CRS risk factors found that occupational exposure to dust and occupational exposure to poisonous gas were significantly associated with self-reported CRS, but these imprecise exposure data are challenging to interpret. For example, the survey referenced "poisonous gas" exposure without explaining what constitutes a poisonous gas, so study participants responded based on their own interpretations of this variable.[23] The relationship between occupational exposures and CRS subtypes (CRSwNP, CRSsNP, and aspirin-exacerbated respiratory disease [AERD]) was recently analyzed by the authors' group to evaluate this knowledge gap. Exposures included vapors, gases, dusts, fumes, fibers, and mists (VGDFFiM) and diesel fumes. Instead of using spatial modeling based on patients' addresses, occupational exposures were estimated based on patients' reported occupations and the occupational airborne chemical exposure matrix described by Sadhra and colleagues.[24] Exposure to VGDFFiM was significantly higher among CRSsNP patients compared with CRSwNP and AERD patients, but there was no significant difference in diesel fume exposure between these groups. VGDFFiM and diesel fume exposure both were associated with higher steroid doses, and VGDFFiM was associated with an increased risk of proceeding to FESS. A subgroup analysis of exposure outcomes between CRSwNP, CRSsNP, and AERD was not significant.[25] Subgroup analysis based on CRS phenotypes, however, is likely an oversimplification, with a growing number of studies using cluster analysis to identify unique CRS endotypes demonstrating a spectrum of unique inflammatory and clinical behaviors.[26–29] Mechanisms of VGDFFiM exposure may be related to disruptions in the epithelial barrier and ciliary dysfunction. Ciliary dyskinesia has been described after occupational exposures, and a recent cross-sectional study of gas station employees found a positive correlation between length of work and nasal mucociliary transport time.[30]

Tobacco smoke exposure also may modify CRS disease severity, with a recent meta-analysis showing that 11 of 13 studies described a significant association between exposure and CRS prevalence.[31] Another study found that current and former smokers had higher odds of CRS than never smokers, but this study relied on self-reported symptoms without support from objective examination.[32] CRS severity also has been associated with both amount and duration of smoke exposure.[33] Secondhand smoke exposure is relevant as well, and a review of 112 studies found an association between CRS and both passive and active smoking, attributing this relationship to decreased ciliary beat frequency and increased sinonasal epithelial inflammation on smoke exposure.[34] A recent prospective cross-sectional study compared CRS severity among tobacco cigarette smokers and tobacco smokers who also habitually use cannabis and found that health-related quality of life burden and Lund-Kennedy endoscopic scores were significantly higher among patients who use a combination of tobacco and cannabis.[35] This data are particularly interesting in light of the increasing number of states that are legalizing cannabis for recreational and medical use.[36]

MECHANISMS OF POLLUTANT EXPOSURE IN CHRONIC RHINOSINUSITIS

Several studies have linked air pollution exposure to both systemic inflammation and local epithelial dysfunction. Epithelial cells release proinflammatory cytokines on PM exposure, and these circulating inflammatory markers sustain a systemic inflammatory state.[37–40] One study examined the biomarkers of systemic inflammation after PM exposure in young, healthy patients. A significant association was found between PM exposure and inflammatory cytokines, including tumor necrosis factor (TNF)-α, interleukin (IL)-8, and IL-6.[41] Another study found similar results when looking at the association between chronic residential PM exposure and C-reactive protein, an acute-phase protein and inflammatory marker that increases after IL-6 secretion.[42] In addition to these systemic effects, similar inflammatory profiles were seen in upper airway epithelium after exposure. With regard to diesel exhaust particles (DEPs), a traffic-related pollutant, 1 study found increased IL-6 and IL-8 expression in human inferior turbinate fibroblasts after DEP exposure, and DEP exposure has been shown to decrease sinonasal epithelial integrity in mice, providing another mechanistic explanation for DEPs' proinflammatory properties.[43,44] A study using RPMI 2650 cells from human nasal septum tissue found increased expression of TNF-α, IL-13, IL-6, and IL-8 after PM exposure, and another reported that $PM_{2.5}$ was associated with tight junction protein degradation and epithelial barrier disruption.[45,46]

The aforementioned effects of pollutant exposure on inflammation and epithelial dysfunction were demonstrated in vivo in a murine model of $PM_{2.5}$ exposure by Ramanathan and colleagues.[47] Mice were subjected to $PM_{2.5}$ inhalation over the course of 16 weeks with mean airborne PM concentrations approximating the values found in many global cities. Examination of the epithelial integrity after PM exposure showed that claudin-1 and E-cadherin, 2 proteins that contribute to intercellular tight junctions, were significantly lower in PM-treated mice. Eosinophils, neutrophils, macrophages, and lymphocytes also were higher in nasal airway lavage fluid from exposed mice compared with controls, and nasal mucosa PCR demonstrated higher expression of several inflammatory cytokines including IL-1β and IL-13.[47] Although several studies describe increased IL-6 and IL-8 in epithelial tissues after pollutant exposure[41–43,45,46], Ramanathan and colleagues describe an eosinophilic inflammatory profile.[47] Nonallergic eosinophilic inflammation also was described, which recapitulates a unique clinical entity found in patients who suffer from NAR with eosinophilia syndrome.[47] These findings may explain the relationship between PM exposure and disease severity among nonallergic CRSsNP patients, which is consistent with the findings from the authors' group's earlier studies.[1,18]

In addition to its impact on inflammation and epithelial dysfunction, air pollutants may have an impact on the nasal microbiome, contributing to the dysbiosis seen in CRS. Black carbon has been shown to affect bacterial colonization, and both *Streptococcus pneumoniae* and *Staphylococcus aureus* biofilms develop more thick and complex structures when exposed to black carbon. *S pneumoniae* and *Staphylococcus aureus* also are more resistant to antibiotics after black carbon exposure.[48] Given the proposed role of bacterial infection, colonization, and *S aureus* superantigens in the pathophysiology of CRS, this information provides additional data that can provide further insight into the links between chronic inflammation, microbiome disturbances, and environmental exposures.[49]

FUTURE CONSIDERATIONS AND SUMMARY

CRS is a complex disorder with several factors contributing to disease expression and progression, but recent studies on the relationship between environmental exposures and CRS suggest that pollution has an impact on disease prevalence and severity. In addition to clinical studies that describe an association between pollutants and CRS, molecular studies about effects on epithelial integrity, chronic inflammation, and nasal dysbiosis provide further mechanistic influences on CRS pathophysiology.

The studies currently described in the literature, including the studies conducted by the authors' group, are limited by the currently available means of quantifying exposure in an individual patient. Spatial modeling based on patients' home addresses and surrogate measures based on occupation or job title likely relate to exposure but fail to address several important variables (eg, real-time exposures, time spent outdoors, and mixed-environment jobs). It may be helpful to compare the exposure data collected from local pollutant modeling sites with data collected from personalized, wearable monitors from patients in that region. A study that utilizes wearable pollutant monitors would be helpful to collect more high-fidelity data. Most studies on this topic also have been cross-sectional, and prospective analyses are needed. By longitudinally following diseased populations and healthy populations over time, the associations between exposure and disease progression and new CRS incidence in previously healthy people could be examined. Tissue samples from patients also could be collected and analyzed to examine the relationship between molecular indications of exposure and clinical outcomes.

From an advocacy and public health standpoint, it would be useful to longitudinally evaluate CRS severity following the enforcement of new environmental exposure legislation. These studies could evaluate macroscopic exposure at the state or national level in addition to examining smaller populations after regional policies or workplace policies are implemented. If these studies demonstrated a significant decrease in disease burden, this information would be valuable to support future clean air legislation. Even without these future studies, the currently available literature on the relationship between air pollution and CRS suggests that exposure is associated with both disease prevalence and severity, and public health initiatives to further decrease ambient pollutant levels are warranted.

DISCLOSURE

S.E. Lee: clinical trial funding: Sanofi Aventis Regeneron, GlaxoSmithKline, and AstraZeneca; Advisory boards: Sanofi Aventis Regeneron and Novartis.

REFERENCES

1. Mady LJ, Schwarzbach HL, Moore JA, et al. The association of air pollutants and allergic and nonallergic rhinitis in chronic rhinosinusitis. Int Forum Allergy Rhinol 2018;8(3):369–76.
2. Ross K, Chmiel JF, Ferkol T. The impact of the clean air act. J Pediatr 2012;161(5): 781–6.
3. Nonattainment areas for criteria pollutants (green book). Available at: https://www.epa.gov/green-book. Accessed September 9, 2019.
4. Shepherd A, Mullins JT. Arthritis diagnosis and early-life exposure to air pollution. Environ Pollut 2019;253:1030–7.
5. Miller JG, Gillette JS, Manczak EM, et al. Fine particle air pollution and physiological reactivity to social stress in adolescence: the moderating role of anxiety and depression. Psychosom Med 2019;81(7):641–8.
6. Lo YC, Lu YC, Chang YH, et al. Air pollution exposure and cognitive function in taiwanese older adults: a repeated measurement study. Int J Environ Res Public Health 2019;16(16) [pii:E2976].
7. Pothirat C, Chaiwong W, Liwsrisakun C, et al. Acute effects of air pollutants on daily mortality and hospitalizations due to cardiovascular and respiratory diseases. J Thorac Dis 2019;11(7):3070–83.
8. Yan P, Liu P, Lin R, et al. Effect of ambient air quality on exacerbation of COPD in patients and its potential mechanism. Int J Chron Obstruct Pulmon Dis 2019;14: 1517–26.
9. Li J, Sun S, Tang R, et al. Major air pollutants and risk of COPD exacerbations: a systematic review and meta-analysis. Int J Chron Obstruct Pulmon Dis 2016;11: 3079–91.
10. Qu F, Liu F, Zhang H, et al. The hospitalization attributable burden of acute exacerbations of chronic obstructive pulmonary disease due to ambient air pollution in Shijiazhuang, China. Environ Sci Pollut Res Int 2019;26(30):30866–75.
11. Bajpai J, Kant S, Bajaj DK, et al. Clinical, demographic and radiological profile of smoker COPD versus nonsmoker COPD patients at a tertiary care center in North India. J Family Med Prim Care 2019;8(7):2364–8.
12. Kim H, Kim H, Lee JT. Effect of air pollutant emission reduction policies on hospital visits for asthma in Seoul, Korea; Quasi-experimental study. Environ Int 2019;132:104954.
13. Park M, Lee JS, Park MK. The effects of air pollutants on the prevalence of common ear, nose, and throat diseases in South Korea: a national population-based study. Clin Exp Otorhinolaryngol 2019;12(3):294–300.
14. Yi S-J, Shon C, Min K-D, et al. Association between exposure to traffic-related air pollution and prevalence of allergic diseases in children, Seoul, Korea. Biomed Res Int 2017;2017:4216107.
15. Nicolussi FH, Santos AP, André SC, et al. Air pollution and respiratory allergic diseases in schoolchildren. Rev Saude Publica 2014;48(2):326–30.
16. Jang A-S, Jun YJ, Park MK. Effects of air pollutants on upper airway disease. Curr Opin Allergy Clin Immunol 2016;16(1):13–7.
17. Atkinson R, Barregard L, Bellander T. Review of evidence on health aspects of air pollution REVIHAAP project technical report. Copenhagen: World Health Organization Regional Office for Europe; 2013.
18. Mady LJ, Schwarzbach HL, Moore JA, et al. Air pollutants may be environmental risk factors in chronic rhinosinusitis disease progression. Int Forum Allergy Rhinol 2018;8(3):377–84.

19. Philpott CM, Erskine S, Hopkins C, et al. Prevalence of asthma, aspirin sensitivity and allergy in chronic rhinosinusitis: data from the UK national chronic rhinosinusitis epidemiology study. Respir Res 2018;19(1):129.

20. Fokkens WJ, Lund VJ, Mullol J, et al. European position paper on rhinosinusitis and nasal polyps 2012. Rhinol Suppl 2012;23. 3 p preceding table of contents, 1-298.

21. Gelincik A, Buyukozturk S, Aslan I, et al. Allergic vs nonallergic rhinitis: which is more predisposing to chronic rhinosinusitis? Ann Allergy Asthma Immunol 2008; 101(1):18–22.

22. Sundaresan AS, Hirsch AG, Storm M, et al. Occupational and environmental risk factors for chronic rhinosinusitis: a systematic review. Int Forum Allergy Rhinol 2015;5(11):996–1003.

23. Gao W-X, Ou C-Q, Fang S-B, et al. Occupational and environmental risk factors for chronic rhinosinusitis in China: a multicentre cross-sectional study. Respir Res 2016;17(1):54.

24. Sadhra SS, Kurmi OP, Chambers H, et al. Development of an occupational airborne chemical exposure matrix. Occup Med (Lond) 2016;66(5):358–64.

25. Smith TL. Scientific abstracts for RhinoWorld 2019. Int Forum Allergy Rhinol 2019; 9(S2):S49–124.

26. Workman AD, Kohanski MA, Cohen NA. Biomarkers in chronic rhinosinusitis with nasal polyps. Immunol Allergy Clin North Am 2018;38(4):679–92.

27. Hoggard M, Waldvogel-Thurlow S, Zoing M, et al. Inflammatory endotypes and microbial associations in chronic rhinosinusitis. Front Immunol 2018;9:2065.

28. Tomassen P, Vandeplas G, Van Zele T, et al. Inflammatory endotypes of chronic rhinosinusitis based on cluster analysis of biomarkers. J Allergy Clin Immunol 2016;137(5):1449–56.e4.

29. Liao B, Liu J-X, Li Z-Y, et al. Multidimensional endotypes of chronic rhinosinusitis and their association with treatment outcomes. Allergy 2018;73(7):1459–69.

30. Rianto BUD, Yudhanto D, Herdini C. The correlation between length of work and nasal mucociliary transport time of gas/fuel station workers. Kobe J Med Sci 2018;64(1):E6–10.

31. Christensen DN, Franks ZG, McCrary HC, et al. A systematic review of the association between cigarette smoke exposure and chronic rhinosinusitis. Otolaryngol Head Neck Surg 2018;158(5):801–16.

32. Hirsch AG, Stewart WF, Sundaresan AS, et al. Nasal and sinus symptoms and chronic rhinosinusitis in a population-based sample. Allergy 2017;72(2):274–81.

33. Shi JB, Fu QL, Zhang H, et al. Epidemiology of chronic rhinosinusitis: results from a cross-sectional survey in seven Chinese cities. Allergy 2015;70(5):533–9.

34. Hoehle LP, Phillips KM, Caradonna DS, et al. A contemporary analysis of clinical and demographic factors of chronic rhinosinusitis patients and their association with disease severity. Ir J Med Sci 2018;187(1):215–21.

35. Awad OGA. Impact of habitual marijuana and tobacco smoke on severity of chronic rhinosinusitis. Am J Otolaryngol 2019;40(4):583–8.

36. Weinberger AH, Delnevo CD, Wyka K, et al. Cannabis use is associated with increased risk of cigarette smoking initiation, persistence, and relapse among adults in the US. Nicotine Tob Res 2019. https://doi.org/10.1093/ntr/ntz085.

37. Sun Q, Wang A, Jin X, et al. Long-term air pollution exposure and acceleration of atherosclerosis and vascular inflammation in an animal model. JAMA 2005; 294(23):3003–10.

38. Anderson JO, Thundiyil JG, Stolbach A. Clearing the air: a review of the effects of particulate matter air pollution on human health. J Med Toxicol 2012;8(2):166–75.

39. Zhao R, Chen S, Wang W, et al. The impact of short-term exposure to air pollutants on the onset of out-of-hospital cardiac arrest: a systematic review and meta-analysis. Int J Cardiol 2017;226:110–7.

40. Scheers H, Jacobs L, Casas L, et al. Long-term exposure to particulate matter air pollution is a risk factor for stroke: meta-analytical evidence. Stroke 2015;46(11): 3058–66.

41. Pope CA, Bhatnagar A, McCracken JP, et al. Exposure to fine particulate air pollution is associated with endothelial injury and systemic inflammation. Circ Res 2016;119(11):1204–14.

42. Hoffmann B, Moebus S, Dragano N, et al. Chronic residential exposure to particulate matter air pollution and systemic inflammatory markers. Environ Health Perspect 2009;117(8):1302–8.

43. Kim JA, Cho JH, Park IH, et al. Diesel exhaust particles upregulate interleukins il-6 and il-8 in nasal fibroblasts. PLoS One 2016;11(6):e0157058.

44. Fukuoka A, Matsushita K, Morikawa T, et al. Diesel exhaust particles exacerbate allergic rhinitis in mice by disrupting the nasal epithelial barrier. Clin Exp Allergy 2016;46(1):142–52.

45. Hong Z, Guo Z, Zhang R, et al. Airborne fine particulate matter induces oxidative stress and inflammation in human nasal epithelial cells. Tohoku J Exp Med 2016; 239(2):117–25.

46. Zhao R, Guo Z, Zhang R, et al. Nasal epithelial barrier disruption by particulate matter </=2.5 mum via tight junction protein degradation. J Appl Toxicol 2018; 38(5):678–87.

47. Ramanathan M Jr, London NR Jr, Tharakan A, et al. Airborne particulate matter induces nonallergic eosinophilic sinonasal inflammation in mice. Am J Respir Cell Mol Biol 2017;57(1):59–65.

48. Hussey SJK, Purves J, Allcock N, et al. Air pollution alters Staphylococcus aureus and Streptococcus pneumoniae biofilms, antibiotic tolerance and colonisation. Environ Microbiol 2017;19(5):1868–80.

49. Bachert C, Zhang N, Patou J, et al. Role of staphylococcal superantigens in upper airway disease. Curr Opin Allergy Clin Immunol 2008;8(1):34–8.

Olfactory Dysfunction and Chronic Rhinosinusitis

Omar G. Ahmed, MD, Nicholas R. Rowan, MD*

KEYWORDS

- Olfaction • Chronic rhinosinusitis • Olfactory loss • Olfactory dysfunction

KEY POINTS

- The overall prevalence of olfactory dysfunction in patients with chronic rhinosinusitis (CRS) is high and imparts significant impact on patient quality of life.
- Olfactory dysfunction is caused by a combination of physical obstruction of odorant molecules to the olfactory cleft and an inflammatory response of the olfactory epithelium.
- Both subjective and objective measures olfaction are important for clinicians managing patients with CRS.
- Oral steroids and endoscopic sinus surgery are associated with posttreatment improvements in olfactory dysfunction for patients with CRS with nasal polyposis.

INTRODUCTION

Chronic rhinosinusitis (CRS) is a common disease affecting 12% of the population of western countries[1] and a leading cause of olfactory dysfunction in the general population.[2] It is estimated that from 60% to 80% of patients with CRS have some form of olfactory impairment, which is 1 of the 4 cardinal symptoms of CRS.[3–5] Although olfaction plays an important role in quality of life (QOL) and safety functions for patients, only recently has there been an increasing focus of clinicians and researchers alike on olfactory dysfunction in patients with CRS. This review first aims to summarize and review the epidemiology and risk factors of olfactory dysfunction in CRS. Then, the pathophysiology, clinical features, and differences between patients with CRS with nasal polyposis (CRSwNP) and patients with CRS without nasal polyposis (CRSsNP) are reviewed. Next, the authors describe both subjective and objective measures used to assess olfaction as well as the impact of olfactory dysfunction in CRS on QOL. Finally, the authors review the impact of both medical and surgical management of olfactory dysfunction in CRS.

Department of Otolaryngology–Head and Neck Surgery, Johns Hopkins Hospital, 601 North Caroline Street, 6th floor, Suite 6164, Baltimore, MD 21287, USA
* Corresponding author.
E-mail address: nrowan1@jhmi.edu

Immunol Allergy Clin N Am 40 (2020) 223–232
https://doi.org/10.1016/j.iac.2019.12.013
0889-8561/20/© 2019 Elsevier Inc. All rights reserved.

EPIDEMIOLOGY

CRS is defined by both subjective and objective criteria, with a subjective change in the sense of smell as 1 of the 4 defining symptoms.[1,6] In general, olfactory dysfunction can be classified as either qualitative or quantitative. Qualitative measures include phantosmias, dysosmias, parosmias, and agnosias. Qualitative dysfunction are somewhat rare manifestations in CRS, but have been reported.[2] Reden and colleagues[2] reported 7% of 392 patients with CRS having some form of phantosmia or parosmia. However, quantitative measures of olfaction, which identify hyposmia and anosmia, are more commonly affected in patients in CRS, with 60% to 80% of patients with CRS overall reporting some form of olfactory dysfunction.[2-4] In a recent metaanalysis reviewing objective measures of olfaction in the CRS population, the overall prevalence of olfactory dysfunction was found to be 67% using the 40-item smell identification test (SIT-40), and 78% using the total Sniffin' Sticks score.[7] Interestingly, up to one-fourth of patients with olfactory loss may not recognize their loss, which is hypothesized to be secondary to a prolonged gradual decline in loss of smell.[8]

Although often overlooked, olfactory dysfunction can have potentially dire consequences for patients, including environmental and safety-related risks, impaired nutritional status, and decreased QOL. Pinto and colleagues[9] demonstrated that older, anosmic patients had a 3-fold increased odds ratio of death compared with normosmic patients, even when controlled for chronic diseases, and that olfactory function was one of the strongest predictors of 5-year mortality. The association between smell loss and depression is also well documented.[10] Similarly, and presumably interrelated, there is also a well-established correlation between CRS and depression. It is estimated that from 11% to 40% of CRS patients have depression.[11] Other studies have specifically evaluated the relationship among olfactory dysfunction, CRS, and depression.[12]

In addition to disruptions in the ability to smell, the sense of taste also appears to be impaired in patients with CRS and should be considered when evaluating olfaction in patients with CRS. A recent prospective investigation demonstrated dysgeusia in 28% of a CRS patient population.[13] Moreover, impaired flavor identification also appears to be a strong predictor for QOL, life satisfaction, depressive symptoms, and health assessment in patients with CRS.[14] Nonetheless, orthonasal olfactory dysfunction has also been shown to directly correlate with poor eating-related QOL,[15,16] and the role of retronasal olfaction in the perception of food may also be implicated.[17,18] Overall, the importance of chemosensory dysfunction in patients with CRS should not be overlooked given its critical importance for the enjoyment of food and the socially shared experience of eating.

RISK FACTORS FOR OLFACTORY DYSFUNCTION IN CHRONIC RHINOSINUSITIS PATIENTS

CRS is multifactorial in nature, although the exact pathophysiology is not completely understood. As one of the hallmark symptoms of the disease, olfactory dysfunction is currently thought to be a manifestation of an immense inflammatory response. Specific, independent risks factors for olfactory dysfunction in CRS include a comorbid diagnosis of smoking, nasal polyposis, and asthma.[19]

Patients with CRSwNP have several potential risk factors and mechanisms of olfactory dysfunction. First, physical obstruction of the olfactory cleft by nasal polyps is an intuitive risk factor for impaired olfaction. In addition to mechanical obstruction, increased tissue eosinophilia appears to have a local, damaging impact by release cytotoxic substances to the olfactory neuroepithelium.[20] Moreover, systemic eosinophilia in patients with CRSwNP and comorbid asthma appears to impart and increased overall systemic inflammatory response, which also affects the olfactory cleft.

Alternatively, patients with CRSsNP also present with olfactory dysfunction, although the overall prevalence and severity of disruption of olfaction in these patients may be less than those patients with CRSwNP.[21] Lower rates of olfactory dysfunction in patients with CRSsNP may be secondary to a less robust inflammatory response and lack of obstructive polyps of the olfactory cleft. Although most CRSsNP patients have subjective olfactory dysfunction, only 17% were found to have objective olfactory dysfunction.[19] These patients are typically less responsive to medical and surgical therapy.[22]

PATHOPHYSIOLOGY OF OLFACTORY DYSFUNCTION IN CHRONIC RHINOSINUSITIS

The 2 leading theories of the pathogenesis of olfactory dysfunction in patients with CRS include, first, a conductive loss, limiting the ability of odorants to present to the olfactory cleft, and second, an inflammatory reaction near the olfactory cleft leading to decreased transmission to olfactory neurons, and a resultant decrease in size of the olfactory bulb.[23] It is likely that both theories play a role in olfactory dysfunction in CRS.

Chronic inflammation of the olfactory cleft may lead to damage to the olfactory epithelium via olfactory sensory neuron apoptosis, leading to the loss of sensory neurons.[24] Chronic inflammation may potentially inhibit olfactory neurogenesis and thus poor recovery of the neuroepithelium, ultimately leading to a transition of this specialized neuroepithelium to squamous or respiratory epithelium.[25] However, this does not explain entirely how inflammation leads to olfactory loss. Clinically, patients may have fluctuating olfactory loss that may be transiently reversed with systemic corticosteroids.[26] There are specific inflammatory mediators that may play a role in the temporary loss of smell associated with CRS. Eosinophils and its inflammatory cytokines (interleukin-2 [IL-2], IL-5, IL-6, IL-10, and IL-13) have been implicated in olfactory loss in CRS.[27] It is hypothesized that perturbations in this cytokine milieu may affect the intracellular tumor necrosis factor-α/c-Jun-N-terminal kinases pathway. Activation of this pathway effects neuronal function and may lead to apoptosis and cell death, and inhibition of this pathway may have neuroprotective effects.[28]

In addition to inflammatory-related issues, investigators have demonstrated an inverse relationship between CRS severity and olfactory bulb size. Chronic sensory deprivation of olfactory neurons appears to be associated with a decrease in function and decrease in size of the olfactory bulb.[29] Similar findings have been reported in patients with postviral anosmia.[30] However, it is unclear if olfactory bulb volume is a consequence or cause of olfactory dysfunction.

SUBJECTIVE MEASURES OF OLFACTORY DYSFUNCTION IN CHRONIC RHINOSINUSITIS

The first step in measurement of olfactory dysfunction in patients with CRS is a subjective assessment. Subjective measures of smell loss may range from limited assessments such as those found as single items in the sinonasal outcome test (SNOT-22) and rhinosinusitis disability index to more sophisticated, olfactory-specific, QOL measures, such as the questionnaire of olfactory disorders-negative statements (QOD-NS).[31]

Although the SNOT-22 questionnaire is the gold standard used to describe sinonasal QOL in patients with CRS, this survey has a single item dedicated to olfactory (and taste) function. The use of a single item limits the ability to identify varying degrees of olfactory dysfunction. In order to provide a more sensitive and detailed assessment, the QOD has been validated and shows good internal consistency and test-retest reliability.[32] This olfactory-specific questionnaire and its abbreviated version, the QOD-NS, delineate subjective olfaction and can be used to assess the impact of olfactory loss and measure the impact of therapeutic interventions.[12] Despite the critical importance of subjective measures in patient QOL, caution should be used in using subjective olfaction metrics alone because subjective assessments may have poor correlation with objective measures of olfaction.[23,33,34]

OBJECTIVE MEASURES OF OLFACTORY DYSFUNCTION IN CHRONIC RHINOSINUSITIS

Objective olfactory function can be grouped into 3 general categories, including psychophysical assessments, imaging modalities, and electrophysiologic tests. In the setting of CRS, psychophysical tests are the most commonly used and readily accessible. Although imaging is also readily accessible, electrophysiologic testing is generally reserved for academic purposes.[35]

There are more than 20 objective psychophysical smell identification tests described in the literature.[23] However, traditionally in the United States, the 40-item SIT-40, also known as the UPSIT, is the most commonly used validated objective measure of olfactory loss. SIT-40 was introduced at the University of Pennsylvania by Doty and colleagues[36] in 1984, which includes a booklet of 40 scratch-and-sniff items, from which a patient has to choose from 1 of 4 proposed smells in a multiple-choice format. This final score is normalized over age. In Europe, and increasingly in the United States, the Sniffin' Sticks test is more commonly used. This test battery assesses odor threshold (T), odor discrimination (D), and odor identification (I), as well as a composite "threshold-discrimination-identification" (TDI) score by using 16 different odorant-containing pens.[37,38] This system also normalizes for gender and age in order to give a more accurate assessment of olfaction. Both of these measures have been used to evaluate olfactory loss in CRS patients. A recent metaanalysis of olfactory function in patients with CRS demonstrated average SIT-40 and TDI scores in the moderate hyposmia range.[7]

Olfactory function can be assessed both orthonasally and retronasally. Orthonasal olfaction is the process in which olfaction is most commonly discussed, with an odorant passing from anterior to posterior from the air, through the nose to the olfactory mucosa. Retronasal olfaction, however, occurs when odorants move from the oral cavity to the nasal cavity through the nasopharynx and to the olfactory mucosa. Retronasal olfactory testing is performed by presenting odorized powders to the oral cavity. Although patients with CRSwNP may have increased retronasal olfaction as compared with traditional orthonasal measures, retronasal olfaction is diminished across patients with CRS.[39]

Beyond psychophysical assessments, imaging of the olfactory cleft and the olfactory bulb can be helpful diagnostic tools to assess olfactory dysfunction in CRS. Computed tomography (CT) imaging is traditionally used to assess the degree of sinonasal mucosal inflammation in patients with CRS. Recent reports have demonstrated that the degree of radiologic opacification in the olfactory cleft on CT correlates with the degree of olfactory loss in CRS.[40] This correlation was stronger in patients with CRSwNP compared with patients with CRSsNP. In line with this, the olfactory cleft endoscopy scale is a validated endoscopic scoring system shown to reliably correlate with objective olfactory function that can easily be performed in routine evaluations for patients with CRS.[41]

MRI is also a useful tool in evaluating patients with olfactory loss and CRS. It can provide detailed imaging of the olfactory apparatus, which includes the olfactory bulb, olfactory tract, sulcus, and the central olfactory projection areas. There is evidence that olfactory bulb size on MRI correlated with olfactory loss in patients with

CRS.[29] There is also evidence of olfactory bulb plasticity, demonstrated by changes in size of the olfactory bulb in accordance with the current olfactory status in patients with CRS.[42] Gudziol and colleagues[42] found that patients with CRSwNP undergoing endoscopic sinus surgery (ESS) had objectively improved olfaction and postoperative increase in olfactory bulb volume size.

OUTCOMES IN OLFACTION AFTER MEDICAL THERAPY

Medical treatment plays an important role in the overall CRS treatment algorithm. Many studies have demonstrated the utility of medical therapy in improving disease severity, overall QOL measures, as well as the utility of medical therapy in improving olfactory outcomes in patients with CRS. Herein, the authors discuss specific olfactory outcomes following various medication therapies, including antibiotics, oral steroids, topical steroids, and combined oral and topical steroids. Most of these studies specifically evaluated patients CRS with polyposis.

The metaanalysis of Banglawala and colleagues[43] of randomized controlled trials (RCTs) specifically evaluating olfactory outcomes after oral steroid treatment in patients with CRSwNP pooled 4 RCTs and found that all studies showed a subjective improvement in olfaction compared with placebo.[44–47] With follow-up limited to a maximum of 6 months, durability of response could not be assessed. Meanwhile, 2 RCTs evaluating objective olfactory outcomes after oral steroids demonstrated short-term improvement with a 2-week follow-up.[45] Emerging evidence also suggests that the degree of olfactory response following the use of oral glucocorticoids correlates with the degree of olfactory improvement following ESS.[48] Although improvements in olfaction following oral steroid administration are certain, the long-term efficacy and sustainability of response are less clear.

Topical steroids may also play a role in the medical management of olfactory dysfunction in CRS. In the metaanalysis by Banglawala and colleagues,[43] 12 RCTs specifically evaluated olfactory outcomes after various topical steroid use in CRS patients. These studies evaluated various forms of topical steroids, including fluticasone, budesonide, and mometasone compared with placebo. These investigators found there was overall subjective improvement in subjective measures, but no objective improvement. As such, it is unclear if the use of topical steroids alone for patients with CRS improves olfactory outcomes, especially given the possible poor correlation between subjective and objective measures.

Meanwhile, 5 clinical trials evaluated the combination of both oral and topical steroids compared with placebo to assess olfaction in CRS patients.[43] In the 5 studies, patients received oral prednisolone for 2 weeks followed by various durations of topical steroid sprays. One-half of the subgroups showed statistical improvement in subjective olfaction, whereas 1 of 3 subgroups demonstrated improvement in objective olfaction.

The use of monoclonal antibodies for patients with CRSwNP may also improve olfactory function.[49,50] Presumably these treatments reduce overall polyposis burden throughout the sinonasal cavities, including the olfactory cleft. Emerging evidence from the postinfectious olfactory loss literature suggests that intranasal sodium citrate may promote improvements in olfaction; however, further investigation is needed to fully elucidate the effects of intranasal sodium citrate, especially as it applied to the CRS patient population.[35]

There have been various other medical treatments to assess olfactory dysfunction in CRS patients that have been studied in the literature, including antibiotics, antifungals, and immune modulators. Although doxycycline and azithromycin may have anti-inflammatory properties, investigations with both of these medications found no significant improvement in olfaction after treatment compared with placebo.[51,52] Similarly, an investigation of intranasal amphotericin B for 3 months compared with placebo also failed to detect an improvement in posttreatment olfaction.[53]

Although there is much literature evaluating olfactory outcomes after medical therapy in CRSwNP patients, there is significantly less available literature specifically investigating patients with CRSsNP. There is some evidence that oral steroids in combination with antibiotics and nasal steroids improve symptoms of CRS, including olfaction with short-term follow-up.[54] However, only 1 of these studies specifically examined olfactory outcomes as the primary endpoint.[54] Other than steroids, low-dose macrolide therapy can be used for CRSsNP patients. It is hypothesized that the potentially anti-inflammatory effects of the antibiotic may reduce inflammation. However, Videler and colleagues[51] found no significant difference in objective smell testing after 11 weeks of low-dose macrolide therapy.

It can be concluded that, although many medical treatments have been shown to have some efficacy in the treatment of CRSwNP, only oral steroids have been shown consistently to improve short-term olfactory outcomes. Evidence is lacking, however, for CRSsNP patients. Long-term outcomes need to be further studied.

OUTCOMES IN OLFACTION AFTER SURGICAL THERAPY

There has been ample research evaluating olfactory outcomes after ESS for CRS. However, one must be cautious in interpreting the data for olfactory outcomes because most studies do not define the extent of surgery.

Objective olfactory function on objective testing generally improves following ESS, with the potential for most significant improvements in women, patients with significant nasal polyposis, and patients with aspirin intolerance.[55,56] Moreover, in a study that specifically evaluated factors associated with recovery of olfactory function after ESS for CRS, patients with more dramatic preoperative loss were more likely to regain postoperative olfactory function in the form of improved UPSIT scores.[19] This study also demonstrated more dramatic olfactory improvement in patients with CRSwNP as compared with patients with CRSsNP after ESS.

One of the first studies to specifically evaluate olfactory-specific QOL outcomes in CRS was published by Soler and colleagues[31] and demonstrated a significant improvement in postoperative QOD-NS scores. Moreover, in this study, baseline radiologic scores predicted postoperative changes in QOD-NS scores. Now, with a growing interest and body of literature examining olfactory-specific outcomes after ESS, a recent metaanalysis evaluated 24 studies on this topic.[57] This review demonstrates postoperative improvements in measures of olfaction in 23 out of the 24 studies, with either objective or subjective testing. Although 50% of nearly 1500 patients reported some improvement in olfaction, several studies did report some degree of worsening of olfaction after ESS.

In addition to ESS alone, there have been studies that specifically evaluated olfactory outcomes after septoplasty and septorhinoplasty for nasal obstruction. In theory, a septoplasty can potentially improve access for odorant molecules to the olfactory cleft. The studies show there is at least short-term improvement in objective olfactory outcomes.[58,59] It is unclear, however, if adding septoplasty to ESS compared with ESS alone improves olfactory outcomes in the CRS population.

Overall, ESS for CRS patients may have a potential benefit in improving olfaction in a subset of patients, including those with nasal polyposis and anosmia. ESS should be performed within established guidelines.

Finally, comparisons between medical and surgical management of CRS have yet to be fully elucidated, but a prospective, multi-institutional study by DeConde and colleagues[60] examined this comparison in 281 medically refractory CRS patients who were candidates for ESS. In this study, 20% of patients elected to continue medical management, whereas 80% chose to undergo ESS. Both groups experienced statistically significant improvement in objective testing for olfactory dysfunction, whereas prior ESS was the only risk factor associated with failure of postoperative olfaction.

SUMMARY AND FUTURE CONSIDERATIONS

Olfactory dysfunction is highly prevalent in the CRS population. This finding is likely related to both an obstructive and an inflammatory response in the olfactory cleft. However, the fluctuating nature of olfactory loss in CRS is still not completely understood. Understanding the importance of inflammatory mediators and their downstream effects in the olfactory epithelium can lead to future targeted therapies, such as stem cell therapy,[61] or even novel treatment strategies, such as electrical stimulation of the olfactory epithelium.[62] Currently, oral steroids and ESS have both demonstrated some degree of efficacy in improving olfactory dysfunction in the short term, especially in patients with CRSwNP; however, durability of response of these therapies remains unclear.

The QOL impacts of olfactory dysfunction in patients with CRS are increasingly understood and are paramount to this patient population. Both validated objective and subjective assessments of olfaction should be performed in patients with CRS. Given the increasing recognition of the role of taste and flavor in QOL, measures of gustation should be considered in future investigations.

DISCLOSURE STATEMENT

The authors have nothing to disclose.

REFERENCES

1. Orlandi RR, Kingdom TT, Hwang PH, et al. International consensus statement on allergy and rhinology: rhinosinusitis. Int Forum Allergy Rhinol 2016;6(Suppl 1):22.
2. Reden J, Maroldt H, Fritz A, et al. A study on the prognostic significance of qualitative olfactory dysfunction. Eur Arch Otorhinolaryngol 2007;264:139–44.
3. Jiang R, Lu F, Liang K, et al. Olfactory function in patients with chronic rhinosinusitis before and after functional endoscopic sinus surgery. Am J Rhinol 2008;22: 445–8.
4. Soler ZM, Mace J, Smith TL. Symptom-based presentation of chronic rhinosinusitis and symptom-specific outcomes after endoscopic sinus surgery. Am J Rhinol 2008;22:297–301.
5. Croy I, Nordin S, Hummel T. Olfactory disorders and quality of life–an updated review. Chem Senses 2014;39:185–94.
6. Fokkens WJ, Lund VJ, Mullol J, et al. EPOS 2012: European position paper on rhinosinusitis and nasal polyps 2012. A summary for otorhinolaryngologists. Rhinology 2012;50:1–12.
7. Kohli P, Naik AN, Harruff EE, et al. The prevalence of olfactory dysfunction in chronic rhinosinusitis. Laryngoscope 2017;127:309–20.
8. Doty RL, Frye R. Influence of nasal obstruction on smell function. Otolaryngol Clin North Am 1989;22:397–411.
9. Pinto JM, Wroblewski KE, Kern DW, et al. Olfactory dysfunction predicts 5-year mortality in older adults. PLoS One 2014;9:e107541.

10. Kohli P, Soler ZM, Nguyen SA, et al. The association between olfaction and depression: a systematic review. Chem Senses 2016;41:479–86.
11. Schlosser RJ, Gage SE, Kohli P, et al. Burden of illness: a systematic review of depression in chronic rhinosinusitis. Am J Rhinol Allergy 2016;30:250–6.
12. Mattos JL, Schlosser RJ, Storck KA, et al. Understanding the relationship between olfactory-specific quality of life, objective olfactory loss, and patient factors in chronic rhinosinusitis. Int Forum Allergy Rhinol 2017;7:734–40.
13. Othieno F, Schlosser RJ, Rowan NR, et al. Taste impairment in chronic rhinosinusitis. Int Forum Allergy Rhinol 2018;8:783–9.
14. Oleszkiewicz A, Park D, Resler K, et al. Quality of life in patients with olfactory loss is better predicted by flavor identification than by orthonasal olfactory function. Chem Senses 2019;44:371–7.
15. Bojanowski V, Hummel T. Retronasal perception of odors. Physiol Behav 2012; 107:484–7.
16. Rowan NR, Soler ZM, Storck KA, et al. Impaired eating-related quality of life in chronic rhinosinusitis. Int Forum Allergy Rhinol 2019;9:240–7.
17. Othieno F, Schlosser RJ, Storck KA, et al. Retronasal olfaction in chronic rhinosinusitis. Laryngoscope 2018;128:2437–42.
18. Ganjaei KG, Soler ZM, Storck KA, et al. Variability in retronasal odor identification among patients with chronic rhinosinusitis. Am J Rhinol Allergy 2018;32:424–31.
19. Litvack JR, Mace JC, Smith TL. Olfactory function and disease severity in chronic rhinosinusitis. Am J Rhinol Allergy 2009;23:139–44.
20. Apter AJ, Mott AE, Cain WS, et al. Olfactory loss and allergic rhinitis. J Allergy Clin Immunol 1992;90:670–80.
21. Alt JA, Mace JC, Buniel MCF, et al. Predictors of olfactory dysfunction in rhinosinusitis using the brief smell identification test. Laryngoscope 2014;124:259.
22. Frasnelli J, Hummel T. Olfactory dysfunction and daily life. Eur Arch Otorhinolaryngol 2005;262:231–5.
23. Hummel T, Whitcroft KL, Andrews P, et al. Position paper on olfactory dysfunction. Rhinology 2016;56:1–30.
24. Kern RC. Chronic sinusitis and anosmia: pathologic changes in the olfactory mucosa. Laryngoscope 2000;110:1071–7.
25. Yee KK, Pribitkin EA, Cowart BJ, et al. Neuropathology of the olfactory mucosa in chronic rhinosinusitis. Am J Rhinol Allergy 2010;24:110–20.
26. Stevens MH. Steroid-dependent anosmia. Laryngoscope 2001;111:200–3.
27. Wu J, Chandra RK, Li P, et al. Olfactory and middle meatal cytokine levels correlate with olfactory function in chronic rhinosinusitis. Laryngoscope 2018;128: E304–10.
28. Victores AJ, Chen M, Smith A, et al. Olfactory loss in chronic rhinosinusitis is associated with neuronal activation of c-Jun N-terminal kinase. Int Forum Allergy Rhinol 2018;8:415–20.
29. Rombaux P, Duprez T, Hummel T. Olfactory bulb volume in the clinical assessment of olfactory dysfunction. Rhinology 2009;47:3–9.
30. Rombaux P, Potier H, Bertrand B, et al. Olfactory bulb volume in patients with sinonasal disease. Am J Rhinol 2008;22:598–601.
31. Soler ZM, Smith TL, Alt JA, et al. Olfactory-specific quality of life outcomes after endoscopic sinus surgery. Int Forum Allergy Rhinol 2016;6:407–13.
32. Simopoulos E, Katotomichelakis M, Gouveris H, et al. Olfaction-associated quality of life in chronic rhinosinusitis: adaptation and validation of an olfaction-specific questionnaire. Laryngoscope 2012;122:1450–4.

33. Landis BN, Hummel T, Hugentobler M, et al. Ratings of overall olfactory function. Chem Senses 2003;28:691–4.

34. Lötsch J, Hummel T. Clinical usefulness of self-rated olfactory performance-a data science-based assessment of ·6000 patients. Chem Senses 2019;44: 357–64.

35. Whitcroft KL, Hummel T. Clinical diagnosis and current management strategies for olfactory dysfunction: a review. JAMA Otolaryngol Head Neck Surg 2019. https://doi.org/10.1001/jamaoto.2019.1728.

36. Doty RL, Shaman P, Kimmelman CP, et al. University of Pennsylvania Smell Identification Test: a rapid quantitative olfactory function test for the clinic. Laryngoscope 1984;94:176–8.

37. Hummel T, Kobal G, Gudziol H, et al. Normative data for the "Sniffin' Sticks" including tests of odor identification, odor discrimination, and olfactory thresholds: an upgrade based on a group of more than 3,000 subjects. Eur Arch Otorhinolaryngol 2007;264:237–43.

38. Hummel T, Sekinger B, Wolf SR, et al. 'Sniffin' sticks': olfactory performance assessed by the combined testing of odor identification, odor discrimination and olfactory threshold. Chem Senses 1997;22:39–52.

39. Heilmann S, Strehle G, Rosenheim K, et al. Clinical assessment of retronasal olfactory function. Arch Otolaryngol Head Neck Surg 2002;128:414–8.

40. Kohli P, Schlosser RJ, Storck K, et al. Olfactory cleft computed tomography analysis and olfaction in chronic rhinosinusitis. Am J Rhinol Allergy 2016;30:402–6.

41. Soler ZM, Hyer JM, Karnezis TT, et al. The Olfactory Cleft Endoscopy Scale correlates with olfactory metrics in patients with chronic rhinosinusitis. Int Forum Allergy Rhinol 2016;6:293–8.

42. Gudziol V, Buschhüter D, Abolmaali N, et al. Increasing olfactory bulb volume due to treatment of chronic rhinosinusitis–a longitudinal study. Brain 2009;132: 3096–101.

43. Banglawala SM, Oyer SL, Lohia S, et al. Olfactory outcomes in chronic rhinosinusitis with nasal polyposis after medical treatments: a systematic review and meta-analysis. Int Forum Allergy Rhinol 2014;4:986–94.

44. Alobid I, Benitez P, Valero A, et al. Oral and intranasal steroid treatments improve nasal patency and paradoxically increase nasal nitric oxide in patients with severe nasal polyposis. Rhinology 2012;50:171–7.

45. Vaidyanathan S, Barnes M, Williamson P, et al. Treatment of chronic rhinosinusitis with nasal polyposis with oral steroids followed by topical steroids: a randomized trial. Ann Intern Med 2011;154:293–302.

46. Alobid I, Benitez P, Pujols L, et al. Severe nasal polyposis and its impact on quality of life. The effect of a short course of oral steroids followed by long-term intranasal steroid treatment. Rhinology 2006;44:8–13.

47. Kroflic B, Coer A, Baudoin T, et al. Topical furosemide versus oral steroid in preoperative management of nasal polyposis. Eur Arch Otorhinolaryngol 2006;263: 767–71.

48. Bogdanov V, Walliczek-Dworschak U, Whitcroft KL, et al. Response to glucocorticosteroids predicts olfactory outcome after ess in chronic rhinosinusitis. Laryngoscope 2019. https://doi.org/10.1002/lary.28233.

49. Tsetsos N, Goudakos JK, Daskalakis D, et al. Monoclonal antibodies for the treatment of chronic rhinosinusitis with nasal polyposis: a systematic review. Rhinology 2018;56:11–21.

50. Cavaliere C, Incorvaia C, Frati F, et al. Recovery of smell sense loss by mepolizumab in a patient allergic to dermatophagoides and affected by chronic rhinosinusitis with nasal polyps. Clin Mol Allergy 2019;17:3.
51. Videler WJ, Badia L, Harvey RJ, et al. Lack of efficacy of long-term, low-dose azithromycin in chronic rhinosinusitis: a randomized controlled trial. Allergy 2011;66: 1457–68.
52. Van Zele T, Gevaert P, Holtappels G, et al. Oral steroids and doxycycline: two different approaches to treat nasal polyps. J Allergy Clin Immunol 2010;125: 106–1076.e4.
53. Ebbens FA, Scadding GK, Badia L, et al. Amphotericin B nasal lavages: not a solution for patients with chronic rhinosinusitis. J Allergy Clin Immunol 2006;118: 1149–56.
54. Poetker DM, Jakubowski LA, Lal D, et al. Oral corticosteroids in the management of adult chronic rhinosinusitis with and without nasal polyps: an evidence-based review with recommendations. Int Forum Allergy Rhinol 2013;3:104–20.
55. Minovi A, Hummel T, Ural A, et al. Predictors of the outcome of nasal surgery in terms of olfactory function. Eur Arch Otorhinolaryngol 2008;265:57–61.
56. Ling FTK, Kountakis SE. Important clinical symptoms in patients undergoing functional endoscopic sinus surgery for chronic rhinosinusitis. Laryngoscope 2007;117:1090–3.
57. Haxel BR. Recovery of olfaction after sinus surgery for chronic rhinosinusitis: a review. Laryngoscope 2019;129:1053–9.
58. Randhawa PS, Watson N, Lechner M, et al. The outcome of septorhinoplasty surgery on olfactory function. Clin Otolaryngol 2016;41:15–20.
59. Schriever VA, Gupta N, Pade J, et al. Olfactory function following nasal surgery: a 1-year follow-up. Eur Arch Otorhinolaryngol 2013;270:107–11.
60. DeConde AS, Mace JC, Alt JA, et al. Comparative effectiveness of medical and surgical therapy on olfaction in chronic rhinosinusitis: a prospective, multi-institutional study. Int Forum Allergy Rhinol 2014;4:725–33.
61. Choi R, Goldstein BJ. Olfactory epithelium: cells, clinical disorders, and insights from an adult stem cell niche. Laryngoscope Investig Otolaryngol 2018;3:35–42.
62. Holbrook EH, Puram SV, See RB, et al. Induction of smell through transethmoid electrical stimulation of the olfactory bulb. Int Forum Allergy Rhinol 2019;9: 158–64.

Primary Immunodeficiency and Rhinosinusitis

Camille Huwyler, MD[a], Sandra Y. Lin, MD[b], Jonathan Liang, MD[c],*

KEYWORDS

- Immune deficiency • Antibody deficiency • Immunoglobulin replacement
- Chronic sinusitis

KEY POINTS

- Patients with difficult-to-treat or refractory chronic rhinosinusitis should be evaluated for underlying primary immunodeficiency.
- Initial investigations of humoral immunodeficiency include serum immunoglobulins and specific antibody response.
- B-cell disorders, including selective immunoglobulin (Ig) A deficiency, common variable immune deficiency, and selective IgG subclass deficiency, are the most common primary immunodeficiency disorders in the adult population; congenital agammaglobulinemia is common in children.
- Early aggressive therapy, including prophylactic antibiotics and intravenous immunoglobulin, can improve clinical outcomes in this population. The role of endoscopic sinus surgery in improving clinical outcomes is unclear.

INTRODUCTION

Sinusitis is a common condition that affects 1 in 8 adults in the United States.[1] The definition of acute rhinosinusitis entails purulent nasal drainage, nasal obstruction, and facial pain or pressure for up to 4 weeks. Chronic rhinosinusitis (CRS) is diagnosed for symptoms persisting greater than 12 weeks. Recurrent acute rhinosinusitis is 4 or more episodes of acute bacterial sinusitis per year with resolution of symptoms between episodes.[2] The direct cost of management of both acute rhinosinusitis and CRS totals more than $11 billion per year with additional indirect costs related to lost workdays, reduced productivity, and reduced quality of life.[3] A subset of patients

[a] Department of Head and Neck Surgery, Kaiser Permanente Oakland Medical Center, 3600 Broadway, Suite 40, Oakland, CA 94611, USA; [b] Department of Otolaryngology–Head and Neck Surgery, Johns Hopkins University School of Medicine, 601 North Caroline Street, 6th Floor, Baltimore, MD 21287, USA; [c] Department of Head and Neck Surgery, Kaiser Permanente Oakland Medical Center, Rhinology & Endoscopic Skull Base Surgery, 3600 Broadway, Suite 40, Oakland, CA 94611, USA
* Corresponding author.
E-mail address: jonathan.liang@kp.org

Immunol Allergy Clin N Am 40 (2020) 233–249
https://doi.org/10.1016/j.iac.2019.12.003
0889-8561/20/© 2019 Elsevier Inc. All rights reserved.

with CRS have refractory disease that persists despite medical and surgical intervention. Underlying conditions that contribute to refractory CRS include allergic rhinitis, granulomatosis with polyangiitis, cystic fibrosis, aspirin-exacerbated respiratory disease, and immunodeficiency.

Primary immunodeficiency represents a multitude of genetic mutations that result in impairment of either the adaptive or innate immune response. This condition is in contrast with secondary immunodeficiency, which results from comorbid medical conditions, including primary illness, human immunodeficiency virus (HIV), and malnutrition, or iatrogenic causes, such as chemotherapy and immune-modulating medication.[4,5] Immunodeficiency manifests in more frequent infections, infections of increased severity, or infections with atypical microorganisms. Defects of immunity can be categorized based on impairment of the humoral, cellular, or innate immune systems. The innate immune system is antigen independent and is involved in pathogen phagocytosis, complement-mediated opsonization, and antigen presentation to activate the adaptive immune system.[6] The adaptive immune system can be categorized into humoral immunity and cellular immunity. With humoral immunity, an extracellular antibody-mediated response occurs against a specific antigen with the assistance of B and helper T lymphocytes. Antibody isotypes are determined by the constant region of the immunoglobulin heavy chain. Serum immunoglobulin (Ig) M is produced in initial infection before class switching to IgG, which has the highest opsonization and neutralization activity. Serum IgA is monomeric but dimerizes on secretion at mucosal surfaces, where it binds microbes to prevent invasion. IgE plays a role in defense against parasitic infection, although increased levels of IgE are seen in atopic and allergic conditions. With cellular immunity, an intracellular response occurs with release of cytokines and activation of cytotoxic T lymphocytes. The activation and function these two arms of the adaptive immune response are summarized in **Table 1**.

REVIEW OF PRIMARY IMMUNODEFICIENCIES ASSOCIATED WITH CHRONIC RHINOSINUSITIS

A comprehensive list of primary immunodeficiencies and their clinical manifestations is shown in **Table 2**. Most primary immunodeficiencies affecting the paranasal sinuses are humoral deficits. Antibodies function in protecting mucosal surfaces, including the

Table 1
Review of adaptive immune system

Humoral Immunity	Cell-Mediated Immunity
• B cell receptors internalize antigen and present part of antigen on surface via MHC type II receptor; T cell receptor–MHC type II interaction causes activation and release of IL-2 and IL-4, which contribute to B cell activation and maturation to secrete immunoglobulins • T cell–independent antibody pathogen neutralization, antibody-dependent cell-mediated cytotoxicity, complement fixation, and agglutination	• Antigen-presenting cells phagocytize antigen and present a fragment of antigen on surface via MHC type II receptor, and secrete IL-1; helper T cells recognize this and secrete IL-2; IL-2 upregulates other T cells, including killer T cells, macrophages, and natural killer cells • Killer T cells attack the infected cells via MHC type I receptor • Natural killer cells are granular lymphocytes that kill infected cells, activated by IL-2 with resulting nonspecific cytotoxic activity

Abbreviations: IL, interleukin; MHC, major histocompatibility complex.

Table 2
Primary immunodeficiency disorders

Disease	Pathogenesis	Clinical Presentation	Treatment
B-cell Disorders			
Congenital agammaglobulinemia[a]	Sporadic or X linked (Bruton) Low immunoglobulin level (<10%) after maternal immunoglobulin is catabolized Presents 6–9 mo of age	Otitis media, sinusitis Sepsis: encapsulated pyogenic organisms Hypoplastic tonsils and adenoids	Prophylactic antibiotics Immunoglobulin replacement
Selective IgA deficiency[a]	Most common immunodeficiency disorder (1 in 700) Low IgA level (<5 mg/dL)	Atopy Sinusitis, pneumonia, otitis media Associated with anaphylaxis during blood transfusion (anti-IgA antibodies)	Antibiotics as needed
Selective IgG subclass deficiency[a]	Low IgG1, IgG2, IgG3, or IgG4 levels Total IgG normal	Otitis media, sinusitis, pneumonia	Immunoglobulin replacement
Common variable hypogammaglobulinemia[a]	Low IgG, IgA, IgM levels Bimodal: age 5–15 y, age 25–45 y, M = F Normal quantity but defective B cells	Sinopulmonary infections Increased risk of malignancy and autoimmune disease Normal tonsils and adenoids	Immunoglobulin replacement
T-cell Disorders			
DiGeorge syndrome	Third and fourth pharyngeal pouch anomaly Agenesis of thymus and parathyroid glands Deletion in 22q11 in >80% Decreased T cells, normal number of B cells	Hypocalcemia and tetany Hypertelorism, mandibular hypoplasia, bifid uvula, short philtrum Fungal infections (thrush), *Pneumocystis jirovecii* pneumonia	Fetal thymus transplant is experimental
Chronic mucocutaneous candidiasis	T cells Defect specific to *Candida*	Thrush Infection of nails and skin	Antifungals

(continued on next page)

Table 2
(continued)

Disease	Pathogenesis	Clinical Presentation	Treatment
Combined B-cell and T-cell Disorders			
Severe combined immunodeficiency disease[a]	X linked or recessive Severe lack of T and B cells Associated adenosine deaminase deficiency	Otitis, pneumocystis pneumonia, candida, diarrhea Failure to thrive, death by age 2 y Absence of tonsils and adenoids	Hematopoietic stem cell transplant Immunoglobulin replacement
Wiskott-Aldrich syndrome[a]	X linked Associated with IgM deficiency Abnormal humoral response to polysaccharide antigens	Triad: thrombocytopenia, eczema, recurrent severe infections Increased risk of atopic disorders, leukemia/lymphoma	Antibiotics Platelets High-dose immunoglobulin replacement Bone marrow transplant
Ataxia-telangiectasia	Caused by a DNA repair defect (gene responsible on chromosome 11) Low immunoglobulin level, and CD3 and CD4 T cells	Recurrent sinopulmonary infections Oculocutaneous telangiectasia Progressive cerebellar ataxia High incidence of malignancy	Antibiotics as needed
Phagocytic/Neutrophil Disorders			
Chronic granulomatous disease[a]	X linked or recessive Defect in NADPH oxidase	Chronic pulmonary, GI, urinary infections Infections by catalase-positive organisms	Prophylactic antibiotics
Chédiak-Higashi syndrome	Autosomal recessive Defect in lysosomal transport protein	Oculocutaneous albinism, neuropathy, neutropenia Staphylococcus and pseudomonas infections	Hematopoietic stem cell transplant
Complement Disorders			

C1 esterase deficiency	Autosomal dominant	Recurrent angioedema	Prophylactic danazol
Terminal complement deficiency (C5–C9)	Inability to form membrane attack complex	Associated with lupus and collagen vascular diseases Recurrent meningococcal or gonococcal infections	Meningococcal vaccine Antibiotics as needed

Abbreviations: GI, gastrointestinal; NADPH, nicotinamide adenine dinucleotide phosphate
a Frequently manifest with sinusitis.

upper and lower airways, and affected individuals develop recurrent otitis media, sinusitis, and pneumonia. These patients are also at increased risk of invasive infections, including meningitis, osteomyelitis, and septicemia, because of antibody dysfunction and/or deficiency.[7] Immunoglobulins in nasal secretions provide antibody-mediated defense against microbes and potential irritants.[8] Humoral immunodeficiency can result from impaired B cell development, immunoglobulin production, or immunoglobulin efficacy.

Congenital agammaglobulinemia is a primary humoral immunodeficiency wherein a de novo or X-linked mutation in a tyrosine kinase impairs cell signaling, resulting in impaired B-cell survival. The incidence of X-linked agammaglobulinemia is 1 in 190,000 male births.[9] Clinical manifestations can appear within the first year of life, commonly with infections of encapsulated organisms including Streptococcus pneumoniae, Staphylococcus aureus, Haemophilus influenzae, and Pseudomonas aeruginosa.[9] Although maternally transmitted IgG protect infants in the first few months of life, mucosal membrane infections, particularly sinusitis and otitis media, can be seen with a lack of secreted IgA.[9] Intravenous immunoglobulin (IVIG) is the mainstay of treatment of agammaglobulinemia and has been shown to reduce serious infections and pulmonary disability.[10] Gastrointestinal and sinopulmonary infections can persist in individuals receiving IVIG, in which case chronic antibiotic therapy is indicated.

Severe combined immunodeficiency (SCID) is a combined B cell and T cell deficiency causing marked immunologic impairment. Current estimates of incidence are approximately 1 in 54,000.[11] SCID is characterized by severe, recurrent bacterial, viral, and fungal infections; chronic diarrhea; and failure to thrive. Most patients present in the first year of life and, without intervention, severe infection and mortality occur by age 2 years. Immune reconstitution with hematopoietic stem cell transplant is curative in 90% of cases.[12]

Common variable immune deficiency (CVID) is a common primary immunodeficiency in adults, affecting about 1 in 25,000 individuals.[13] Patients experience variable hypogammaglobulinemia with reductions in IgG and IgA or IgM levels. Presentation of CVID is highly variable, frequently delaying diagnosis.[14,15] Recurrent infections of the upper and lower airway are common and, over time, bronchiectasis may develop. In a study by Oksenhendler and colleagues,[15] sinusitis was present in 63% of patients before study enrollment. Gastrointestinal infections and chronic diarrhea are also common, as is splenomegaly and associated liver disease and portal hypertension.[15] Bondioni and colleagues[16] showed a high prevalence of sinusitis and pulmonary changes in individuals with CVID, although the two did not correlate in severity. In addition, about 25% of patients with CVID develop autoimmune conditions, including thrombocytopenia, hemolytic anemia, and pernicious anemia. Patients with CVID are at increased risk of malignancy, with 6% to 8% developing B cell lymphoma and showing shorter survival than age-matched and sex-matched controls.[15,17] Immunoglobulin replacement is the primary treatment of CVID. It has been shown to reduce the incidence of pneumonia and significantly decrease associated hospitalizations.[18]

Selective IgA deficiency reflects reduced levels of serum IgA with normal levels of IgG and IgM. It is the most common primary immunodeficiency, with an incidence of 1 in 223 to 1 in 1000 in the general population, although the true incidence is unknown because most individuals are asymptomatic.[19] Clinical manifestations of IgA deficiency include recurrent sinopulmonary infections, gastrointestinal infections and inflammatory disorders, and a predisposition to asthma and atopy.[20–22] In addition, anaphylaxis can be seen in the presence of anti-IgA antibodies. A study by Carr and colleagues[23] showed low serum immunoglobulin levels in patients with refractory CRS and inadequate antipneumococcal titers following vaccination. Similarly, Odat and Alqudah[24] showed low serum IgA levels in individuals with refractory CRS compared with age-matched and sex-matched controls. Treatment of IgA deficiency involves treating associated conditions, with consideration of prophylactic antibiotics in the case of recurrent infections. IVIG is not used because these individuals synthetize normal IgG antibodies.

IgG subclass deficiency is characterized by a reduction in the level of one of the 4 IgG isotypes with a normal level of total IgG. Often, IgG subclass deficiency is a laboratory diagnosis, although clinically significant antibody dysfunction can result in recurrent sinopulmonary infections, atopy, associated IgA deficiency, and an inadequate response to vaccination.[25] In 1 study, IgG subclass deficiency was noted in 21% of patients presenting with prolonged or severe infections.[26] IgG subtypes are designated based on the heavy-chain antigenic epitope, with IgG1 and IgG3 active against toxins and viral protein antigens, whereas IgG2 and IgG4 target bacterial capsular polysaccharides.[27] IgG subclass deficiency has been shown in individuals with refractory rhinosinusitis, although the clinical significance is unknown because 2% to 20% of healthy individuals show reduced levels of 1 or more IgG subclasses.[4,28] The normal levels of IgG subclasses vary with age: IgG1 reaches normal adult levels at 5 years of age, whereas IgG2, IgG3, and IgG4 reach adult levels only by adolescence.[29] Because IgG1 comprises about 60% of total serum IgG, low levels of IgG1 are often associated with low total serum IgG. IgG2 subclass deficiency is more prevalent in children than in adults and can be associated with frequent infections given the role of IgG2 in the polysaccharide capsule antigen response.[30] IgG2 subclass deficiency can occur in isolation or also with IgG4 or IgA deficiency. IgG3 subclass deficiency occurs more commonly in adults than in children.[31] Symptomatic patients have recurrent sinopulmonary infections similar to other subclass deficiencies. In addition, IgG4 deficiency is common in the general population and most individuals are asymptomatic. Deficiency of this subclass has been associated with lung infections, bronchiectasis, and autoimmune conditions.[32] Although IgG subclass deficiency can contribute to chronic sinusitis, Seppänen and colleagues[33] showed IgG4 with low IgG1 or IgG2 level to be associated with chronic or recurrent sinusitis. Treatment of IgG subclass deficiency includes vaccination with the conjugated pneumococcal vaccine in the event of a poor response to the unconjugated polysaccharide vaccine. Antibiotic therapy is indicated for sinopulmonary infections, with recurrent infections warranting prophylactic administration. Despite normal levels of total IgG, IVIG can also be considered for individuals with infections persistent despite antibiotics, although this is controversial because not all patients show improvement.[34,35]

Specific antibody deficiency (SAD) is a humoral immune deficiency characterized by normal serum concentrations of IgG, IgM, and IgA with an inadequate response to polysaccharide antigens as with *S pneumoniae* or *H influenzae* vaccination. A diagnosis of SAD can be difficult to establish because an abnormal vaccine response can indicate a more extensive immunologic defect warranting further evaluation. In addition, consensus has not been established as to the number of serotypes and degree of deficiency needed for diagnosis. As determined by Boyle and colleagues,[36] the incidence of SAD in children with recurrent infections is 14.9%, although the prevalence in the general population is not known. SAD has been associated with allergic rhinitis and recurrent infections, including otitis media, sinusitis, and bronchitis.[23,36,37] Carr and colleagues[23] showed the incidence of SAD to be 11.6% of patients with refractory CRS. These patients also had lower levels of serum IgA and preimmunization antipneumococcal titers, suggestive of impaired sinonasal mucosal immunity. Vaccination with the PCV13 (pneumococcal conjugate vaccine 13) is recommended for individuals with SAD. In children with inadequate response to the pneumococcal polysaccharide vaccine, 80% to 90% responded to the conjugate vaccine.[38] Similar to other humoral immunodeficiencies, antibiotics are indicated for active infections with prophylactic administration for recurrent infections. In small studies and a case report, IVIG was shown to decrease the frequency of infections in patients with SAD, although its use remains controversial given the normal levels of total immunoglobulins and monitoring for response because IgG trough levels are not helpful.[39,40]

Wiskott-Aldrich syndrome (WAS) is a rare cause of immunodeficiency, occurring in 1 in 100,000 live births.[41] Classic WAS is associated with innate and adaptive immunodeficiency, thrombocytopenia, and eczema. However, in its less severe form, X-linked thrombocytopenia, the disease can present with thrombocytopenia with or without infections or eczema.[42] Frequent infections in patients with WAS include otitis media, sinusitis, skin abscess, pneumonia, gastrointestinal and genitourinary infections, and meningitis.[43,44] Treatment of WAS includes prophylactic antibiotics to prevent *Pneumocystis jirovecii* pneumonia, prophylactic acyclovir to treat recurrent herpes simplex infections, and platelet transfusions to treat major bleeding episodes.[42] IVIG is indicated for individuals with significant antibody deficiency. Immunosuppression with medication, such as rituximab, can be used to treat autoimmune manifestations such as autoimmune cytopenia. Elective splenectomy can also be performed to address the thrombocytopenia, although this increases the incidence of sepsis and is not routinely recommended. WAS can be cured with hematopoietic cell transplant from human leukocyte antigen–matched donors.[42]

Chronic granulomatous disease (CGD) is an uncommon primary immunodeficiency that occurs in 1 in 200,000 live births. CGD is attributable to a defect in nicotinamide adenine dinucleotide phosphate (NADPH) oxidase, which prevents the generation of oxygen radicals to kill pathogens after phagocytosis. Catalase-positive organisms such as *S aureus*, *Burkholderia cepacia*, and *Aspergillus* are phagocytosed, leading to the generation of granulomas and a chronic inflammatory response. Patients present with recurrent pneumonias, suppurative adenitis, hepatic abscesses, and osteomyelitis. Sinusitis affects 15% of patients with CGD, with frequent fungal sinus infections.[45] Treatment entails lifelong antibacterial and antifungal prophylaxis with aggressive management of infectious complications, whereas curative therapy entails hematopoietic cell transplant.[46]

Individuals with primary immunodeficiency and CRS with nasal polyps (CRSwNP) also warrant special consideration. In a study investigating immunoglobulin levels and genotyping the complement C4 allele, Seppänen and colleagues[33] found that low complement level and IgG subclass and IgA deficiency were more common in those with chronic sinusitis rather than acute sinusitis. In analysis of patients with SAD and chronic sinusitis, the presence of nasal polyposis was not differentially associated with pneumococcal antibody response.[23] Similarly, in a retrospective review of immunodeficiencies associated with refractory CRS, Alqudah and colleagues[47] found that nasal polyposis was present in 28% of the study population and this group tended to show an impaired response to the unconjugated pneumococcal polysaccharide vaccine, although this was not significant. There are limited data on treatment response in individuals with CRSwNP and primary immunodeficiency. In Khalid and colleagues'[48] review of functional endoscopic sinus surgery outcomes in this group, 2 individuals had nasal polyposis, although their clinical courses and outcomes were not specifically delineated.

DIAGNOSTIC WORK-UP FOR PRIMARY IMMUNODEFICIENCY

Current guidelines dictate that immune function should be evaluated in individuals with CRS or recurrent acute rhinosinusitis in the event of failed management or sinusitis associated with otitis media, bronchiectasis, or pneumonia.[2] The European Society for Immunodeficiencies recommends testing for primary immunodeficiency in adults with 4 or more infections requiring antibiotics within 1 year, recurrent or persistent infections necessitating prolonged antibiosis, 2 or more severe bacterial infections (sepsis, osteomyelitis, and so forth), multiple radiographically confirmed pneumonia in 3 years, infections of atypical pathogens or unusual locations, or a family history of primary immunodeficiency.[49] In addition to recurrent infections, pediatric immunodeficiency may present with impaired growth or failure to thrive. Although CRS is a chronic condition with recurring exacerbations and bacterial infections, Sethi and colleagues[50] advocate screening for primary immunodeficiency on meeting the following criteria: persistence of sinus infection after sinus surgery, inadequate response to antibiotic therapy, unusual pathogens on sinonasal culture, recurrent acute sinusitis, or a history of infections at other sites.

Initial laboratory evaluation includes a complete blood count with differential to quantify lymphocytes; quantitative serum immunoglobulins (IgM, IgG, IgA, and IgE); and the specific antibody response to polysaccharide vaccine antigens, including *H influenzae* type b and *S pneumoniae* (**Fig. 1**).[4] IgG subclasses can be quantified with initial testing or after inadequate vaccine response has been documented. A summary of laboratory findings in individuals with antibody deficiencies is seen in **Table 3**. Similar to humoral immunodeficiency, those with complement pathway defects can present with recurrent infections of encapsulated organisms such as *Neisseria* despite normal blood counts

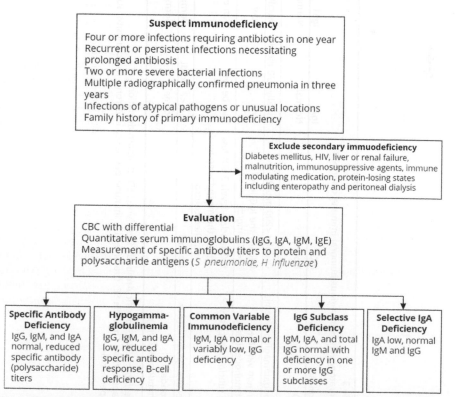

Fig. 1. Flowchart with proposed work-up of patients with CRS and suspected immunodeficiency. CBC, complete blood count.

Table 3
Laboratory values in various humoral immune disorders

Diagnosis	IgG	IgA	IgM	Vaccine Response	B Cells
SAD	Normal	Normal	Normal	Specific antibody titers <1.3 µg/mL	Normal
Hypogammaglobulinemia	Usually <200 mg/dL	Usually <20 mg/dL	Usually <20 mg/dL	Normal	<2% of lymphocytes
Common variable immunodeficiency	Usually the IgG level is <400 mg/dL	Low	Low	Low	Normal or low
IgG subclass deficiency	IgG subclass levels 2 SDs less than the mean for age-matched controls	Can be low	Can be low	Low	Normal
Selective IgA deficiency	Normal	IgA <7 mg/dL	Normal	Normal or low	Normal
Secondary immunodeficiency	Low	Normal	Normal	Normal or low	Normal or low

Abbreviation: SAD, Specific Antibody Deficiency; SD, standard deviation.
Adapted from Chiarella SE, Grammer LC. Immune deficiency in chronic rhinosinusitis: screening and treatment. Expert Rev Clin Immunol 2017;13(2):117-123; with permission.

and immunoglobulin levels and function. In these cases, a total hemolytic complement (CH50) assay is warranted.[51] Individuals infected with usually benign viruses such as cytomegalovirus or Epstein-Barr virus, fungi, or opportunistic infections should be evaluated for T-cell defects because these indicate cellular immune deficiency.[52]

PREVALENCE OF PRIMARY IMMUNODEFICIENCY IN REFRACTORY CHRONIC RHINOSINUSITIS

Primary immunodeficiency is a risk factor in the development of CRS. In a meta-analysis performed by Schwitzguébel and colleagues,[53] the pooled prevalence of CVID, IgA deficiency, and IgG deficiency was 9.4% for recurrent CRS and 18.6% for difficult-to-treat CRS (defined as noncontrolled rhinosinusitis despite sinus surgery and medical management for at least 1 year). A similar incidence of humoral immuno-deficiency was observed by Vanlerberghe and colleagues[28] in which 21.8% of patients with refractory sinusitis showed humoral immune disorders. The prevalence of specific humoral immunodeficiencies has been evaluated in several studies. In a retrospective review of 78 patients with refractory sinusitis, Chee and colleagues[54] showed low serum IgG levels in 17.9%, low IgA levels in 16.7%, and low IgM levels in 5.1%. This study also evaluated the role of cellular immunity in CRS and found the in vitro T-cell response was reduced in 26.3% of patients and 54.8% had abnormal proliferation rates. Similarly, delayed-type hypersensitivity skin testing showed reduced response or anergy in 40% of 55 patients tested. Although the contribution of this finding to the pathogenesis of refractory chronic sinusitis is unknown, aberrant T-cell function could impair normal humoral immunity and the response to viral and fungal pathogens.

Humoral immunodeficiency was further characterized by Vanlerberghe and colleagues[28] in 2006 after patients with refractory sinusitis were subject to humoral immune testing: an incidence of IgA deficiency was detected in 2.2% of individuals, and, in the IgG subclasses evaluated, IgG2 deficiency was noted in 2% and IgG3 deficiency in 17.9% of patients. No patients were found to have CVID, and the distribution of humoral immunodeficiency was not significantly different between adult and child participants. Based on their findings, the investigators recommend screening individuals with refractory CRS for quantitative immunoglobulins as well as IgG subclass deficiency. In addition to evaluation of immunoglobulin isotypes and IgG subclasses, Alqudah and colleagues[47] assessed the humoral response following unconjugated pneumococcal polysaccharide vaccination: inadequate vaccine response was noted if the increase in postvaccination titers was less than 4-fold for at least 7 of the 14 serotypes; this was found in 67% of patients and was not correlated to deficiency in any 1 immunoglobulin isotype or subclass. In addition, although poor responders tended to have more sinus surgeries and sinopulmonary infections, this was not statistically significant from the study population. Given these findings, the investigators recommended quantitative assessment of humoral immunity in addition to functional assessment in patients with refractory CRS and normal immunoglobulin levels. Further study on the humoral response to vaccination was performed by Carr and colleagues,[23] who assessed individuals with CRS for SAD. In their study of 129 individuals, 72% had low baseline antipneumococcal titers and 11.6% were diagnosed with SAD based on antibody titers less than 1.3 μg/mL for at least 7 of the 14 serotypes.[23] These patients had lower serum IgA levels and lower levels of prevaccination pneumococcal titers, suggestive of deficiency in both humoral and innate immune systems.

Bacterial pathogens in acute sinusitis consist of mostly aerobic bacteria, including *S pneumoniae*, *H influenzae*, and *Moraxella catarrhalis*, whereas isolates of chronic sinusitis include anaerobes such as *Prevotella, Porphyromonas, Peptostreptococcus,* and *Fusobacterium* subspecies.[55] In studies of patients with primary immunodeficiency and CRS, bacterial isolates are similar: *M catarrhalis, S pneumoniae, S aureus, H influenzae.*[48,56,57]

TREATMENT

CRS can be difficult to treat in refractory cases and presents lifelong management considerations for patients. Treatment goals include improving quality of life and symptom management through the reduction of mucosal inflammation, maintenance of patent sinus drainage pathways, treating microbial pathogens, and limiting the severity and frequency of acute exacerbations. Initial treatment is designed to minimize symptoms before patients are started on maintenance therapy. Saline irrigation and intranasal glucocorticoids are mainstays of treatment, with antibiotics reserved for initial therapy or acute exacerbations.[2] Recognition of primary immunodeficiency in individuals with CRS allows early and aggressive treatment of acute exacerbations, prophylactic antibiotics, vaccination with the conjugated pneumococcal antigen vaccine, and initiation of IVIG if indicated.

Before a diagnosis of primary immunodeficiency, most patients have already received multiple courses of antibiotics for treatment of sinusitis or even prophylaxis.[50] Early culture-directed therapy is warranted because microbial pathogens may be atypical in this population and a longer duration of antibiotics is often required. Prophylactic antibiotics can reduce the frequency of acute exacerbations and, given the high prevalence of sinus inflammation and colonization reported by Kainulainen and colleagues,[58] they recommend consideration of antibiotic prophylaxis in asymptomatic individuals.[50,59] Ocampo and Peters[60] recommend using β-lactams, trimethoprim-sulfamethoxazole, and azithromycin for prophylaxis in this patient population.

Multiple studies have investigated the role of IVIG in patients with primary immunodeficiency and CRS. Initiation of IVIG can be considered for individuals with recurrent sinonasal infections despite prophylactic antibiosis.[60] In 2006 the US Food and Drug Administration approved subcutaneous immunoglobulin to treat patients with primary immunodeficiency. Subcutaneous administration has been shown to be safe and efficacious with improved tolerance and ease of administration.[61,62] In a study of patients with CVID or SAD, Walsh and colleagues[63] showed a reduction in sinonasal infections from 5 per year to 0.7 per year and discontinuation of prophylactic antibiotic use in 56% of individuals. Improved inflammation as quantified by Lund-Mackay scores was also noted but this was not significant after controlling for prior sinus surgery. Similarly, Roifman and colleagues[31] showed a reduction in sinopulmonary infections necessitating hospitalization and improved inflammation radiographically after administration of IVIG in patients with hypogammaglobulinemia. These data are contested by the findings of Quinti and colleagues,[14] who showed that IVIG therapy in patients with CVID slowed progression of chronic lung disease but its efficacy in treating sinusitis is less clear. Quinti and colleagues[14] showed an increasing prevalence of sinusitis in patients with CVID even after initiation of IVIG.

Endoscopic sinus surgery (ESS) can be considered in individuals with CRS to establish patent sinus drainage pathways and improve ventilation on failure of medical treatment. Few studies have been done to assess the efficacy of sinus surgery on those with primary immunodeficiency. Main outcomes in this population include symptom improvement, antibiotic use, and quality-of-life metrics. An early study of 20 patients with primary immunodeficiency, including IgG subclass deficiency, by Sethi and colleagues[50] examined the various surgical procedures performed to treat

CRS. The most common procedure performed was ethmoidectomy, followed by revision sphenoethmoidectomy. In 7 patients on antibiotic prophylaxis, 5 were downgraded to intermittent antibiotics and only 1 was continued on regular antibiotics after 6 months. Khalid and colleagues[48] evaluated ESS in patients with immune deficiency, both primary and secondary, and autoimmune conditions. Compared with case-matched controls, quality-of-life scores and symptom improvement were similar; on 18-month follow-up, computed tomography and endoscopic examinations were similar as well.

CONSIDERATIONS FOR PEDIATRIC PATIENTS

Children with immunodeficiency constitute a unique subset of patients with CRS. Shapiro and colleagues[64] reviewed the cases of 61 children aged 2 to 13 years with CRS. Thirty-four patients were found to have primary immunodeficiency. Eleven patients had low serum immunoglobulin levels, most commonly IgG3, and 23 had a poor response to vaccination with pneumococcal and H influenzae antigens. Patients were managed with antibiotics and few were enrolled in trials of IVIG. Patients were followed over a 1-year period, so long-term improvement and clinical course are unclear.[64] A large cohort of pediatric patients with CRS and primary immunodeficiency were retrospectively reviewed by Bernatowska and colleagues.[65] Ramesh and colleagues[66] published a trial of IVIG in children with CRS without primary immunodeficiency. Quantitative immunoglobulins were assessed and 2 patients had IgG2 subclass deficiency, 1 had decreased total serum IgG level, and another had reduced total IgG and IgG1 levels. IVIG treatment was initiated after patients failed prophylactic antibiotics. Five of 6 patients showed a significant reduction in daily antibiotic use and a mean reduction in sinusitis exacerbations from 9 to 4 per year. Comorbid asthma also improved in 4 of 5 patients with reduced oral steroid use and frequency of exacerbations. The role of sinus surgery in pediatric patients with primary immunodeficiency was evaluated by Lusk and colleagues,[67] with 5 of 9 patients reporting significant symptom improvement on 2-year follow-up, and prophylactic antibiotics were discontinued in 3 patients.

SUMMARY AND FUTURE CONSIDERATIONS

In patients with refractory CRS, comorbid conditions such as immunodeficiency should be considered. A preliminary work-up, including a complete blood count with differential and quantitative serum immunoglobulins, can aid in diagnosis of commonly occurring primary immunodeficiencies. Treatment with culture-directed or prophylactic antibiotics, IVIG, and ESS if warranted can improve sinopulmonary outcomes and avoid long-term pulmonary complications.

Future research of CRS in the primary immunodeficient population could better define the relationship between the severity of immunodeficiency and CRS symptoms. Research to date has established the prevalence of various primary immunodeficiencies in individuals with recalcitrant CRS, but understanding the degree to which CRS symptoms and quality-of-life impairment are affected by the severity of hypogammaglobulinemia could help identify treatment parameters in this population. Additional investigation could aim to optimize medical and surgical treatment. Immune supplementation has been shown to be beneficial in the progression of pulmonary disease in primary immunodeficient patients, but optimizing medical treatment of sinusitis beyond antibiosis is critical. In addition, because immune-modulating medications are becoming increasingly prevalent, secondary immunodeficiency and CRS may become more common. In addition, although quality of life and symptoms improve with sinus surgery for CRS in patients with immunodeficiency, the timing of and indications for surgery are variable, and best practices remain to be elucidated.

DISCLOSURE

Potential conflicts of interest: none.

REFERENCES

1. Lethbridge-Çejku M, Rose D, Vickerie JL. Summary health statistics for the US adults; National health interview survey, 2004. Vital Health Stat 10 2006;(228): 1–164.
2. Rosenfeld RM, Piccirillo JF, Chandrasekhar SS, et al. Clinical practice guideline (update): adult sinusitis. Otolaryngol Head Neck Surg 2015;152(2_suppl):S1–39.
3. Blackwell DL, Lucas JW, Clarke TC. Summary health statistics for US adults: national health interview survey, 2012. Vital Health Stat 10 2014;(260):1–161.
4. Fried AJ, Bonilla FA. Pathogenesis, diagnosis, and management of primary antibody deficiencies and infections. Clin Microbiol Rev 2009;22(3):396–414.
5. Rosen FS, Cooper MD, Wedgwood RJ. The primary immunodeficiencies. N Engl J Med 1984;311(4):235–42.
6. Warrington R, Watson W, Kim HL, et al. An introduction to immunology and immunopathology. Allergy Asthma Clin Immunol 2011;7(1):S1.
7. Rosen FS, Cooper MD, Wedgwood RJ. The primary immunodeficiencies. N Engl J Med 1995;333(7):431–40.
8. Kirkeby L, Rasmussen TT, Reinholdt J, et al. Immunoglobulins in nasal secretions of healthy humans: structural integrity of secretory immunoglobulin A1 (IgA1) and occurrence of neutralizing antibodies to IgA1 proteases of nasal bacteria. Clin Diagn Lab Immunol 2000;7(1):31–9.
9. Winkelstein JA, Marino MC, Lederman HM, et al. X-linked agammaglobulinemia: report on a United States registry of 201 patients. Medicine 2006;85(4):193–202.
10. Quartier P, Debré M, De Blic J, et al. Early and prolonged intravenous immunoglobulin replacement therapy in childhood agammaglobulinemia: a retrospective survey of 31 patients. J Pediatr 1999;134(5):589–96.
11. Kwan A, Abraham RS, Currier R, et al. Newborn screening for severe combined immunodeficiency in 11 screening programs in the United States. JAMA 2014; 312(7):729–38.
12. Heimall J, Logan BR, Cowan MJ, et al. Immune reconstitution and survival of 100 SCID patients post–hematopoietic cell transplant: a PIDTC natural history study. Blood 2017;130(25):2718–27.
13. Cunningham-Rundles C. How I treat common variable immune deficiency. Blood 2010;116(1):7–15.
14. Quinti I, Soresina A, Spadaro G, et al. Long-term follow-up and outcome of a large cohort of patients with common variable immunodeficiency. J Clin Immunol 2007;27(3):308–16.
15. Oksenhendler E, Gérard L, Fieschi C, et al. Infections in 252 patients with common variable immunodeficiency. Clin Infect Dis 2008;46(10):1547–54.
16. Bondioni MP, Duse M, Plebani A, et al. Pulmonary and sinusal changes in 45 patients with primary immunodeficiencies: computed tomography evaluation. J Comput Assist Tomogr 2007;31(4):620–8.
17. Resnick ES, Moshier EL, Godbold JH, et al. Morbidity and mortality in common variable immune deficiency over 4 decades. Blood 2012;119(7):1650–7.

18. Busse PJ, Razvi S, Cunningham-Rundles C. Efficacy of intravenous immunoglobulin in the prevention of pneumonia in patients with common variable immunodeficiency. J Allergy Clin Immunol 2002;109(6):1001–4.

19. Cunningham-Rundles C. Physiology of IgA and IgA deficiency. J Clin Immunol 2001;21(5):303–9.

20. Yel L. Selective IgA deficiency. J Clin Immunol 2010;30(1):10–6.

21. Urm SH, Yun HD, Fenta YA, et al. Asthma and risk of selective IgA deficiency or common variable immunodeficiency: a population-based case-control study. Paper presented at: Mayo Clinic Proceedings. Elsevier: 2013;88(8). p. 813–21.

22. Ludviksson B, Eiriksson T, Ardal B, et al. Correlation between serum immunoglobulin A concentrations and allergic manifestations in infants. J Pediatr 1992; 121(1):23–7.

23. Carr TF, Koterba AP, Chandra R, et al. Characterization of specific antibody deficiency in adults with medically refractory chronic rhinosinusitis. Am J Rhinol Allergy 2011;25(4):241–4.

24. Odat H, Alqudah M. Prevalence and pattern of humoral immunodeficiency in chronic refractory sinusitis. Eur Arch Otorhinolaryngol 2016;273(10):3189–93.

25. de Moraes Lui C, Oliveira LC, Diogo CL, et al. Immunoglobulin G subclass concentrations and infections in children and adolescents with severe asthma. Pediatr Allergy Immunol 2002;13(3):195–202.

26. Aucouturier P, Lacombe C, Bremard C, et al. Serum IgG subclass levels in patients with primary immunodeficiency syndromes or abnormal susceptibility to infections. Clin Immunol Immunopathol 1989;51(1):22–37.

27. Schroeder HW Jr, Cavacini L. Structure and function of immunoglobulins. J Allergy Clin Immunol 2010;125(2):S41–52.

28. Vanlerberghe L, Joniau S, Jorissen M. The prevalence of humoral immunodeficiency in refractory rhinosinusitis: a retrospective analysis. B-ENT 2006;2(4): 161–6.

29. Agarwal S, Cunningham-Rundles C. Assessment and clinical interpretation of reduced IgG values. Ann Allergy Asthma Immunol 2007;99(3):281–3.

30. Javier FC III, Moore CM, Sorensen RU. Distribution of primary immunodeficiency diseases diagnosed in a pediatric tertiary hospital. Ann Allergy Asthma Immunol 2000;84(1):25–30.

31. Roifman C, Levison H, Gelfand E. High-dose versus low-dose intravenous immunoglobulin in hypogammaglobulinaemia and chronic lung disease. Lancet 1987; 329(8541):1075–7.

32. Kim J-H, Park H-J, Choi G-S, et al. Immunoglobulin G subclass deficiency is the major phenotype of primary immunodeficiency in a Korean adult cohort. J Korean Med Sci 2010;25(6):824–8.

33. Seppänen M, Suvilehto J, Lokki ML, et al. Immunoglobulins and complement factor C4 in adult rhinosinusitis. Clin Exp Immunol 2006;145(2):219–27.

34. Olinder-Nielsen A-M, Granert C, Forsberg P, et al. Immunoglobulin prophylaxis in 350 adults with IgG subclass deficiency and recurrent respiratory tract infections: a long-term follow-up. Scand J Infect Dis 2007;39(1):44–50.

35. Abdou NI, Greenwell CA, Mehta R, et al. Efficacy of intravenous gammaglobulin for immunoglobulin G subclass and/or antibody deficiency in adults. Int Arch Allergy Immunol 2009;149(3):267–74.

36. Boyle R, Le C, Balloch A, et al. The clinical syndrome of specific antibody deficiency in children. Clin Exp Immunol 2006;146(3):486–92.

37. Cheng YK, Decker PA, O'Byrne MM, et al. Clinical and laboratory characteristics of 75 patients with specific polysaccharide antibody deficiency syndrome. Ann Allergy Asthma Immunol 2006;97(3):306–11.
38. Sorensen RU, Leiva LE, Giangrosso PA, et al. Response to a heptavalent conjugate Streptococcus pneumoniae vaccine in children with recurrent infections who are unresponsive to the polysaccharide vaccine. Pediatr Infect Dis J 1998;17(8): 685–91.
39. Cohn JA, Skorpinski E, Cohn JR. Prevention of pneumococcal infection in a patient with normal immunoglobulin levels but impaired polysaccharide antibody production. Ann Allergy Asthma Immunol 2006;97(5):603–5.
40. Zora J, Silk H, Tinkelman D. Evaluation of postimmunization pneumococcal titers in children with recurrent infections and normal levels of immunoglobulin. Ann Allergy 1993;70(4):283–8.
41. Stray-Pedersen A, Abrahamsen TG, Frøland SS. Primary immunodeficiency diseases in Norway. J Clin Immunol 2000;20(6):477–85.
42. Ochs HD, Filipovich AH, Veys P, et al. Wiskott-Aldrich syndrome: diagnosis, clinical and laboratory manifestations, and treatment. Biol Blood Marrow Transplant 2009;15(1):84–90.
43. Imai K, Morio T, Zhu Y, et al. Clinical course of patients with WASP gene mutations. Blood 2004;103(2):456–64.
44. Sullivan KE, Mullen CA, Blaese RM, et al. A multiinstitutional survey of the Wiskott-Aldrich syndrome. J Pediatr 1994;125(6):876–85.
45. Towbin AJ, Chaves I. Chronic granulomatous disease. Pediatr Radiol 2010;40(5): 657–68.
46. Seger RA. Modern management of chronic granulomatous disease. Br J Haematol 2008;140(3):255–66.
47. Alqudah M, Graham SM, Ballas ZK. High prevalence of humoral immunodeficiency patients with refractory chronic rhinosinusitis. Am J Rhinol Allergy 2010; 24(6):409–12.
48. Khalid AN, Mace JC, Smith TL. Outcomes of sinus surgery in ambulatory patients with immune dysfunction. Am J Rhinol Allergy 2010;24(3):230–3.
49. European Society for Immunodeficiencies. The 6 ESID warning signs for ADULT primary immunodeficiency diseases. 2019. Available at: https://esid.org/Education/6-Warning-Signs-for-PID-in-Adults. Accessed August 28, 2019.
50. Sethi DS, Winkelstein JA, Lederman H, et al. Immunologic defects in patients with chronic recurrent sinusitis: diagnosis and management. Otolaryngol Head Neck Surg 1995;112(2):242–7.
51. Wen L, Atkinson JP, Giclas PC. Clinical and laboratory evaluation of complement deficiency. J Allergy Clin Immunol 2004;113(4):585–93.
52. Dropulic LK, Cohen JI. Severe viral infections and primary immunodeficiencies. Clin Infect Dis 2011;53(9):897–909.
53. Schwitzguébel AJ-P, Jandus P, Lacroix J-S, et al. Immunoglobulin deficiency in patients with chronic rhinosinusitis: Systematic review of the literature and meta-analysis. J Allergy Clin Immunol 2015;136(6):1523–31.
54. Chee L, Graham SM, Carothers DG, et al. Immune dysfunction in refractory sinusitis in a tertiary care setting. Laryngoscope 2001;111(2):233–5.
55. Brook I. Bacteriology of chronic sinusitis and acute exacerbation of chronic sinusitis. Arch Otolaryngol Head Neck Surg 2006;132(10):1099–101.
56. Gabra N, Alromaih S, Endam LM, et al. Clinical features of cytotoxic CD8+ T-lymphocyte deficiency in chronic rhinosinusitis patients: a demographic and functional study. InInternational forum of allergy & rhinology 2014;4(6):495–501.

57. Buehring I, Friedrich B, Schaaf J, et al. Chronic sinusitis refractory to standard management in patients with humoral immunodeficiencies. Clin Exp Immunol 1997;109(3):468–72.
58. Kainulainen L, Suonpää J, Nikoskelainen J, et al. Bacteria and viruses in maxillary sinuses of patients with primary hypogammaglobulinemia. Arch Otolaryngol Head Neck Surg 2007;133(6):597–602.
59. Chiarella SE, Grammer LC. Immune deficiency in chronic rhinosinusitis: screening and treatment. Expert Rev Clin Immunol 2017;13(2):117–23.
60. Ocampo CJ, Peters AT. Antibody deficiency in chronic rhinosinusitis: epidemiology and burden of illness. Am J Rhinol Allergy 2013;27(1):34–8.
61. Kobrynski L. Subcutaneous immunoglobulin therapy: a new option for patients with primary immunodeficiency diseases. Biologics 2012;6:277–87.
62. Lucas M, Lee M, Lortan J, et al. Infection outcomes in patients with common variable immunodeficiency disorders: Relationship to immunoglobulin therapy over 22 years. J Allergy Clin Immunol 2010;125(6):1354–60.e4.
63. Walsh JE, Gurrola JG, Graham SM, et al. Immunoglobulin replacement therapy reduces chronic rhinosinusitis in patients with antibody deficiency. Paper presented at: International forum of allergy & rhinology 2017.
64. Shapiro GG, Virant FS, Furukawa CT, et al. Immunologic defects in patients with refractory sinusitis. Pediatrics 1991;87(3):311–6.
65. Bernatowska E, Mikołuć B, Krzeski A, et al. Chronic rhinosinusitis in primary antibody immunodeficient patients. Int J Pediatr Otorhinolaryngol 2006;70(9):1587–92.
66. Ramesh S, Brodsky L, Afshani E, et al. Open trial of intravenous immune serum globulin for chronic sinusitis in children. Ann Allergy Asthma Immunol 1997;79(2):119–24.
67. Lusk RP, Polmar SH, Muntz HR. Endoscopic ethmoidectomy and maxillary antrostomy in immunodeficient patients. Arch Otolaryngol Head Neck Surg 1991;117(1):60–3.

The Microbiome and Chronic Rhinosinusitis

Do-Yeon Cho, MD[a,b], Ryan C. Hunter, PhD[c], Vijay R. Ramakrishnan, MD[d,*]

KEYWORDS

- Microbiome • Sinusitis • Chronic rhinosinusitis • Anaerobe • Mucin fermentation
- Animal model of CRS • Pseudomonas

KEY POINTS

- The dysbiosis hypothesis (alteration of microbial composition associated with perturbation of the local ecological landscape) has been widely implicated in chronic rhinosinusitis (CRS).
- CRS might develop through a defined series of temporally dependent events: Impaired mucus clearance → anaerobic microenvironments → anaerobe proliferation → increased nutrient availability for sinus pathogens.
- There remains a need for continued CRS research with longitudinal sampling prior to and during disease initiation and application of robust preclinical models.

INTRODUCTION

The upper airways play a critical role in the respiratory system by conditioning and clearing contaminants from the inspired airstream before it accesses the lower respiratory system.[1] Large particulate matter is removed from inhaled air in the anterior naris or nasal vestibule, a relatively dry environment lined by skinlike squamous epithelial cells and containing sebaceous glands and vibrissae. Smaller particulate matter, including bacteria and hydrophilic aerosolized compounds, are trapped in a flowing mucus blanket covering the sinonasal mucosa deeper in the nasal cavity and sinuses. Sinonasal mucociliary function is a key host defense mechanism that clears the inhaled particulate matter. Characterized by impaired mucociliary clearance (MCC), bacterial colonization may play some role in the initiation or sustenance of the inflammatory process in chronic rhinosinusitis (CRS).[2]

[a] Department of Otolaryngology-Head & Neck Surgery, University of Alabama at Birmingham, 1155 Faculty Office Tower, 510 20th Street South, Birmingham, AL 35233, USA; [b] Gregory Fleming James Cystic Fibrosis Research Center, University of Alabama at Birmingham, Birmingham, AL, USA; [c] Department of Microbiology & Immunology, University of Minnesota, 3-115 Microbiology Research Facility, 689 23rd Avenue SE, Minneapolis, MN 55455, USA; [d] Department of Otolaryngology-Head and Neck Surgery, University of Colorado, 12631 East 17th Avenue, B205, Aurora, CO 80045, USA
* Corresponding author.
E-mail address: vijay.ramakrishnan@ucdenver.edu

Immunol Allergy Clin N Am 40 (2020) 251–263
https://doi.org/10.1016/j.iac.2019.12.009
0889-8561/20/© 2019 Elsevier Inc. All rights reserved.
immunology.theclinics.com

In recent years, growing understanding of the fundamental role of the microbiome in the initiation, adaptation, and function of the human immune system has revolutionized the field of mucosal immunology.[3] Although each inflammatory disease can be differentiated by exclusive genetic and biological mechanisms, many inflammatory diseases, including CRS, are associated with significant shifts in the resident microbiota from a healthy to a diseased state.[3] The dysbiosis hypothesis—alteration of microbial composition associated with perturbation of the local ecological landscape—has been widely suggested as a mechanism involved in CRS pathogenesis. This hypothesis is supported by several studies identifying a healthy local environment with particular keystone species, or microbes that normally maintain a stable and interactive community.[4–6] Yet, sinus microbiome studies are in their infancy; many findings have not been replicated due to small study cohorts and variable experimental methods. In addition, results across studies are difficult to interpret in aggregate, and observed associations do not establish causality between the presence of certain microbial communities in the airways and the development of CRS.[7] Many of these difficulties are intrinsically related to the broad diagnostic parameters of CRS and lack of a universally appropriate animal model.

High-impact microbiome studies from other organ systems (eg, gut) have been conceptually applied to the respiratory field.[8] Although seemingly reasonable, nucleic acid–based surveys of airway microbial communities and their proposed role(s) in CRS remain to be addressed using appropriate model systems. Should an etiological role of specific community structures hold true, opportunities will arise for novel therapeutic interventions with potential for personalized, microbiome-based treatment strategies. This review discusses major concepts that highlight the complex role of the microbiota in sinus health and disease and explores future directions for study.

CONSIDERATIONS IN SINUS MICROBIOME INVESTIGATION

Sampling locations vary between studies, reflecting subtly different microenvironments throughout the upper airway, and making cross-study meta-analyses a challenge.[9] It is clear that the anterior nasal cavity microbiome is distinct from the middle meatus and sphenoethmoid recess in the healthy state,[10] but the most representative single sampling site in the nasal cavity is often argued.[4,11] How can a single site encompass the complexities of the many anatomic niches and account for differences in local immune and disease properties? The middle meatus often is used as a representative sampling site for the deeper sinuses, given

1. Its high agreement in culture comparison studies with the maxillary sinus[12]
2. Its location as a common drainage pathway of the 3 major (maxillary, anterior ethmoid, and frontal) sinuses
3. Its accessibility for sampling[9,13]

In the gastrointestinal (GI) microbiome field, stool often is studied as a convenient single sample that overrepresents the cecal contribution, acknowledging there are likely biogeographical differences between the upper GI tract, duodenum, jejunum, ileum, and large intestine. To address this concern in the context of CRS, the authors compared 12 sites from 8 subjects with CRS at the time of surgical intervention and found a fair concordance between the middle meatus and underlying sinuses. These data suggest that, if there is interested in single-site representation, then the middle meatus would be a reasonable proxy for the entire upper airway.[14]

In terms of bacterial detection, it is clear that molecular methods are superior to traditional culture-based approaches in CRS, because identification of even the most fastidious of organisms can be achieved with DNA-based detection and classification by variable regions with the 16S ribosomal RNA (rRNA).[15–17] Hauser and colleagues[16] demonstrated that bacterial detection using 16S rRNA gene sequencing allows for greater sensitivity and provides more information on bacterial diversity than standard clinical swab culture in CRS. Although clinical laboratory culture has been the gold standard for decades and offers useful information, these techniques are unique to institutional laboratories and may miss bacteria that are present in disease. The true clinical utility of culture-independent molecular techniques remains, however, to be determined. The ability to detect bacteria that are present more accurately may allow for more effective treatment regimens and allow for an improved basis for clinical and laboratory research into CRS. Nevertheless, there are some shortcomings of culture-independent molecular techniques. 16S rRNA gene sequencing measures total or relative abundance of bacterial DNA and does not differentiate between actively growing, dormant, or dead biomass.[18] As with all tests, it is important to be aware of such biases. To better understand in vivo bacterial activity, culture-independent approaches must be improved and new innovative techniques should continue to be integrated, for instance, by separating active cells from extracellular DNA and inactive microbial subpopulations.[19,20]

Currently, there are 2 main gene sequencing approaches used for studying microbial communities:

1. Targeted sequencing of specific marker genes (ie, 16S rRNA gene for bacteria and 18S rRNA or internal transcribed spacer regions for fungi)
2. Shotgun sequencing of the metagenome

16S rRNA gene sequencing currently is the most widely used approach for characterizing bacterial community membership and comparing phylogeny between samples. This method is based on the premise that 9 hypervariable regions within the 16S rRNA gene harbor sufficient sequence diversity to differentiate bacterial taxa down to the genus or species level. Flanking these regions are highly conserved sequences across bacteria and archaea that facilitate the use of universal polymerase chain reaction primer sets.[21,22] Although costlier, shotgun sequencing methods are useful for characterizing microbial communities more broadly, including viruses and fungi that also have been implicated in the development of upper airway disease. Shotgun metagenomics, the study of whole-community DNA extracted directly from samples, increasingly has been used in various settings, particularly as sequencing costs decrease and output increases.[23,24] Furthermore, relative to targeted amplicon assays (eg, 16S rRNA gene sequencing), shotgun metagenomics offers potential for both higher-resolution identification of organisms and the study of microbial communities without introduction of sequencing bias due to unequal amplification of the target gene.[24,25] Moreover, shotgun approaches capture details of the microbial metagenome (ie, antibiotic resistance and virulence factors) not provided using single-marker gene studies.[22,26] Sequencing technologies have undergone rapid advances during the past several years to attempt to resolve biases associated with current methods and to obtain a better balance between data yield, read length, and cost.[22] These efforts have resulted in third-generation sequencing technologies (eg, Oxford Nanopore, Technologies Oxford Science Park, UK and PacBio platforms, Pacific Biosciences, Menlo Park, CA), which are single-molecule and real-time technologies that reduce amplification bias as well as short read length limitations.[22,27,28] Reduction in cost and time presented by these sequencing methods are valuable assets, and certainly future incorporation of new technologies and bioinformatics is expected.

Based on the anatomic location and local disease environment, viruses and fungi have hypothesized interactions with the bacterial community, which have been borne out in a prior study.[29] The relative absence of fungal and viral study at the current time may be a simple lag behind the bacterial microbiome research explosion, because the early microbial detection techniques focused primarily on numerically dominant bacteria. Multiple studies have demonstrated the presence of viruses and fungi in CRS.[30–35] Virus replication can result in epithelial damage and increase bacterial mucosal adhesion, whereas fungi may act synergistically with pathogenic bacteria to play a role in the pathogenesis of CRS.[32,36] The precise roles of these organisms in the pathogenesis of CRS and etiologic importance remains poorly understood.[32]

DYSBIOSIS OF SINUS MICROBIOTA IN CHRONIC RHINOSINUSITIS

Analysis of the normal state of the microbiome in sinus cavities is crucial, because there is a clear role for commensals in pathogen exclusion and in the modulation of the healthy host-microbial immune response.[37] The deeper nasal cavity and sinuses have unique local microenvironments (P_{O_2}, pH, and so forth) and host immune properties.[11,38,39] Although Yan and colleagues[10] recently examined deeper anatomic subsites in healthy human nasal cavities and Ramakrishnan and colleagues[14] compared upper airway subsites and sinuses in CRS, there has been no thorough comparison within normal sinus cavities to date, perhaps owing to the requirement of a more invasive approach.

In the healthy state, commonly identified bacterial genera from the upper airways include   Staphylococcus,   Corynebacterium,   Peptoniphilus,   and Propionibacterium.[2,6,32,36,40,41] Total bacterial load present in healthy and diseased sinuses appear surprisingly alike across adults. Furthermore, high interindividual microbiome variation often is observed in healthy controls and CRS patients.[42,43] Many opportunistic pathogens are found at low abundance in healthy sinuses and, therefore, have the potential to create disease after an acute alteration in the stable baseline microbial community (ie, dysbiosis).[2,32]

Disruption of stable microbiota may contribute to the exacerbation of chronic inflammatory disease in the absence of acute infection.[11,44] Dysbiosis can lead to benign microbial communities becoming proinflammatory or invasive or allowing overgrowth of pathogens. There also is growing evidence that dysbiosis of the sinus microbiota is associated with CRS pathogenesis.[45] Human studies have revealed that the CRS microbiome is characterized by loss of diversity compared with healthy controls,[5,43,46] indicating the opportunity for prosperity of pathogens.[47] Results from these and other sequence-based studies have transformed understanding of the role of microbial community composition and dynamics in CRS pathogenesis.

Disruption of healthy commensal interactions with the local immune system seems to be a critical determinant of CRS progression. Linear discriminant analysis identified the genus Corynebacterium as a potential biomarker that was significantly increased in abundance in CRS patients; however, this genus also was omnipresent in healthy subjects from other studies.[4,11] Using a murine model challenged with C tuberculostearicum after antibiotic-mediated microbial depletion, Abreu and colleagues[48] demonstrated goblet cell hyperplasia and mucin hypersecretion, 2 important histologic hallmarks of CRS. In this study, however, there were only 7 samples from CRS patients, and another study subsequently reported opposing findings that CRS patients with enriched C tuberculostearicum colonization at the time of endoscopic sinus surgery showed improved surgical outcomes.[6,49] Regarding host interaction with local immune system, another group found that nasal lavage samples of microbiota collected from CRS patients stimulated the induction of proinflammatory cytokines, such as interleukin 5, in peripheral leukocytes isolated from healthy controls.[11,50] Together, these data suggest that the CRS state represents an altered ecological landscape interacting with an aberrant immune response. To this concept, a recent cross-sectional study of CRS and non-CRS patients who underwent endoscopic sinus surgery demonstrated a correlation between the loss of bacterial species richness and diversity and the severity of inflammation and tissue eosinophilia.[51] Whether dysbiosis is causative or a result of the disrupted local immune system remains to be determined.

A preponderance of anaerobes has been consistently observed in studies of CRS, which may be explained

1. By selective pressure of antimicrobial agents enabling anaerobic organisms to flourish[52]
2. From the existence of conditions appropriate for anaerobic growth (ie, sinus hypoxia)[53]

Anaerobic taxa, such as *Peptoniphilus, Anaerococcus*, and *Prevotella*, have been reported as abundant taxa in multiple CRS studies.[4,42,54–56] Ambient conditions within the sinus cavities may not be hypoxic, especially after endoscopic sinus surgery has opened the cavities. Expansion of anaerobes in CRS may be indicative, however, of underlying tissue hypoxia, or may suggest that discrete microenvironments within mucus or bacterial biofilms in CRS also can be oxygen limited, allowing anaerobes to thrive.[4,53,57] It is likely that, similar to mucus plugs in the lower airways of individuals with cystic fibrosis (CF), oxygen levels within sinus mucus are dynamic and driven by both host and microbial processes.[58] Whether anaerobic bacteria have an etiologic role in CRS disease progression has been addressed only marginally and is an emerging area of research in chronic airway disease.

MICROBIAL INTERACTIONS IN CHRONIC RHINOSINUSITIS

Understanding the complexity and dynamics of interspecies and interkingdom relationships represents a major challenge in microbiome research but has the potential to help clarify effects in several chronic respiratory diseases including CRS.[8] Symbiosis in healthy microbial ecosystems allows for efficient nutrient utilization and results in decreased pathogen colonization.[47] Most microorganisms face a constant battle for resources, and there are diverse mechanisms by which bacterial species can coexist with, or dominate, other organisms competing for the same pool of resources.[59] Understanding of microbial interactions will be crucial in establishing the function of microbial communities in CRS and implementing new therapeutic strategies.

Yan and colleagues[10] studied the interaction between *S aureus* and *Corynebacterium* in the healthy human nasal cavity and showed that *Corynebacterium* spp are involved in both mutualistic and inhibitory interactions with *S aureus*. *C accolens* and *S aureus* appear to be adapted to each other and mutually promote each other's growth in vitro, whereas *C pseudodiphtheriticum* may interfere with colonization of *S aureus* and was observed to inhibit *S aureus* growth in vitro. Within the nasal cavity, these reciprocal interactions suggest the possibility for niche competition and possible protection against *S aureus* nasal colonization.

Pseudomonas aeruginosa also is an important respiratory pathogen and often carries intrinsic and/or acquired resistance to many classes of antibiotics. Its appearance and recalcitrance in a portion of CRS subjects is an ongoing clinical challenge. Flynn and colleagues[60] investigated the role of airway mucins as the microbial carbon source in the CF airway and characterized their potential to stimulate the growth of *Pseudomonas*. Their group demonstrated that coculture of *P aeruginosa* with an anaerobic bacterial consortium facilitates robust growth of *P aeruginosa* using mucins as a sole nutritional carbon source. These data support an ecological role for anaerobes in shaping the landscape of the human airway for progression of chronic disease (eg, CRS) and these data a model for the role of anaerobes in disease pathogenesis.[60] In this model, potential pathogens that cannot degrade mucins (eg, *P aeruginosa* and *S aureus*) do not establish an airway infection until mucin-fermenting bacteria (anaerobes) have colonized (**Fig. 1**). Numerous 16S rRNA gene sequencing studies in CRS have demonstrated a previously unrecognized abundance of anaerobes in the disease state.[6,48] Based on this hypothesis, chronic airway disease could develop through a defined series of dependent events:

1. Impaired mucus clearance
2. Generation of anaerobic microenvironments
3. Dysbiosis with mucin-fermenting anaerobes
4. Mucin degradation to carbon source nutrients (eg, short-chain fatty acids [SCFAs])
5. Proliferation of sinus pathogens

In this context, the authors preliminarily tested whether there is evidence of mucin fermentation in human CRS by analyzing the presence of SCFAs in the mucus of subjects during acute exacerbations. Using gas chromatography–mass spectrometry, 3 SCFAs (acetate, propionate, and butyrate) were quantified in human mucus

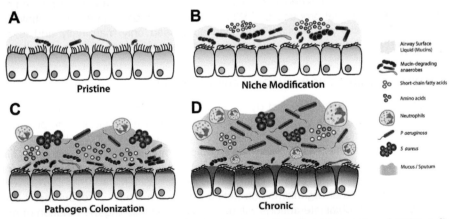

Fig. 1. Model for the role of mucin-fermenting bacteria in the progression of CF lung disease, as applied to CRS. (*A*) In early life, airway surface liquid harbors a low number of bacteria. Numerous factors allow for establishment of personal local microbiota. (*B*) Local insult resulting in impaired MCC and defective immune responses results in hypoxic environment ideal for expansion of anaerobes. In turn, their ability to degrade and ferment respiratory mucins further modifies the airway environment for secondary colonizers. (*C*) The abundance of fermentation byproducts facilitates pathogen colonization, heightened inflammation, neutrophil recruitment, and further hypoxia. (*D*) In late stages of disease, host inflammatory responses and epithelial damage increase the abundance of pathogens, whereas healthy commensals are eliminated by the host and via broad-spectrum antibiotic therapies. (*Data from* Flynn JM, Niccum D, Dunitz JM, et al. Evidence and Role for Bacterial Mucin Degradation in Cystic Fibrosis Airway Disease. PLoS Pathog 2016;12(8):e1005846.)

samples collected from 6 controls and 9 CRS patients during acute exacerbation episodes. SCFAs were found at millimolar concentrations in all mucus samples and at significantly higher concentrations in CRS compared with healthy subjects (**Fig. 2**). Given that SCFAs are derived predominately from bacterial fermentation, this evidence suggests that mucin-fermenting bacteria are able to generate carbon source nutrients for pathogenic bacteria in CRS, similar to proposed mechanisms of disease progression in the lower airways.[60] Based on these data, it is intriguing to consider that the growth of canonical airway pathogens (eg, *S aureus* and *P aeruginosa*) might be inhibited by targeting co-colonizing microbiota that potentiate their growth and virulence.

DEVELOPING PRECLINICAL MODELS

The study of dysbiosis in human CRS is especially challenging because medical therapies used in disease treatment are likely to affect resident bacterial communities.[45,61,62] Observed alterations in CRS local microbiota in cross-sectional studies have been unable to account for the repeated and prolonged medical therapies that are common in study subjects. Unfortunately, small animals are not universally accepted in CRS because they do not develop upper airway phenotypes (eg, CF murine models), possibly from absence of submucosal glands,[63] and their small size precludes thorough examination of sinus pathology.[64] Thus, there remains a need for a robust preclinical model of CRS for longitudinal sampling prior to and during disease initiation. Although there are some limitations when applying animal findings to human pathophysiology, preclinical models have played a significant role in the process of understanding CRS pathophysiology.[65–67]

Many different animals (eg, murine, rabbit, sheep, and pigs) have been used to establish acute and chronic sinus inflammation in prior studies. Small animal models used in CRS microbiome research include the murine model of sinusitis described previously in investigation of *C tuberculostearicum* as a potential pathogen on the sinus microbiota. By inoculating *C tuberculostearicum* into the nasal cavity with and without preceding antibiotic treatment, this study showed the capability of *C tuberculostearicum* to induce a CRS phenotype, particularly in conjunction with a depleted host commensal community. Co-inoculation of *C tuberculostearicum* with *Lactobacillus sakei*, a putative probiotic, resulted in a reduced abundance of *C tuberculostearicum*.[48] In addition, mice have been used to understand the dynamics of sinonasal infection and the role of the mucosal microbiome in short-term and long-term responses after topical inoculation of human pathogens (eg, *P aeruginosa*).[68] Mice are

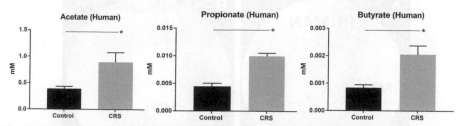

Fig. 2. Concentrations of SCFAs in human mucus samples from CRS with acute exacerbation versus healthy controls. All 3 SCFAs were significantly higher in CRS (n = 9) compared with control (n = 6): (left) acetate = 0.89 mM ± 0.19 mM versus 0.39 ± 0.04 mM (*P*<.05); (middle) propionate = 0.01 mM ± 0.00 mM versus 0.0045 mM ± 0.00 mM (*P*<.0001); and (right) butyrate = 0.002 mM ± 0.00 mM versus 0.0008 mM ± 0.00 mM (*P*<.01). * indicates as P<0.05.

easy to work with in the laboratory and carry many advantages of experimental application that have been extensively documented. Murine CRS models are limited, however, due to animal size, unclear similarity of commensal microbes to human counterparts, and poorly defined ecological properties of stability and resilience and because mice do not reproduce key aspects of human airway physiology. They do not have true sinuses, for instance, essential for the analysis of the pathophysiologic mechanisms of CRS.[69] Furthermore, immune responses in mice are notably different from those in humans.[70] Compared with mice, rat models are much larger, which makes acquiring larger tissue specimens easier and ameliorates the technical limitations of smaller models.[71] Transgenic rat models useful for CRS are rare, however, and the CF transmembrane conductance regulator (CFTR) knockout rat model (*Rattus norvegicus*; SD-CFTRtm1sage) does not develop spontaneous sinusitis.[64]

As an alternative small animal model, the in vivo rabbit sinusitis model is established and may be well suited for studies of therapeutic intervention. The rabbit sinusitis model

1. Can recapitulate histopathologic features of sinusitis
2. Is of sufficient size to study spatial and temporal microbial changes
3. Has been used to explore experimental ostial obstruction and/or microbial inoculation in the development of the disease[72]

Cho and colleagues[73] developed a rabbit model of sinusitis by blocking the maxillary sinus ostium for 2 weeks in the absence of infection to create an anaerobic environment with decreased MCC, resulting in the infiltration of sinus epithelium with acute inflammatory cells (neutrophils). When followed for another 12 weeks after removal of ostial obstruction, those rabbits exhibited a chronic inflammatory phenotype at week 14 (**Fig. 3**). In this model, the mucin-fermenting anaerobic phyla *Firmicutes* and *Bacteroidetes* dominated at week 2 but were followed by a significant microbial shift to pathogenic Proteobacteria (eg, Burkholderiales, and Pseudomonadales) during the development of chronic inflammation by week 14. Such a model provides the opportunity to study microbial host interactions with a level of experimental control that is not achievable in mouse or humans and also permits multiple longitudinal samplings because the nasal cavity is accessible by nasal endoscopy.

FUTURE DIRECTIONS IN CHRONIC RHINOSINUSITIS MICROBIOME RESEARCH
Standardization in Sampling Procedures

Many protocols have been utilized and advocated for different reasons. The ideal sampling protocol depends on the question being addressed. Mucus swab of the middle

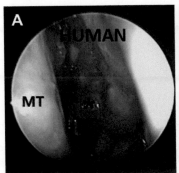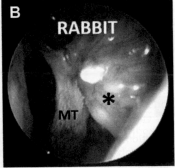

Fig. 3. Middle meatus (*asterisk*) of human (*A*) versus rabbit (*B*) CRS. Similar significant polypoid mucosal changes (*asterisk*). MT, middle turbinate.

meatus or ethmoid cavity may be the simplest approach for longitudinal study of the sinus microbiome, considering that it can be obtained from a wide range of subjects and does not require invasive procedures. Whether microbes are sampled by swab, brush, or tissue biopsy, sequencing provides a general picture of the composition of the bacterial community, while an accompanying clinically meaningful and functional physiologic approach is still required.

Healthy Microbiome Patterns

What is the healthy sinus microbiome consortium and what defines "normal"? How do healthy microbiota protect against potential pathogens, either passively through niche competition or actively through or metabolic processes or secretion of antimicrobial compound? Are these organisms susceptible to changes that occur in the sinus environment as a result of the CRS disease process or iatrogenic manipulation? Normality patterns for viruses and fungi still need to be defined in the upper respiratory system.

Further Characterization of Nonculturable and/or Nonpathogenic Bacteria

16S rRNA gene analyses have shown discrete patterns of nonculturable microorganisms obtained from patients with CRS. Conventional sequencing methods do not differentiate, however, between actively growing, dormant, or dead biomass nor do they capture in situ activity at the transcriptional and/or protein level. Detailed characterization of CRS-associated microbial communities therefore requires further innovative assessment. As an example, bioorthogonal noncanonical amino acid tagging (BONCAT) can be used to fluorescently label actively growing bacteria within samples prior to gene sequencing and has the potential to enhance traditional sequencing methods by characterizing bacterial activity at the protein level.[19] Other methods, such as stable isotope probing or single-cell transcriptional analyses coupled with in situ imaging, also carry potential for generating unprecedented insights into the microbial basis of CRS disease progression.[74,75]

Local versus Systemic Microbial Interactions

Future studies may need to address the contributions of both local and systemic microbial communities (ie, local and GI occupants). New studies, including bacteriophage, viral, and fungal contributions to functional host immune processes, are eagerly anticipated.

Interventions

Bacterial supplementation and modulation of the microbiota through prebiotics or probiotics and equivalents are opportunities for thoughtful and ethical clinical research. Whether probiotics directly target inflammatory processes within the sinonasal epithelium or aim to restore normal upper airway microbiota by mucus transfer, novel strategies to address pathogens in CRS are needed.

ACKNOWLEDGMENTS

Research reported in this publication was supported by the National Institute on Deafness and Other Communication Disorders of the National Institutes of Health under award number K23DC014747 (V.R. Ramakrishnan), National Institute of Allergy and Infectious Diseases K08AI146220 (D-.Y. Cho), Flight Attendant Medical Research Institute grant CIA130066 (Daniel Frank and V.R. Ramakrishnan), American Rhinologic Society New Investigator Award (D-.Y. Cho), Cystic Fibrosis Foundation Research Development Pilot grant (ROWE15R0) (D-.Y. Cho), Cystic Fibrosis Foundation postdoctoral fellowship (FLYNN16F0), and National Center for Advancing Translational Sciences grant (UL1TR000114) to R.C. Hunter. The content is solely the responsibility of the authors and does not necessarily represent the official views of the National Institutes of Health.

REFERENCES

1. Shusterman D. The effects of air pollutants and irritants on the upper airway. Proc Am Thorac Soc 2011;8(1):101–5.
2. Ramakrishnan VR, Feazel LM, Gitomer SA, et al. The microbiome of the middle meatus in healthy adults. PLoS One 2013;8(12):e85507.
3. Belkaid Y, Hand TW. Role of the microbiota in immunity and inflammation. Cell 2014;157(1):121–41.
4. Copeland E, Leonard K, Carney R, et al. Chronic rhinosinusitis: potential role of microbial dysbiosis and recommendations for sampling sites. Front Cell Infect Microbiol 2018;8:57.
5. Wagner Mackenzie B, Waite DW, Hoggard M, et al. Bacterial community collapse: a meta-analysis of the sinonasal microbiota in chronic rhinosinusitis. Environ Microbiol 2017;19(1):381–92.
6. Ramakrishnan VR, Hauser LJ, Feazel LM, et al. Sinus microbiota varies among chronic rhinosinusitis phenotypes and predicts surgical outcome. J Allergy Clin Immunol 2015;136(2):334–42.e1.
7. Ramakrishnan VR, Frank DN. Microbiome in patients with upper airway disease: moving from taxonomic findings to mechanisms and causality. J Allergy Clin Immunol 2018;142(1):73–5.
8. Faner R, Sibila O, Agusti A, et al. The microbiome in respiratory medicine: current challenges and future perspectives. Eur Respir J 2017;49(4) [pii:1602086].
9. Ramakrishnan VR, Hauser LJ, Frank DN. The sinonasal bacterial microbiome in health and disease. Curr Opin Otolaryngol Head Neck Surg 2016;24(1):20–5.
10. Yan M, Pamp SJ, Fukuyama J, et al. Nasal microenvironments and interspecific interactions influence nasal microbiota complexity and S. aureus carriage. Cell Host Microbe 2013;14(6):631–40.
11. Proctor DM, Relman DA. The landscape ecology and microbiota of the human nose, mouth, and throat. Cell Host Microbe 2017;21(4):421–32.
12. Dubin MG, Ebert CS, Coffey CS, et al. Concordance of middle meatal swab and maxillary sinus aspirate in acute and chronic sinusitis: a meta-analysis. Am J Rhinol 2005;19(5):462–70.
13. Lund VJ, Stammberger H, Fokkens WJ, et al. European position paper on the anatomical terminology of the internal nose and paranasal sinuses. Rhinol Suppl 2014;24:1–34.
14. Ramakrishnan VR, Gitomer S, Kofonow JM, et al. Investigation of sinonasal microbiome spatial organization in chronic rhinosinusitis. Int Forum Allergy Rhinol 2017;7(1):16–23.
15. Feazel LM, Frank DN, Ramakrishnan VR. Update on bacterial detection methods in chronic rhinosinusitis: implications for clinicians and research scientists. Int Forum Allergy Rhinol 2011;1(6):451–9.
16. Hauser LJ, Feazel LM, Ir D, et al. Sinus culture poorly predicts resident microbiota. Int Forum Allergy Rhinol 2015;5(1):3–9.
17. Rhoads DD, Cox SB, Rees EJ, et al. Clinical identification of bacteria in human chronic wound infections: culturing vs. 16S ribosomal DNA sequencing. BMC Infect Dis 2012;12:321.

18. Willis AL, Calton JB, Carr TF, et al. Dead or alive: deoxyribonuclease I sensitive bacteria and implications for the sinus microbiome. Am J Rhinol Allergy 2016; 30(2):94–8.

19. Couradeau E, Sasse J, Goudeau D, et al. Probing the active fraction of soil microbiomes using BONCAT-FACS. Nat Commun 2019;10(1):2770.

20. Nelson MT, Pope CE, Marsh RL, et al. Human and extracellular DNA depletion for metagenomic analysis of complex clinical infection samples yields optimized viable microbiome profiles. Cell Rep 2019;26(8):2227–40.e5.

21. Bent SJ, Pierson JD, Forney LJ, et al. Measuring species richness based on microbial community fingerprints: the emperor has no clothes. Appl Environ Microbiol 2007;73(7):2399–401 [author reply: 2399-2401].

22. Malla MA, Dubey A, Kumar A, et al. Exploring the human microbiome: the potential future role of next-generation sequencing in disease diagnosis and treatment. Front Immunol 2018;9:2868.

23. Manichanh C, Chapple CE, Frangeul L, et al. A comparison of random sequence reads versus 16S rDNA sequences for estimating the biodiversity of a metagenomic library. Nucleic Acids Res 2008;36(16):5180–8.

24. Yang X, Noyes NR, Doster E, et al. Use of metagenomic shotgun sequencing technology to detect foodborne pathogens within the microbiome of the beef production chain. Appl Environ Microbiol 2016;82(8):2433–43.

25. Shah N, Tang H, Doak TG, et al. Comparing bacterial communities inferred from 16S rRNA gene sequencing and shotgun metagenomics. Pac Symp Biocomput 2011;165–76. https://doi.org/10.1142/9789814335058_0018.

26. Tessler M, Neumann JS, Afshinnekoo E, et al. Large-scale differences in microbial biodiversity discovery between 16S amplicon and shotgun sequencing. Sci Rep 2017;7(1):6589.

27. Fichot EB, Norman RS. Microbial phylogenetic profiling with the Pacific Biosciences sequencing platform. Microbiome 2013;1(1):10.

28. Kasianowicz JJ, Brandin E, Branton D, et al. Characterization of individual polynucleotide molecules using a membrane channel. Proc Natl Acad Sci U S A 1996;93(24):13770–3.

29. Robinson CM, Pfeiffer JK. Viruses and the microbiota. Annu Rev Virol 2014;1: 55–69.

30. Liao B, Hu CY, Liu T, et al. Respiratory viral infection in the chronic persistent phase of chronic rhinosinusitis. Laryngoscope 2014;124(4):832–7.

31. Ramadan HH, Farr RW, Wetmore SJ. Adenovirus and respiratory syncytial virus in chronic sinusitis using polymerase chain reaction. Laryngoscope 1997;107(7): 923–5.

32. Sivasubramaniam R, Douglas R. The microbiome and chronic rhinosinusitis. World J Otorhinolaryngol Head Neck Surg 2018;4(3):216–21.

33. Wood AJ, Antoszewska H, Fraser J, et al. Is chronic rhinosinusitis caused by persistent respiratory virus infection? Int Forum Allergy Rhinol 2011;1(2):95–100.

34. Zhao YC, Bassiouni A, Tanjararak K, et al. Role of fungi in chronic rhinosinusitis through ITS sequencing. Laryngoscope 2018;128(1):16–22.

35. Zhang I, Pletcher SD, Goldberg AN, et al. Fungal microbiota in chronic airway inflammatory disease and emerging relationships with the host immune response. Front Microbiol 2017;8:2477.

36. Gevers D, Knight R, Petrosino JF, et al. The Human Microbiome Project: a community resource for the healthy human microbiome. PLoS Biol 2012;10(8): e1001377.

37. Lee JT, Frank DN, Ramakrishnan V. Microbiome of the paranasal sinuses: Update and literature review. Am J Rhinol Allergy 2016;30(1):3–16.

38. Seshadri S, Rosati M, Lin DC, et al. Regional differences in the expression of innate host defense molecules in sinonasal mucosa. J Allergy Clin Immunol 2013;132(5):1227–30.e5.

39. White LC, Weinberger P, Coulson H, et al. Why sinonasal disease spares the inferior turbinate: An immunohistochemical analysis. Laryngoscope 2016;126(5): E179–83.

40. Kaspar U, Kriegeskorte A, Schubert T, et al. The culturome of the human nose habitats reveals individual bacterial fingerprint patterns. Environ Microbiol 2016;18(7):2130–42.

41. Mahdavinia M, Engen PA, LoSavio PS, et al. The nasal microbiome in patients with chronic rhinosinusitis: analyzing the effects of atopy and bacterial functional pathways in 111 patients. J Allergy Clin Immunol 2018;142(1):287–90.e4.

42. Biswas K, Hoggard M, Jain R, et al. The nasal microbiota in health and disease: variation within and between subjects. Front Microbiol 2015;9:134.

43. Hoggard M, Biswas K, Zoing M, et al. Evidence of microbiota dysbiosis in chronic rhinosinusitis. Int Forum Allergy Rhinol 2017;7(3):230–9.

44. Dickson RP, Martinez FJ, Huffnagle GB. The role of the microbiome in exacerbations of chronic lung diseases. Lancet 2014;384(9944):691–702.

45. Orlandi RR, Kingdom TT, Hwang PH, et al. International consensus statement on allergy and rhinology: rhinosinusitis. Int Forum Allergy Rhinol 2016;6(Suppl 1): S22–209.

46. Wilson MT, Hamilos DL. The nasal and sinus microbiome in health and disease. Curr Allergy Asthma Rep 2014;14(12):485.

47. Cardinale BJ, Duffy JE, Gonzalez A, et al. Biodiversity loss and its impact on humanity. Nature 2012;486(7401):59–67.

48. Abreu NA, Nagalingam NA, Song Y, et al. Sinus microbiome diversity depletion and Corynebacterium tuberculostearicum enrichment mediates rhinosinusitis. Sci Transl Med 2012;4(151):151ra124.

49. Chalermwatanachai T, Vilchez-Vargas R, Holtappels G, et al. Chronic rhinosinusitis with nasal polyps is characterized by dysbacteriosis of the nasal microbiota. Sci Rep 2018;8(1):7926.

50. Aurora R, Chatterjee D, Hentzleman J, et al. Contrasting the microbiomes from healthy volunteers and patients with chronic rhinosinusitis. JAMA Otolaryngol Head Neck Surg 2013;139(12):1328–38.

51. Rom D, Bassiouni A, Eykman E, et al. The association between disease severity and microbiome in chronic rhinosinusitis. Laryngoscope 2019;129(6):1265–73.

52. Barenfanger J, Drake CA, Lawhorn J, et al. Outcomes of improved anaerobic techniques in clinical microbiology. Clin Infect Dis 2002;35(Suppl 1):S78–83.

53. Brook I. The role of anaerobic bacteria in sinusitis. Anaerobe 2006;12(1):5–12.

54. Cleland EJ, Bassiouni A, Vreugde S, et al. The bacterial microbiome in chronic rhinosinusitis: Richness, diversity, postoperative changes, and patient outcomes. Am J Rhinol Allergy 2016;30(1):37–43.

55. Stephenson MF, Mfuna L, Dowd SE, et al. Molecular characterization of the polymicrobial flora in chronic rhinosinusitis. J Otolaryngol Head Neck Surg 2010; 39(2):182–7.

56. Ivanchenko OA, Karpishchenko SA, Kozlov RS, et al. The microbiome of the maxillary sinus and middle nasal meatus in chronic rhinosinusitis. Rhinology 2016;54(1):68–74.

57. Kim YJ, Cho HJ, Shin WC, et al. Hypoxia-mediated mechanism of MUC5AC production in human nasal epithelia and its implication in rhinosinusitis. PLoS One 2014;9(5):e98136.
58. Cowley ES, Kopf SH, LaRiviere A, et al. Pediatric cystic fibrosis sputum can be chemically dynamic, anoxic, and extremely reduced due to hydrogen sulfide formation. MBio 2015;6(4):e00767.
59. Hibbing ME, Fuqua C, Parsek MR, et al. Bacterial competition: surviving and thriving in the microbial jungle. Nat Rev Microbiol 2010;8(1):15–25.
60. Flynn JM, Niccum D, Dunitz JM, et al. Evidence and role for bacterial mucin degradation in cystic fibrosis airway disease. PLoS Pathog 2016;12(8):e1005846.
61. Dethlefsen L, Huse S, Sogin ML, et al. The pervasive effects of an antibiotic on the human gut microbiota, as revealed by deep 16S rRNA sequencing. PLoS Biol 2008;6(11):e280.
62. Liu CM, Soldanova K, Nordstrom L, et al. Medical therapy reduces microbiota diversity and evenness in surgically recalcitrant chronic rhinosinusitis. Int Forum Allergy Rhinol 2013;3(10):775–81.
63. Wine JJ, Joo NS. Submucosal glands and airway defense. Proc Am Thorac Soc 2004;1(1):47–53.
64. Tipirneni KE, Cho DY, Skinner DF, et al. Characterization of primary rat nasal epithelial cultures in CFTR knockout rats as a model for CF sinus disease. Laryngoscope 2017;127(11):E384–91.
65. Jia M, Chen Z, Du X, et al. A simple animal model of Staphylococcus aureus biofilm in sinusitis. Am J Rhinol Allergy 2014;28(2):e115–9.
66. London NR Jr, Lane AP. Innate immunity and chronic rhinosinusitis: what we have learned from animal models. Laryngoscope Investig Otolaryngol 2016;1(3): 49–56.
67. Shin HW. Animal models in CRS and pathophysiologic insights gained: a systematic review. Laryngoscope Investig Otolaryngol 2016;1(5):116–23.
68. Cope EK, Goldberg AN, Pletcher SD, et al. A chronic rhinosinusitis-derived isolate of Pseudomonas aeruginosa induces acute and pervasive effects on the murine upper airway microbiome and host immune response. Int Forum Allergy Rhinol 2016;6(12):1229–37.
69. Lindsay R, Slaughter T, Britton-Webb J, et al. Development of a murine model of chronic rhinosinusitis. Otolaryngol Head Neck Surg 2006;134(5):724–30 [discussion: 731–2].
70. Liang KL, Jiang RS, Wang J, et al. Developing a rabbit model of rhinogenic chronic rhinosinusitis. Laryngoscope 2008;118(6):1076–81.
71. Mashimo T, Serikawa T. Rat resources in biomedical research. Curr Pharm Biotechnol 2009;10(2):214–20.
72. Al-Sayed AA, Agu RU, Massoud E. Models for the study of nasal and sinus physiology in health and disease: a review of the literature. Laryngoscope Investig Otolaryngol 2017;2(6):398–409.
73. Cho DY, Mackey C, Van Der Pol WJ, et al. Sinus microanatomy and microbiota in a rabbit model of rhinosinusitis. Front Cell Infect Microbiol 2017;7:540.
74. DePas WH, Starwalt-Lee R, Van Sambeek L, et al. Exposing the three-dimensional biogeography and metabolic states of pathogens in cystic fibrosis sputum via hydrogel embedding, clearing, and rRNA labeling. MBio 2016;7(5) [pii:e00796-16].
75. Kopf SH, Sessions AL, Cowley ES, et al. Trace incorporation of heavy water reveals slow and heterogeneous pathogen growth rates in cystic fibrosis sputum. Proc Natl Acad Sci U S A 2016;113(2):E110–6.

Measuring Success in the Treatment of Patients with Chronic Rhinosinusitis

Naweed Chowdhury, MD[a],*, Timothy L. Smith, MD, MPH[b],
Daniel M. Beswick, MD[c]

KEYWORDS

- Chronic rhinosinusitis • Outcomes • Endoscopic sinus surgery • Quality of life
- Olfaction • Endoscopy

KEY POINTS

- Because chronic rhinosinusitis (CRS) primarily affects quality of life (QOL), patient-reported outcome measures are the main determinants of treatment success.
- Objective data from imaging, endoscopy, and olfactory testing are useful adjunct measures to diagnose and prevent progression of disease, although these metrics have mixed correlations with symptoms and QOL.
- Molecular biology and multiomics techniques may change how successful CRS treatment is defined in the future.

INTRODUCTION

Chronic rhinosinusitis (CRS) is one of the most common health care diagnoses in the United States, with an estimated $10 billion to $13 billion per year spent in direct costs.[1,2] Endoscopic sinus surgery (ESS) is also one of the most frequently performed surgical procedures in otolaryngology, with more than 250,000 cases annually.[3] However, these numbers underestimate the true economic cost of CRS, because its substantial effects on quality of life (QOL)[4–7] and productivity[8–10] lead to an additional indirect impact of $20 billion.[1] As the cost of treatment increases, it is becoming critical to balance cost with quality outcomes to improve value. This balance requires careful, methodical measurement of quality through both subjective and objective outcomes measures.

[a] Department of Otolaryngology/Head and Neck Surgery, Vanderbilt University Medical Center, Vanderbilt University, 1215 21st Avenue South, Nashville, TN 37232, USA; [b] Department of Otolaryngology/Head and Neck Surgery, Oregon Health and Science University, 3303 Southwest Bond Avenue, Portland, OR 97239, USA; [c] Department of Otolaryngology/Head and Neck Surgery, University of Colorado, 12631 East 17th Avenue, MSB-205, Aurora, CO 80045, USA
* Corresponding author.
E-mail address: Naweed.chowdhury@vumc.org

Immunol Allergy Clin N Am 40 (2020) 265–279
https://doi.org/10.1016/j.iac.2019.12.004
immunology.theclinics.com

Despite its importance, determining success in the management of CRS remains challenging. First, many symptoms of CRS overlap with other disease states, such as migraine,[11] depression,[12,13] and allergic rhinitis.[14] Second, objective measures of disease such as computed tomography (CT) and nasal endoscopy have inconsistent correlations with patient-reported disease experiences,[15–20] potentially leading to asymmetric perspectives for physicians and patients. In addition, because CRS is a chronic process with potential for relapse or recurrence,[21] patients often require lifelong medical management of their disease, which may not seem like a success to many.

This article seeks to understand what it means to measure and achieve success in the management of CRS through several current physician-reported and patient-reported outcomes measures, and looks ahead to understand the next-generation tools that will help define success in the future.

THE MINIMAL CLINICALLY IMPORTANT DIFFERENCE

There is a fundamental problem with using any continuous, linear measure of disease such as a survey score to measure success: although any change or improvement of the measure is assuredly positive, a marginal improvement in an outcome may not be clinically noticeable. Recognizing this issue, the minimal clinically important difference (MCID)[22,23] was developed, which identifies a threshold of improvement by which the average patient reports a change in health status. In rhinology, this concept has been applied to the 22-item Sinonasal Outcomes Test (SNOT-22),[24] its 5 subdomains,[25,26] the Brief Smell Identification Test (BSIT),[27] the Questionnaire of Olfactory Disorders (QOD),[28] and the 5-dimensional EuroQol (EQ-5D),[29] making the MCID the most widely used statistical measure of clinical success in rhinologic research.

There are several ways to compute the MCID that have been described.[30,31] Briefly, these can be grouped into distribution-based methods, which use statistical methods to describe/summarize the variance of an instrument to infer an appropriate MCID value, and anchor-based methods, which link change scores to externally validated metrics of change. Although both have been used for clinical purposes, anchor-based methods are generally preferred because they incorporate patient preferences better than distribution-based methods.[30]

However, from a patient perspective, achieving only a minimal improvement after an invasive procedure or expensive medical treatment may not be acceptable.[32] The concept of the patient-acceptable symptom score (PASS)[33] has been used in other chronic disease states to determine the threshold at which the average patient reports an acceptable symptom burden, and may be an even more patient-centered measure of successful CRS treatment than the MCID. In addition, outcomes measures that focus on symptom control[34] rather than absolute improvement may be more useful in this regard.

PHYSICIAN-OBSERVED OUTCOMES MEASURES

Over the past 40 years, beginning with the parallel adoption of nasal endoscopy and CT for evaluation and management of sinonasal disease,[35] otolaryngologists have sought to encapsulate the information present in these examinations into various quantitative metrics. Although the clinical utility of these tests is undeniable, there have been mixed results when attempting to link these objective disease scores with subjective patient measures of success.[18,20,36] Nevertheless, they remain useful to manage exacerbations or recurrence of CRS ahead of their impact on patient QOL.

Nasal Endoscopy

In 1995, the Lund-Kennedy (LK) endoscopic grading system[37] was introduced, which quantifies endoscopic findings on a 0 to 2 scale across 5 categories: polyps, edema, drainage, crusting, and scarring. Each side is scored independently, for a maximum score of 20. The LK score continues to be the primary endoscopic scoring system used for outcomes research, although it has been criticized for having limited correlations with patient outcomes.[17,20] Alternative endoscopic scoring systems have been proposed, including the Discharge, Inflammation, Polyp (DIP) score,[38] the Perioperative Sinus Endoscopy (POSE) score,[39] and, most recently, the modified Lund-Kennedy score (MLK),[40] which drops the crusting and scarring scores from the original system. Both the DIP and the MLK scores been shown to have improved responsiveness, validity, and reliability compared with LK scores,[41] but correlations with subjective symptom scores remained weak.[40,41] A recent canonical correlation analysis–derived alternative weighting of the LK score further improved correlations with SNOT-22 and rhinologic domain scores,[42] although use of this has been limited.

For patients with CRS with nasal polyps, a polyp grading score developed for use in clinical trials has been described.[43] This grades polyp severity on a 0 to 4 scale: 0, absent; 1, confined to the middle meatus; 2, multiple polyps within the middle meatus; 3, extending beyond the middle meatus; and 4, completely filling the nasal cavity. Several recent randomized studies have used percentage and absolute reduction of this polyp score as a primary outcome measure of successful treatment.[44,45]

Computed Tomography Staging

Similar to nasal endoscopic staging systems, CT scores compress three-dimensional imaging data into a composite number for research and quality-improvement purposes. However, because CT scans are not routinely performed postoperatively to monitor for recurrence or progression because of radiation concerns, there are fewer data about changes in CT scores as a measure of clinical success. The most common system is the Lund-Mackay (LM) score,[46] which grades 6 sinonasal areas bilaterally on a 0 to 2 scale (the osteomeatal complex, maxillary, anterior ethmoid, posterior ethmoid, sphenoid, and frontal sinuses) for a total maximum score of 24. A score of 0 indicates no opacification, 1 indicates partial opacification, and 2 indicates complete opacification, with the sole exception of the osteomeatal complex, which is only graded as 0 for no inflammation and 2 for any opacification.

Because of this semiquantitative approach, the LM score is reliable and easy to use in clinical practice, but is criticized for not capturing enough granularity, resulting in conflicting correlations between radiographic evidence of disease and patient-reported outcomes in the literature.[16,18,47] Alternate staging systems have been devised, most notably the Zinreich score, which expands scoring from 0 to 5 by including additional gradations for partial opacification.[48] There has also been promising work with volumetric systems, which require significant manual effort to obtain but more comprehensively capture sinonasal inflammation.[49] Interestingly, a study comparing both pretreatment and posttreatment CT scans showed significantly improved correlations between CT score change and symptom outcomes using volumetric analysis, suggesting the clinical link between radiographic disease and symptom burden is real.[50] In addition, volumetric analysis of the olfactory cleft seems to correlate with objective measures of olfaction.[51] However, even in volumetric studies that show significant associations with subjective outcomes, the effect size of these relationships may be small,[52] and the work required to acquire volumetric data limits its present clinical utility. In the near future, automated techniques for CT segmentation[53] and interpretation by artificial intelligence algorithms[54] may solve the latter problem, allowing more widespread use of radiographic inflammation as a clinical biomarker to measure treatment response.

Olfactory Testing

Several objective tests are commonly used to measure olfactory outcomes in CRS. The most widely used test is the University of Pennsylvania Smell Identification Test (SIT), a 40-item scratch-and-sniff test that measures olfactory function by scoring the patient's ability to identify odorants released from a microencapsulated strip.[55] In general, a score of more than 35 for women and 34 for men indicates normal olfaction. Because of the time required to administer the test, a 12-item version of the SIT, known as the BSIT, was also developed.[56] In patients with CRS, the BSIT and SIT are both highly correlated, but a cut point of 9 or less for abnormal olfaction is suggested to improve sensitivity,[57] because the BSIT is less reliable than the SIT.[58] The BSIT also has the advantage of a defined MCID value of 1.0 in patients with surgically treated CRS,[27] and it has been shown to improve following endoscopic sinus surgery.[59]

For more comprehensive evaluations of olfaction, identification testing should be supplemented by threshold and discrimination tests. The Sniffin' Sticks instrument[60] uses a series of odorant-impregnated felt pens to assess all 3 components of olfaction, reporting subscores for each as well as the combined threshold, discrimination, identification (TDI) score. A recent assessment of olfactory function in patients with CRS showed dysfunction across all 4 domains, particularly within threshold testing.[61] Identification scores seemed to significantly underreport olfactory dysfunction in patients without polyposis, suggesting that TDI testing may be the measure of choice in those with CRS.

Endotypes and Inflammatory Biomarkers

As molecular biology and multiomics techniques become more accessible for research purposes, there has been increased attention on identifying endotypes[62] of CRS based on quantitative analysis of inflammatory biomarkers from tissue[63,64] and mucus.[65,66] In the future, these biomarkers could represent new, objective measures of outcome once translated into clinical practice, especially for biologic therapies designed to blockade cytokine signals thought to contribute to the pathogenesis of CRS.[67] Preliminary evidence suggests that patient QOL measures[68] and postsurgical outcomes[69] may be associated with baseline inflammatory markers, but much work is needed to develop and validate these tools as indicators of successful treatment.

PATIENT-REPORTED OUTCOME MEASURES

Patient-reported outcome measures (PROMs) are an important means to evaluate outcomes in CRS management and have been receiving increasing focus recently.[70,71] These instruments are designed to prioritize the patients' own views of their health statuses and disease states.[72] PROMs may be disease specific, focusing on QOL related to CRS, sinonasal disorder, or other diseases, or generalized, centering on overall health-related QOL.[72] Optimal attributes of a PROM include strong reliability, high validity, broad assessment of the impacts of disease on QOL, and minimal time burden.[73,74] Clinicians and researchers are increasingly using PROMs to evaluate outcomes of CRS based on findings such as that QOL impairment is often the primary force compelling patients to seek out treatment of CRS.[75]

Many different disease-specific and generalized PROMs exist. CRS-specific instruments include the SNOT-22, Rhinosinusitis Disability Index (RSDI), and Sinus Control

Test (SCT). The SNOT-22 questionnaire was developed via enhancements of prior surveys, including the 16-question and 20-question versions of the Sinonasal Outcome Tests, as well as the 31-question Rhinosinusitis Severity Outcome Measure (RSOM-31). Two questions on nasal obstruction and olfaction/dysgeusia were added to the SNOT-20, the immediate precursor version, to arrive at the SNOT-22.[24] Looking forward, a 25-item version of this test, the SNOT-25, has been described and validated in 2019, with 3 additional questions on productivity included.[76]

PROMs that evaluate related conditions affected by CRS are also available, including olfactory-specific instruments, such as the QOD; surveys that measure sleep quality, such as the Pittsburgh Sleep Quality Index (PSQI); and questionnaires that focus on asthma control, such as the Mini Asthma QOL Questionnaire and the Asthma Control Test.[77] In addition to these disease-specific PROMs, there are numerous instruments that evaluate generalized, health-related QOL. Fifteen validated PROMs for use in adult sinusitis were identified in a recent systematic review and meta-analysis (**Table 1**).[24,34,72–74,78–89]

Details of PROMs used to assess outcomes in patients with CRS are reviewed next. Based on developmental attributes, psychometric properties, and validation studies, the SNOT-22, QOD, and SCT are the highest-quality disease-specific measures available, and the EQ-5D is the best-quality general QOL instrument available.[78]

Twenty-two–question Sinonasal Outcome Test

The SNOT-22 questionnaire is one of the highest-quality and most widely used PROMs used to evaluate outcomes in CRS.[72] This questionnaire has been thoroughly validated, is available in multiple languages,[24] and predicts symptom control as perceived by patients following ESS.[90] Some researches have noted that this questionnaire does not contain elements to assess the duration of disease or medication burden,[91] and these areas must be assessed separately.[72] Analysis of the symptom-based questions in the SNOT-22 survey Identified several distinct subdomains.[5,19,92] These subdomains show the impact of CRS on separate symptom areas: rhinologic, extranasal rhinologic, ear/facial, psychological distress, and sleep limitations according to one research group[5]; and nasal, sleep distress, otologic/facial, and emotion according to another research group.[92] The MCID for the SNOT-22 total score is 8.9, and MCID values for individual subdomains have also been defined.[24–26]

Multiple reports have shown that patients with refractory CRS who undergo ESS experience improvements in QOL as measured by the SNOT-22.[93,94] A systematic review and meta-analysis evaluating 40 studies on this topic over 9 years showed that the mean improvement after surgery was 24.4 points, well exceeding the MCID.[94] In contrast, patients with refractory CRS who do not undergo ESS but instead elect to continue medical therapy experience stability or minimal improvement in SNOT-22 scores[95]; however, these patients also tend to be less symptomatic at baseline.[96] Impairment in specific SNOT-22 subdomains also seems to predict patient choice of treatment of refractory CRS, with patients who select ESS being more likely to report sleep and psychological limitations.[4]

Questionnaire of Olfactory Disorders

Olfactory dysfunction is a defining symptom of CRS and adversely affects QOL.[97,98] The QOD is a validated survey used to assess the impact of olfactory dysfunction on patients with sinonasal disease.[89] First described in 2005, this instrument evaluates olfactory dysfunction using questionnaires, compared with objective olfactory testing.[99] The average MCID for the negative statements version of the QOD is 5.2.[28] Similar to the SNOT-22, distinct subdomains of the QOD have been identified,

Table 1
Validated patient-reported outcome measures used in chronic rhinosinusitis

Instrument	Year Developed	Questions (N)	Domains (N)	Domains Assessed	Time To Complete (min)
CSS	1995	6	2	CRS symptoms; medication use	5
RSOM-31	1995	31	7	Nasal; eye; ear; sleep; general; emotional; functional	15
RSDI	1997	30	3	Physical; functional; emotional	5–10
SNOT-16	1999	16	0	NA	5
SNOT-20	2002	20	0	NA	5
RSI	2003	20	3	CRS symptoms; medication use; work and social	5
RhinoQoL	2005	17	3	Symptom severity; bothersomeness; impact scale	7
RSTF	2007	14	0	NA	3
SNOT-22	2009	22	0	Rhinologic; extranasal rhinologic; ear/facial; psychosocial; sleep	7
SNQ	2009	5	0	NA	<2
DyNaChron	2012	78	6	Nasal obstruction; anterior rhinorrhea; posterior rhinorrhea; sense of smell difficulty; facial pain; cough	15
QOD	2012	25	3	Negative items; positive items; social items	7–10
DSS	2013	6	2	Symptoms; HRQoL	<2
EQ-5D	2015	15	5	Mobility; self-care; usual activity; pain/discomfort; anxiety/depression	<2
SCT	2015	4	3	Symptoms; productivity; rescue medication use	1

Abbreviations: CSS, chronic sinusitis survey; DSS, disease severity score; DyNaChron, questionnaire for chronic nasal dysfunction; HRQoL, health-related quality of life; NA, not available/applicable; RhinoQoL, rhinosinusitis quality of life questionnaire; RSI, rhinosinusitis severity inventory; RSTF, rhinosinusitis task force; SNQ, sinonasal 5-item questionnaire.

Adapted from Rudmik L, Hopkins C, Peters A, et al. Patient-reported outcome measures for adult chronic rhinosinusitis: A systematic review and quality assessment. J Allergy Clin Immunol 2015; 136(6):1535; with permission.

corresponding largely to social-related, eating-related, stress/depression-related, and QOL-related questions.[100] An abbreviated version of the QOD has also shown excellent correlations with both total and domain-specific scores.[93] Subsequent research has shown that olfactory impairment identified via the QOD correlates with SNOT-22 results and composite TDI score, with discrimination having the strongest correlation.[101] In patients with refractory CRS, olfaction-specific QOL as measured by the QOD is more severe in patients with nasal polyposis and allergy and is significantly improved in patients who undergo ESS and, in certain cases, medical therapy.[93,94]

Sinus Control Test

The SCT was developed to determine control of CRS. Validated measures of disease control exist for other inflammatory airway diseases, but not until 2016 was a validated PROM developed for CRS control.[34] This instrument contains 4 questions and categorizes patients' CRS as well controlled, partially controlled, or uncontrolled.[34] Research has shown that the SCT is a reliable instrument to monitor change in CRS control and is responsive to surgical intervention.[102] Patients with refractory CRS who undergo ESS also have improvements in SCT.[93] However, given the recency of development of this PROM, limited data have been published using it.

Pittsburgh Sleep Quality Index

The PSQI is an 18-item measure of sleep duration and quality that has been widely used and has high internal consistency, reliability, and construct validity.[103] This self-reported survey assesses sleep quality over the preceding 4 weeks. The PSQI has 7 domains (total score range, 0–21) with higher scores ($\geq$5) indicating poor sleep.[104] Most patients with CRS experience impaired sleep, as assessed by this validated instrument, and sleep impairment associates with QOL, gender, depression, and certain cytokines, but not radiologic (LM) or endoscopic (LK) scores.[104,105] Beyond PROM-based assessment of sleep quality, patients with CRS also have worse clinical parameters related to sleep compared with controls, including mean oxygen saturation, rapid eye movement sleep latency, and snoring.[106] Multiple research groups using international patient cohorts have shown that, for patients with refractory CRS who undergo ESS, sleep quality is improved postoperatively.[93,103,106] In contrast, in patients with refractory CRS who pursue medical therapy as opposed to ESS, sleep quality as assessed by the PSQI failed to improve.[107]

EuroQol Five-dimensional Instrument

EQ-5D is the highest-quality generalized health-related QOL metric for CRS and consists of 5 domains.[78] This standardized instrument was developed by the EuroQol group and includes 5 domains: mobility, self-care, usual activities, pain/discomfort, and anxiety/depression. EQ-5D responses can be computed into health utility values (HUVs), which are preference values that patients attach to their overall health status. These values range from 0.0 (representing death) to 1.0 (representing perfect health), with the mean utility for the US population reported as 0.81 to 0.85.[108] Conversion from EQ-5D response to HUV is accomplished using a crosswalk link function based on existing country-specific value sets, which indicates overall health utility as one of 3125 distinct health states.[109] The MCID for HUV changes calculated from the EQ-5D is 0.04.[29] In patients with CRS, otologic/facial and sleep-related symptoms have the biggest effect on generalized QOL as assessed by the EQ-5D, and better control of CRS symptoms correlates with higher QOL.[6,110] Patients with refractory CRS who undergo ESS have improvements in EQ-5D–derived HUV.[108]

Short-form Surveys

The Medical Outcome Study Short Form (SF)-36 is a well-validated set of QOL measures that includes a total score and 8 domains scores.[111] Like the EQ-5D, short-form surveys are measures of general health-related QOL. The SF-36 has been frequently used in CRS outcome studies and has consistently shown that ESS improves general QOL.[112–114] More recently, abbreviated versions of the SF-36 that maintain the validity of the questionnaire have been used, including the SF-12, SF-8, and SF-6D; the SF-6D uses 6 of the initial 8 domains and permits calculations of HUV.[115,116] Analyses using SF-8 and other scores have shown QOL is associated with certain inflammatory cytokines as well as postoperative pain.[68,117] Following ESS, SF-8 scores improve with some variation based on patient age,[7] and SF-6D–derived HUVs increase in a clinically significant manner in patients with CRS and remain increased toward population norms through 10 years following surgery.[118,119] In patients with CRS who maintain a medical treatment regimen, SF-6D–calculated HUV values remain stable.[120]

Productivity Loss

Calculating productivity loss caused by CRS and changes in this measure following treatment is another important method of assessing outcomes. The indirect cost of a disease is frequently referred to as productivity loss because the components of this indirect cost are primarily missed work time (absenteeism) and impairments in efficiency or performance while working (presenteeism).[10] For CRS, these indirect societal costs have been estimated at $12 billion to $20 billion per year.[1,2] Two methods of calculating productivity loss are the human capital approach (HCA) and the friction cost method. Most studies evaluating productivity loss in CRS use the HCA. PROM-type questionnaires that quantify the components of the HCA include the Quality and Quantity survey and the Work Productivity and Activity Impairment survey.[121] The lost time caused by disease calculated by these instruments can then be monetized by applying census wage rates.[1]

Productivity losses are significant among patients with medically refractory CRS and have been estimated at more than $10,000 per patient per year.[10] Productivity loss is worse among patients with worse disease-specific and olfactory QOL, active smokers, those with more frequent acute exacerbations in patients with comorbid asthma, and in patients with greater impairment in the sleep, otologic/facial, and emotional/psychological SNOT-22 domains.[8,10,122,123] In general, medical therapy for CRS maintains a degree of productivity loss without major improvements or detriments.[124] Patients who undergo ESS experience an improvement in mean productivity loss, and this productivity improvement is distributed across symptomatic gains in all SNOT-22 domains.[9,93,125]

SUMMARY

The prior 3 decades of outcomes research in CRS have generated a variety of validated measures to determine success, and, with the help of technological advances, clinicians will continue to refine both patient-reported and physician-reported metrics of change in the years to come. However, regardless of the approach used, relief of patient symptoms and improvement of QOL should be the primary objectives of any treating physician.

DISCLOSURE

The authors have no disclosures.

REFERENCES

1. Rudmik L. Economics of chronic rhinosinusitis. Curr Allergy Asthma Rep 2017; 17(4):20.
2. Smith KA, Orlandi RR, Rudmik L. Cost of adult chronic rhinosinusitis: a systematic review. Laryngoscope 2015;125(7):1547–56.
3. Bhattacharyya N. Ambulatory sinus and nasal surgery in the United States: demographics and perioperative outcomes. Laryngoscope 2010;120(3):635–8.
4. DeConde AS, Mace JC, Bodner T, et al. SNOT-22 quality of life domains differentially predict treatment modality selection in chronic rhinosinusitis. Int Forum Allergy Rhinol 2014;4(12):972–9.
5. DeConde AS, Bodner TE, Mace JC, et al. Response shift in quality of life after endoscopic sinus surgery for chronic rhinosinusitis. JAMA Otolaryngol Head Neck Surg 2014;140(8):712–9.
6. Hoehle LP, Phillips KM, Bergmark RW, et al. Symptoms of chronic rhinosinusitis differentially impact general health-related quality of life. Rhinology 2016;54(4): 316–22.
7. Yancey KL, Lowery AS, Chandra RK, et al. Advanced age adversely affects chronic rhinosinusitis surgical outcomes. Int Forum Allergy Rhinol 2019;9(10): 1125–34.
8. Chowdhury NI, Mace JC, Smith TL, et al. What drives productivity loss in chronic rhinosinusitis? A SNOT-22 subdomain analysis. Laryngoscope 2018;128(1): 23–30.
9. Beswick DM, Mace JC, Rudmik L, et al. Productivity changes following medical and surgical treatment of chronic rhinosinusitis by symptom domain. Int Forum Allergy Rhinol 2018;8(12):1395–405.
10. Rudmik L, Smith TL, Schlosser RJ, et al. Productivity costs in patients with refractory chronic rhinosinusitis. Laryngoscope 2014;124(9):2007–12.
11. Hsueh WD, Conley DB, Kim H, et al. Identifying clinical symptoms for improving the symptomatic diagnosis of chronic rhinosinusitis. Int Forum Allergy Rhinol 2013;3(4):307–14.
12. Cox DR, Ashby S, Mace JC, et al. The pain-depression dyad and the association with sleep dysfunction in chronic rhinosinusitis. Int Forum Allergy Rhinol 2017;7(1):56–63.
13. Schlosser RJ, Hyer JM, Smith TL, et al. Depression-specific outcomes after treatment of chronic rhinosinusitis. JAMA Otolaryngol Head Neck Surg 2016; 142(4):370–6.
14. Koskinen A, Numminen J, Markkola A, et al. Diagnostic accuracy of symptoms, endoscopy, and imaging signs of chronic rhinosinusitis without nasal polyps compared to allergic rhinitis. Am J Rhinol Allergy 2018;32(3):121–31.
15. Smith TL, Rhee JS, Loehrl TA, et al. Objective testing and quality-of-life evaluation in surgical candidates with chronic rhinosinusitis. Am J Rhinol 2003;17(6): 351–6.
16. Hopkins C, Browne JP, Slack R, et al. The Lund-Mackay staging system for chronic rhinosinusitis: how is it used and what does it predict? Otolaryngol Head Neck Surg 2007;137(4):555–61.
17. Ryan WR, Ramachandra T, Hwang PH. Correlations between symptoms, nasal endoscopy, and in-office computed tomography in post-surgical chronic rhinosinusitis patients. Laryngoscope 2011;121(3):674–8.
18. Brooks SG, Trope M, Blasetti M, et al. Preoperative Lund-Mackay computed tomography score is associated with preoperative symptom severity and predicts

quality-of-life outcome trajectories after sinus surgery. Int Forum Allergy Rhinol 2018;8(6):668–75.

19. Sedaghat AR, Gray ST, Caradonna SD, et al. Clustering of chronic rhinosinusitis symptomatology reveals novel associations with objective clinical and demographic characteristics. Am J Rhinol Allergy 2015;29(2):100–5.

20. Mace JC, Michael YL, Carlson NE, et al. Correlations between endoscopy score and quality-of-life changes after sinus surgery. Arch Otolaryngol Head Neck Surg 2010;136(4):340–6.

21. DeConde AS, Mace JC, Levy JM, et al. Prevalence of polyp recurrence after endoscopic sinus surgery for chronic rhinosinusitis with nasal polyposis. Laryngoscope 2017;127(3):550–5.

22. Copay AG, Subach BR, Glassman SD, et al. Understanding the minimum clinically important difference: a review of concepts and methods. Spine J 2007; 7(5):541–6.

23. Jaeschke R, Singer J, Guyatt GH. Measurement of health status. Ascertaining the minimal clinically important difference. Control Clin Trials 1989;10(4):407–15.

24. Hopkins C, Gillett S, Slack R, et al. Psychometric validity of the 22-item sinonasal outcome test. Clin Otolaryngol 2009;34(5):447–54.

25. Chowdhury NI, Mace JC, Bodner TE, et al. Investigating the minimal clinically important difference for snot-22 symptom domains in surgically managed chronic rhinosinusitis. Int Forum Allergy Rhinol 2017;7(12):1149–55.

26. Chowdhury NI, Mace JC, Bodner TE, et al. Does medical therapy improve sinonasal outcomes test-22 domain scores? An analysis of clinically important differences. Laryngoscope 2019;129(1):31–6.

27. Levy JM, Mace JC, Bodner TE, et al. Defining the minimal clinically important difference for olfactory outcomes in the surgical treatment of chronic rhinosinusitis. Int Forum Allergy Rhinol 2017;7(8):821–6.

28. Mattos JL, Schlosser RJ, Mace JC, et al. Establishing the minimal clinically important difference for the questionnaire of olfactory disorders. Int Forum Allergy Rhinol 2018;8(9):1041–6.

29. Hoehle LP, Phillips KM, Speth MM, et al. Responsiveness and minimal clinically important difference for the EQ-5D in chronic rhinosinusitis. Rhinology 2019; 57(2):110–6.

30. Jayadevappa R, Cook R, Chhatre S. Minimal important difference to infer changes in health-related quality of life-a systematic review. J Clin Epidemiol 2017;89:188–98.

31. Crosby RD, Kolotkin RL, Williams GR. Defining clinically meaningful change in health-related quality of life. J Clin Epidemiol 2003;56(5):395–407.

32. Tubach F, Dougados M, Falissard B, et al. Feeling good rather than feeling better matters more to patients. Arthritis Rheum 2006;55(4):526–30.

33. Kvien TK, Heiberg T, Hagen KB. Minimal clinically important improvement/difference (MCII/MCID) and patient acceptable symptom state (PASS): what do these concepts mean? Ann Rheum Dis 2007;66(Suppl 3):iii40–1.

34. Banglawala SM, Schlosser RJ, Morella K, et al. Qualitative development of the sinus control test: a survey evaluating sinus symptom control. Int Forum Allergy Rhinol 2016;6(5):491–9.

35. Tajudeen BA, Kennedy DW. Thirty years of endoscopic sinus surgery: what have we learned? World J Otorhinolaryngol Head Neck Surg 2017;3(2):115–21.

36. Stewart MG, Smith TL. Objective versus subjective outcomes assessment in rhinology. Am J Rhinol 2005;19(5):529–35.

37. Lund VJ, Kennedy DW. Quantification for staging sinusitis. Ann Otol Rhinol Laryngol 1995;104(10_suppl):17–21.
38. Durr ML, Pletcher SD, Goldberg AN, et al. A novel sinonasal endoscopy scoring system: the discharge, inflammation, and polyps/edema (DIP) score. Int Forum Allergy Rhinol 2013;3(1):66–72.
39. Wright ED, Agrawal S. Impact of perioperative systemic steroids on surgical outcomes in patients with chronic rhinosinusitis with polyposis: evaluation with the novel perioperative sinus endoscopy (POSE) scoring system. Laryngoscope 2007;117(S115):1–28.
40. Psaltis AJ, Li G, Vaezeafshar R, et al. Modification of the lund-kennedy endoscopic scoring system improves its reliability and correlation with patient-reported outcome measures. Laryngoscope 2014;124(10):2216–23.
41. Zhang L, Zhang LH. Comparison of different endoscopic scoring systems in patients with chronic rhinosinusitis: reliability, validity, responsiveness and correlation. Rhinology 2017;55(4):363–8.
42. DeConde AS, Bodner TE, Mace JC, et al. Development of a clinically relevant endoscopic grading system for chronic rhinosinusitis using canonical correlation analysis. Int Forum Allergy Rhinol 2016;6(5):478–85.
43. Meltzer EO, Hamilos DL, Hadley JA, et al. Rhinosinusitis: developing guidance for clinical trials. J Allergy Clin Immunol 2006;118(5):S17–61.
44. Bachert C, Mannent L, Naclerio RM, et al. Effect of subcutaneous dupilumab on nasal polyp burden in patients with chronic sinusitis and nasal polyposis: a randomized clinical trial. JAMA 2016;315(5):469–79.
45. Bachert C, Sousa AR, Lund VJ, et al. Reduced need for surgery in severe nasal polyposis with mepolizumab: randomized trial. J Allergy Clin Immunol 2017;140(4):1024–31.e14.
46. Lund VJ, Mackay IS. Staging in rhinosinusitus. Rhinology 1993;31(4):183–4.
47. Bhattacharyya N. Radiographic stage fails to predict symptom outcomes after endoscopic sinus surgery for chronic rhinosinusitis. Laryngoscope 2006;116(1):18–22.
48. Zinreich SJ. Imaging for staging of rhinosinusitis. Ann Otol Rhinol Laryngol Suppl 2004;193:19–23.
49. Garneau J, Ramirez M, Armato SG, et al. Computer-assisted staging of chronic rhinosinusitis correlates with symptoms. Int Forum Allergy Rhinol 2015;5(7):637–42.
50. Pallanch JF, Yu L, Delone D, et al. Three-dimensional volumetric computed tomographic scoring as an objective outcome measure for chronic rhinosinusitis: clinical correlations and comparison to Lund-Mackay scoring. Int Forum Allergy Rhinol 2013;3(12):963–72.
51. Soler ZM, Pallanch JF, Sansoni ER, et al. Volumetric computed tomography analysis of the olfactory cleft in patients with chronic rhinosinusitis. Int Forum Allergy Rhinol 2015;5(9):846–54.
52. Lim S, Ramirez M, Garneau JC, et al. 3D image analysis for staging chronic rhinosinusitis. Int Forum Allergy Rhinol 2017;7(11):1052–7.
53. Lenchik L, Heacock L, Weaver AA, et al. Automated segmentation of tissues using CT and MRI: a systematic review. Acad Radiol 2019;26(12):1695–706.
54. Chowdhury NI, Smith TL, Chandra RK, et al. Automated classification of osteomeatal complex inflammation on computed tomography using convolutional neural networks. Int Forum Allergy Rhinol 2019;9(1):46–52.

55. Doty RL, Shaman P, Kimmelman CP, et al. University of Pennsylvania smell identification test: a rapid quantitative olfactory function test for the clinic. Laryngoscope 1984;94(2 Pt 1):176–8.

56. Doty RL, Marcus A, Lee WW. Development of the 12-item cross-cultural smell identification test (CC-SIT). Laryngoscope 1996;106(3 Pt 1):353–6.

57. El Rassi E, Mace JC, Steele TO, et al. Sensitivity analysis and diagnostic accuracy of the brief smell identification test in patients with chronic rhinosinusitis. Int Forum Allergy Rhinol 2016;6(3):287–92.

58. Doty RL, McKeown DA, Lee WW, et al. A study of the test-retest reliability of ten olfactory tests. Chem Senses 1995;20(6):645–56.

59. Levy JM, Mace JC, Sansoni ER, et al. Longitudinal improvement and stability of olfactory function in the evaluation of surgical management for chronic rhinosinusitis. Int Forum Allergy Rhinol 2016;6(11):1188–95.

60. Hummel T, Sekinger B, Wolf SR, et al. 'Sniffin' Sticks': olfactory performance assessed by the combined testing of odor identification, odor discrimination and olfactory threshold. Chem Senses 1997;22(1):39–52.

61. Soler ZM, Kohli P, Storck KA, et al. Olfactory impairment in chronic rhinosinusitis using threshold, discrimination, and identification scores. Chem Senses 2016; 41(9):713–9.

62. Succar EF, Turner JH. Recent advances in understanding chronic rhinosinusitis endotypes. F1000Res 2018;7 [pii:F1000 Faculty Rev-1909].

63. Tomassen P, Vandeplas G, Van Zele T, et al. Inflammatory endotypes of chronic rhinosinusitis based on cluster analysis of biomarkers. J Allergy Clin Immunol 2016;137(5):1449–56.e4.

64. Tan BK, Klingler AI, Stevens WW, et al. Heterogenous inflammatory patterns in chronic rhinosinusitis without nasal polyps in Chicago, Illinois. J Allergy Clin Immunol 2017;139(2):699–703.e7.

65. Turner JH, Chandra RK, Li P, et al. Identification of clinically relevant chronic rhinosinusitis endotypes using cluster analysis of mucus cytokines. J Allergy Clin Immunol 2018;141(5):1895–7.e7.

66. Miyake MM, Workman AD, Nocera AL, et al. Discriminant analysis followed by unsupervised cluster analysis including exosomal cystatins predict presence of chronic rhinosinusitis, phenotype, and disease severity. Int Forum Allergy Rhinol 2019;9(9):1069–76.

67. Jonstam K, Swanson BN, Mannent LP, et al. Dupilumab reduces local type 2 pro-inflammatory biomarkers in chronic rhinosinusitis with nasal polyposis. Allergy 2019;74(4):743–52.

68. Chowdhury NI, Chandra RK, Li P, et al. Investigating the correlation between mucus cytokine levels, inflammatory cell counts, and baseline quality-of-life measures in chronic rhinosinusitis. Int Forum Allergy Rhinol 2019;9(5):538–44.

69. Chowdhury NI, Li P, Chandra RK, et al. Baseline mucus cytokines predict 22-item sino-nasal outcome test results after endoscopic sinus surgery. Int Forum Allergy Rhinol 2019. https://doi.org/10.1002/alr.22449.

70. Noon E, Hopkins C. Review article: outcomes in endoscopic sinus surgery. BMC Ear Nose Throat Disord 2016;16:9.

71. Hopkins C, Philpott C, Crowe S, et al. Identifying the most important outcomes for systematic reviews of interventions for rhinosinusitis in adults: working with patients, public and practitioners. Rhinology 2016;54(1):20–6.

72. Beswick D, Soler Z, Hopkins C, et al. Chronic rhinosinusitis: outcomes of medical and surgical treatment. Chapter 43. 7th edition. Elsevier; 2020.

73. Ling FTK, Kountakis SE. Rhinosinusitis task force symptoms versus the sinonasal outcomes test in patients evaluated for chronic rhinosinusitis. Am J Rhinol 2007;21(4):495–8.

74. Piccirillo JF, Merritt MG, Richards ML. Psychometric and clinimetric validity of the 20-item sino-nasal outcome test (SNOT-20). Otolaryngol Head Neck Surg 2002;126(1):41–7.

75. Soler ZM, Smith TL. Quality of life outcomes after functional endoscopic sinus surgery. Otolaryngol Clin North Am 2010;43(3):605–12.

76. Tait SD, Kallogjeri D, Chidambaram S, et al. Psychometric and clinimetric validity of the modified 25-item sino-nasal outcome test. Am J Rhinol Allergy 2019; 33(5):577–85.

77. Schlosser RJ, Smith TL, Mace J, et al. Asthma quality of life and control after sinus surgery in patients with chronic rhinosinusitis. Allergy 2017;72(3):483–91.

78. Rudmik L, Hopkins C, Peters A, et al. Patient-reported outcome measures for adult chronic rhinosinusitis: a systematic review and quality assessment. J Allergy Clin Immunol 2015;136(6):1532–40.e2.

79. Anderson ER, Murphy MP, Weymuller EA. Clinimetric evaluation of the sinonasal outcome test-16. Student research award 1998. Otolaryngol Head Neck Surg 1999;121(6):702–7.

80. Atlas SJ, Metson RB, Singer DE, et al. Validity of a new health-related quality of life instrument for patients with chronic sinusitis. Laryngoscope 2005;115(5): 846–54.

81. Benninger MS, Senior BA. The development of the rhinosinusitis disability index. Arch Otolaryngol Head Neck Surg 1997;123(11):1175–9.

82. Bhattacharyya N. The economic burden and symptom manifestations of chronic rhinosinusitis. Am J Rhinol 2003;17(1):27–32.

83. Dixon AE, Sugar EA, Zinreich SJ, et al. Criteria to screen for chronic sinonasal disease. Chest 2009;136(5):1324–32.

84. Gliklich RE, Metson R. Economic implications of chronic sinusitis. Otolaryngol Head Neck Surg 1998;118(3 Pt 1):344–9.

85. Brooks R. EuroQol: the current state of play. Health Policy 1996;37(1):53–72.

86. Kacha S, Guillemin F, Jankowski R. Development and validity of the DyNaChron questionnaire for chronic nasal dysfunction. Eur Arch Otorhinolaryngol 2012; 269(1):143–53.

87. Naidoo Y, Tan N, Singhal D, et al. Chronic rhinosinusitis assessment using the adelaide disease severity score. J Laryngol Otol 2013;127(Suppl 2):S24–8.

88. Remenschneider AK, D'Amico L, Gray ST, et al. The EQ-5D: a new tool for studying clinical outcomes in chronic rhinosinusitis. Laryngoscope 2015;125(1):7–15.

89. Simopoulos E, Katotomichelakis M, Gouveris H, et al. Olfaction-associated quality of life in chronic rhinosinusitis: adaptation and validation of an olfaction-specific questionnaire. Laryngoscope 2012;122(7):1450–4.

90. Gray ST, Phillips KM, Hoehle LP, et al. The 22-item sino-nasal outcome test accurately reflects patient-reported control of chronic rhinosinusitis symptomatology. Int Forum Allergy Rhinol 2017;7(10):945–51.

91. Jafari A, DeConde AS. Outcomes in medical and surgical treatment of nasal polyps. Adv Otorhinolaryngol 2016;79:158–67.

92. Feng AL, Wesely NC, Hoehle LP, et al. A validated model for the 22-item Sino-Nasal Outcome Test subdomain structure in chronic rhinosinusitis. Int Forum Allergy Rhinol 2017;7(12):1140–8.

93. Smith TL. Scientific abstracts for RhinoWorld 2019. Int Forum Allergy Rhinol 2019;9(S2):S49–124.

94. Soler ZM, Jones R, Le P, et al. Sino-Nasal outcome test-22 outcomes after sinus surgery: a systematic review and meta-analysis. Laryngoscope 2018;128(3): 581–92.

95. Steele TO, Rudmik L, Mace JC, et al. Patient-centered decision making: the role of the baseline SNOT-22 in predicting outcomes for medical management of chronic rhinosinusitis. Int Forum Allergy Rhinol 2016;6(6):590–6.

96. Soler ZM, Rudmik L, Hwang PH, et al. Patient-centered decision making in the treatment of chronic rhinosinusitis. Laryngoscope 2013;123(10):2341–6.

97. Rosenfeld RM, Piccirillo JF, Chandrasekhar SS, et al. Clinical practice guideline (update): adult sinusitis. Otolaryngol Head Neck Surg 2015;152(2 Suppl): S1–39.

98. Rombaux P, Huart C, Levie P, et al. Olfaction in chronic rhinosinusitis. Curr Allergy Asthma Rep 2016;16(5):41.

99. Frasnelli J, Hummel T. Olfactory dysfunction and daily life. Eur Arch Otorhinolaryngol 2005;262(3):231–5.

100. Mattos JL, Schlosser RJ, DeConde AS, et al. Factor analysis of the questionnaire of olfactory disorders in patients with chronic rhinosinusitis. Int Forum Allergy Rhinol 2018;8(7):777–82.

101. Mattos JL, Schlosser RJ, Storck KA, et al. Understanding the relationship between olfactory-specific quality of life, objective olfactory loss, and patient factors in chronic rhinosinusitis. Int Forum Allergy Rhinol 2017;7(7):734–40.

102. Kohli P, Soler ZM, Storck KA, et al. Responsiveness and reliability of the sinus control test in chronic rhinosinusitis. Rhinology 2017;55(1):39–44.

103. Alt JA, Smith TL, Schlosser RJ, et al. Sleep and quality of life improvements after endoscopic sinus surgery in patients with chronic rhinosinusitis. Int Forum Allergy Rhinol 2014;4(9):693–701.

104. Alt JA, Smith TL, Mace JC, et al. Sleep quality and disease severity in patients with chronic rhinosinusitis. Laryngoscope 2013;123(10):2364–70.

105. Alt JA, Sautter NB, Mace JC, et al. Antisomnogenic cytokines, quality of life, and chronic rhinosinusitis: a pilot study. Laryngoscope 2014;124(4):E107–14.

106. Alt JA, Ramakrishnan VR, Platt MP, et al. Impact of chronic rhinosinusitis on sleep: a controlled clinical study. Int Forum Allergy Rhinol 2019;9(1):16–22.

107. Alt JA, Ramakrishnan VR, Platt MP, et al. Sleep quality outcomes after medical and surgical management of chronic rhinosinusitis. Int Forum Allergy Rhinol 2017;7(2):113–8.

108. Remenschneider AK, Scangas G, Meier JC, et al. EQ-5D-derived health utility values in patients undergoing surgery for chronic rhinosinusitis. Laryngoscope 2015;125(5):1056–61.

109. van Reenen M, Janssen B. EQ-5D-5L user guide. Basic information on how to use the EQ-5D-5L instrument.

110. Gray ST, Hoehle LP, Phillips KM, et al. Patient-reported control of chronic rhinosinusitis symptoms is positively associated with general health-related quality of life. Clin Otolaryngol 2017;42(6):1161–6.

111. 36-Item Short Form Survey (SF-36). RAND Health Care.

112. Chester AC, Sindwani R. Symptom outcomes in endoscopic sinus surgery: a systematic review of measurement methods. Laryngoscope 2007;117(12): 2239–43.

113. Macdonald KI, McNally JD, Massoud E. Quality of life and impact of surgery on patients with chronic rhinosinusitis. J Otolaryngol Head Neck Surg 2009;38(2): 286–93.

114. Smith TL, Litvack JR, Hwang PH, et al. Determinants of outcomes of sinus surgery: a multi-institutional prospective cohort study. Otolaryngol Head Neck Surg 2010;142(1):55–63.
115. Brazier JE, Roberts J. The estimation of a preference-based measure of health from the SF-12. Med Care 2004;42(9):851–9.
116. Brazier J, Roberts J, Tsuchiya A, et al. A comparison of the EQ-5D and SF-6D across seven patient groups. Health Econ 2004;13(9):873–84.
117. Chowdhury NI, Turner JH, Dorminy C, et al. Preoperative quality-of-life measures predict acute postoperative pain in endoscopic sinus surgery. Laryngoscope 2019;129(6):1274–9.
118. Rudmik L, Mace J, Soler ZM, et al. Long-term utility outcomes in patients undergoing endoscopic sinus surgery. Laryngoscope 2014;124(1):19–23.
119. Smith TL, Schlosser RJ, Mace JC, et al. Long-term outcomes of endoscopic sinus surgery in the management of adult chronic rhinosinusitis. Int Forum Allergy Rhinol 2019;9(8):831-41.
120. Luk LJ, Steele TO, Mace JC, et al. Health utility outcomes in patients undergoing medical management for chronic rhinosinusitis: a prospective multiinstitutional study. Int Forum Allergy Rhinol 2015;5(11):1018–27.
121. Zhang W, Bansback N, Anis AH. Measuring and valuing productivity loss due to poor health: a critical review. Soc Sci Med 2011;72(2):185–92.
122. Schlosser RJ, Storck KA, Rudmik L, et al. Association of olfactory dysfunction in chronic rhinosinusitis with economic productivity and medication usage. Int Forum Allergy Rhinol 2017;7(1):50–5.
123. Phillips KM, Bergmark RW, Hoehle LP, et al. Chronic rhinosinusitis exacerbations are differentially associated with lost productivity based on asthma status. Rhinology 2018;56(4):323–9.
124. Rudmik L, Soler ZM, Smith TL, et al. Effect of continued medical therapy on productivity costs for refractory chronic rhinosinusitis. JAMA Otolaryngol Head Neck Surg 2015;141(11):969–73.
125. Rudmik L, Smith TL, Mace JC, et al. Productivity costs decrease after endoscopic sinus surgery for refractory chronic rhinosinusitis. Laryngoscope 2016;126(3):570–4.

Personalized Medicine in Chronic Rhinosinusitis
Phenotypes, Endotypes, and Biomarkers

Ashley M. Bauer, MD, Justin H. Turner, MD, PhD*

KEYWORDS

- Cytokine • Inflammation • Rhinosinusitis • Phenotype • Endotype

KEY POINTS

- Understanding the molecular basis behind the clinical manifestations of chronic rhinosinusitis (CRS) can potentially provide a more comprehensive and personalized approach to treating individual patients.
- Studies incorporating CRS endotyping have used different variations of biomarkers, resulting in a variable number of disease clusters; however, the studies have largely produced consistent results with respect to the underlying characteristics of identified endotypes.
- The ideal CRS biomarker should be highly specific and have the ability to facilitate diagnosis, differentiate phenotypes and endotypes, indicate treatment responsiveness, and monitor disease control.

INTRODUCTION

Chronic rhinosinusitis (CRS) is now recognized as a heterogenous disease process with a broad spectrum of clinical presentations and pathogenic mechanisms. Identification of specific drivers of disease has become a focus of CRS research and has the potential to predict outcomes and response to treatment, in addition to encouraging development of new and improved biotherapeutics. With this in mind, it is important to note that definitive algorithms for CRS management have remained elusive and at times highly variable. A more personalized approach to care of the patient with CRS will become imperative going forward, given direct costs to the US health care system of more than 10 billion dollars yearly.[1–5] Ultimately, meeting this goal will require improved understanding of disease heterogeneity in relation to clinically observable patient characteristics (phenotypes), underlying cellular or molecular

Department of Otolaryngology–Head and Neck Surgery, Vanderbilt University Medical Center, 1215 21st Avenue South, Suite 7209, Nashville, TN 37232-8605, USA
* Corresponding author.
E-mail address: justin.h.turner@vumc.org

Immunol Allergy Clin N Am 40 (2020) 281–293
https://doi.org/10.1016/j.iac.2019.12.007
0889-8561/20/© 2019 Elsevier Inc. All rights reserved.

immunology.theclinics.com

pathogenic mechanisms (endotypes), and clinically significant outcomes.[6,7] The present review summarizes recent advancements in personalized approaches in CRS, with a focus on disease phenotypes, endotypes, and potential biomarkers.

PATHOPHYSIOLOGY

Although the pathophysiology of CRS is incompletely defined, current evidence suggests that a combination of host and environmental factors play an integrative role. The following factors are thought to play a role in the cycle of anatomic dysfunction and chronic mucosal inflammation that is commonly observed in CRS:

- Innate and epithelial immunity: the upper airways have a unique epithelial barrier characterized by tight and adherens junctions that coordinate to protect underlying immunosensitive tissue from environmental irritants and microbial pathogens.[8] This epithelial barrier is dysregulated in CRS possibly secondary to pathogens such as *Staphylococcus aureus* and *Pseudomonas aeruginosa*, which can directly affect tight junctions, or due to cytokines such as interferon gamma (IFN-γ) and interleukin 4(IL-4), which can interfere with barrier protein expression.[9]
- Mucociliary clearance: among the most essential functions of the upper airway, mucociliary clearance serves as the first line of defense against airborne particles and microbial pathogens.[10] Ciliated sinonasal mucosa is covered with a mobile mucous layer that lays on a less viscous periciliary layer working together to move foreign particles through the nose and into the gastrointestinal tract.[11] A breakdown in mucociliary clearance is characteristic of specific CRS phenotypes, such as cystic fibrosis and primary ciliary dyskinesia, but is also observed in other patients with CRS as well.[12,13] Certain pathogens, including *Haemophilus influenza, Streptococcus pneumoniae, S aureus, P aeruginosa,* and *Aspergillus* secrete proteases that impair ciliary movement. In addition, hypoxia develops due to excess secretions and alters ion transport, resulting in an ineffective mucous layer and uncoordinated ciliary movement.[14–17]
- Tolerance and adaptive immunity: breakdown of the epithelial barrier enables allergens and microbial antigens to transgress physical barriers, culminating in local tissue inflammation and/or allergen sensitization.[6] This induces epithelial cells to secrete inflammatory mediators and cytokines that recruit and activate multiple effector cells.[18(p2),19–21] Microbial pathogens, particulates, and allergens all have the ability to activate antigen-specific T-helper (Th) cells. Multiple subsets of Th and innate immune cells drive inflammation in CRS, including type 1/Th1 cells that produce IFN-γ; type 2/Th2 cells that secrete IL-4, IL-5, and IL-13; and type 3/Th17 cells that produce IL-17 and IL-22. Immune polarization in CRS is highly variable, and a combination of type 1, type 2, and type 3 immune mechanisms drive the production of specific cytokines and results in a persistent inflammatory state.[22–24]
- Microbiome: the diversity and composition of the sinonasal microbiome plays an integrative role in the health of the respiratory environment. Multiple studies have attempted to isolate specific bacteria linked with the pathogenesis of CRS[25–28]; however, even with more recent advances in molecular genetics, a specific causative organism has yet to be identified. Nonetheless, current evidence suggests that imbalance (or dysbiosis) within the microbiome, specifically a decrease in microbial diversity, may be a common characteristic of patients with CRS.[26] This imbalance can lead to an overabundance of opportunistic pathogens such as *S aureus* and *P aeruginosa* and loss of key commensal organisms.[29]

PHENOTYPES

Phenotypic classifications in CRS have largely been driven by clinical practice and have remained largely unchanged. Classically, patients have been differentiated primarily by the presence (chronic rhinosinusitis with nasal polyps [CRSwNP]) or absence (chronic rhinosinusitis without nasal polyps [CRSsNP]) of nasal polyps, as this is among the most clinically observable features in most patients. This classification has largely driven treatment approaches, and dichotomization of patients based on polyp status has long been linked to differences in pathobiology and disease mechanisms. CRSwNP has primarily been linked to type 2 inflammation and eosinophilic tissue infiltration, whereas CRSsNP has typically been linked with elevated type 1-associated cytokines.[30,31] However, this rigid dichotomy is now recognized as overly simplistic, and substantial research now suggests that both CRSsNP and CRSwNP can present with a combination of type 1-, type 2-, and type 3-associated signatures.[23,32–34] Furthermore, there is evidence to suggest that within phenotypes, particularly among patients with nasal polyps, further subgrouping based on other observable qualities or comorbidities (eg, allergy, asthma, aspirin sensitivity) can be associated with unique disease behavior. This can potentially include local aggressiveness, altered responses to therapeutics, and high recurrence rates after surgical treatment. As such, additional subphenotypes such as aspirin-exacerbated respiratory disease, allergic fungal rhinosinusitis, and cystic fibrosis–associated CRS have been described and are used clinically. Unfortunately, within individual phenotypes there is substantial variability in patient demographics, comorbidities, and clinical responses to therapy that make this approach inefficient.

ENDOTYPES

The heterogeneity and complexity of CRS strongly suggests the need for alternatives to phenotype-based classification systems. In contrast to phenotypes, which are based on easily observable features, endotypes are instead derived from assessment of biomarkers that reflect underlying biological mechanisms.[35] Understanding the molecular basis behind the clinical manifestations of CRS can potentially provide a more comprehensive and personalized approach to treating individual patients. Endotyping has advanced treatment paradigms in other heterogeneous inflammatory diseases, particularly in asthma where it has led to improved understanding of treatment-resistant disease, enhanced diagnostic schemes, and facilitated targeting for biological therapies.[36–38] Inflammatory endotyping has only recently been explored for CRS, but early studies have shown consistent findings and advanced understanding of the disease process. Although endotyping can incorporate any biomarker, most studies have focused on cytokines and inflammatory mediators measured in nasal secretions or sinonasal tissue biopsies.[32,33] The use of hierarchical clustering and other unstructured statistical approaches allows for incorporation of an infinite combination of biomarkers without any presumed outcome. This allows for patients with similar inflammatory signatures to be grouped into "clusters," presumably with similar underlying pathophysiologic mechanisms of disease.[32,33,39,40] To date, studies incorporating CRS endotyping have used different variations of biomarkers resulting in a variable number of disease clusters; however, the studies have largely produced consistent results with respect to the underlying characteristics of identified endotypes. In a landmark European study, Tomassen and colleagues[32] used hierarchical cluster analysis using 14 different inflammatory markers to identify putative CRS inflammatory endotypes. They identified 10 distinct clusters characterized by the following:

1. Eosinophilic and Th2-related markers (IL-5 and immunoglobulin E [IgE]),
2. Neutrophilic or proinflammatory mediators or both (IL-1β, IL-6, IL-8, and myeloperoxidase),
3. Th17/Th22 markers (IL-17A, IL-22, and tumor necrosis factor-alpha), and
4. IFN-γ.[32]

In a smaller cohort study, Divekar and colleagues[39] used a similar approach with a commercially available immunoassay of 41 cytokine/chemokines in tissue from 26 patients from a North American population. They identified 3 distinct clusters driven by Th1/Th17-type mediators (IL-17A, granulocyte-colony stimulating factor, IL-8, and IFN-γ), type 2-associated mediators (IL-5, IL-9, IL-13 and eotaxin) and finally a third cluster characterized by elevated growth factors (platelet-derived growth factor and vascular endothelial growth factor). Finally, Turner and colleagues[33] performed hierarchical cluster analysis on 90 patients using 18 different biomarkers measured in mucus to identify 5 to 6 distinct clusters.[41] Individual clusters were primarily characterized by type 2 inflammation, proinflammatory and neutrophilic inflammation, or clusters with minimal to low overall inflammation. All of these studies show similar patterns of inflammatory burden and suggest that type 2-associated inflammation is present in most European and North American patients with CRS but only dominant in a small minority.

In a different geographic demographic, Liao and colleagues[40] analyzed 246 Chinese patients with CRS and incorporated both inflammatory biomarkers and clinical/demographic variables in the clustering model. Seven distinct clusters were identified. Similar to other published studies, some clusters were characterized by mild inflammatory burden or neutrophilic inflammation, whereas only 20% of patients were assigned to clusters dominated by type 2 inflammation, further highlighting potential geographic differences in disease characteristics. This study also analyzed treatment outcomes with respect to disease clusters and found that "difficult-to-treat" CRS was mainly associated with neutrophilic endotypes and those associated with elevated proinflammatory profiles, whereas a smaller group with severe disease and poor treatment outcomes was associated with the type 2 endotype.

It is important to recognize that endotypic classification is largely a representation of individual inflammatory mechanisms and not a clearly definable entity with a direct biological basis. There is likely a continuum of different types of inflammation within individual patients and thus few patients will be linked directly to a single inflammatory endotype or immune signature. The longitudinal stability of putative CRS endotypes also remains unclear, and it is likely that medical/surgical treatment, environmental factors, geography, and other variables may have significant impacts on endotypic assignment. In support of this hypothesis, a recent study found that most of the patients undergoing endoscopic sinus surgery moved to a different inflammatory endotype postoperatively.[42]

BIOMARKERS

The term "biomarker'" refers to any objective measure that reflects the underlying medical condition of a patient or predicts outcomes to treatment. In CRS management, and for the purposes of this review, biomarkers typically refer to biological molecules measured in serum, tissue, or nasal secretions, which reflect underlying disease pathophysiology and aid in diagnostics and treatment algorithms. In general, an ideal biomarker should be highly specific and facilitate diagnosis, differentiate phenotypes and endotypes, indicate treatment responsiveness, and monitor disease control. Although currently explored biomarkers have some ability to classify patients, single biomarkers have generally lacked the ability to accurately characterize patients, largely because each biomarker is involved in unique but complex molecular pathways. The use of multiple biomarkers may ultimately have greater potential to clarify such complex pathophysiology and improve predictive power. The following section is a summary of potential CRS biomarkers.

Eosinophils

Eosinophilic mucin, eosinophilia, and elevated IgE levels are part of the type 2 immune response and have frequently been associated with treatment outcomes and extent of disease. Tissue eosinophilia in CRS is thought to be related to more extensive disease and a decreased likelihood of surgical success.[43–45] Elevated systemic eosinophils may also reflect worse prognosis, increased severity of symptoms, and extensive sinus disease.[46] Conversely, eosinophilic nasal polyps are generally thought to be more glucocorticoid responsive than their noneosinophilic counterparts.[47] Because eosinophilia has clear prognostic and treatment implications, substantial effort has focused on minimally invasive approaches to identify these patients. Importantly, the degree of tissue eosinophilia is extremely difficult to determine based on clinical symptoms and cannot be predicted by the presence of asthma or aspirin-exacerbated respiratory disease.[48] Likewise, phenotypic differentiation of patients with CRS based on polyp status fails to accurately align with presence or absence of eosinophils.[49] Because significant overlap in clinical phenotypes and symptoms exist among patients with and without eosinophilia, direct measurement of tissue and/or serum eosinophils has generally been required to accurately differentiate patients.

Tissue eosinophilia can most accurately be characterized using tissue histopathology; however, indicators and definitions of eosinophilia have been inconsistent. For example, Kountakis and colleagues[50] proposed that greater than 5 eosinophils per high power field (HPF) was diagnostic based primarily on the degree of presumed eosinophil activation. In contrast, Soler and colleagues[51] defined mucosal eosinophilia as greater than 10 eosinophils/HPF, which was predictive of less improvement in disease-specific quality of life scores after surgery. Regardless of the precise definition, most patients fall along a continuum of eosinophil infiltration, making precise grouping difficult. As an alternative, peripheral blood eosinophil levels have been investigated as a potential surrogate marker for tissue eosinophilia, as this does not require analysis of surgical specimens or tissue biopsies. In one study by Sakuma and colleagues,[52] a blood eosinophil percentage of greater than or equal to 6% correlated with tissue eosinophilia. However, various comorbid disorders including allergies, autoimmune diseases, adverse drug reactions, and parasitic infections can alter circulating eosinophil counts, and as such, the utility of blood eosinophil counts as a biomarker remain limited.

Finally, the presence of eosinophils alone does not indicate eosinophilic inflammation or activation. Biomarkers that include byproducts or molecules secreted by eosinophils and key eosinophil-associated cytokines may potentially be more indicative of underlying eosinophil activation.[24] This approach may be superior to histologic approaches, which can be semiquantitative and subject to both interpreter and intraspecimen variation. Examples of eosinophil markers include eosinophil cationic protein (ECP), major basic protein, eotaxins, total IgE, and S aureus enterotoxins (SE-IgE).[53]

Immunoglobulin E

IgE binds to receptors on eosinophils, basophils, mast cells, and other cell types and can amplify the type 2 immune response. IgE has been investigated as a potential biomarker due to frequently elevated levels of serum and local IgE in patients with

CRS and associated atopy and eosinophilic inflammation.[32] Bachert and colleagues[35] found that concentrations of total IgE correlated significantly with levels of ECP and IL-5 and thus local eosinophilic inflammation. In a prospective follow-up, high local IgE ultimately predicted the need for revision surgery.[54] In addition, among patients with nasal polyps, tissue IgE and SE-IgE were identified as risk factors for comorbid asthma.[55]

Type 2 Cytokines

IL-5 is a key cytokine responsible for survival, maturation, and activation of eosinophils within the bone marrow and at sites of inflammation and is a key mediator of type 2 inflammation.[56] Patients with high local and systemic IL-5 also have a higher risk of having asthma comorbidity.[55(p5)] Elevated tissue IL-5 is a common characteristic of nasal polyps, with recent studies suggesting high levels in 80% of European nasal polyp cases and 20% to 60% of Asian nasal polyp cases.[22] Gevaert and colleagues[57] found that elevated IL-5 in nasal secretions predicted clinical response to reslizumab, a humanized anti-IL-5 monoclonal antibody. Likewise, Turner and colleagues[58] found that levels of mucous IL-5, and the related type 2 cytokine IL-13, were associated with greater disease severity and prior surgical intervention.

IL-4 and IL-13 are also essential cytokines that activate the type 2 inflammatory response. They synergistically promote the synthesis of IgE from B cells and stimulate mucous secretion in epithelial cells. In addition to the induction of eosinophilic inflammation, IL-4 plays a role in nasal polyp formation. IL-13 affects epithelial differentiation resulting in decreased ciliation and goblet cell metaplasia as well as increasing hyperreactivity of the airway and subepithelial fibrosis. Although IL-4 was not found to be a reliable biomarker in CRS in mucous samples, it has been found to be significantly elevated in tissue samples of patients with CRS compared with controls.[58–60] Turner and colleagues[58] found that patients with a high IL-13 signature had significantly worse preoperative disease than their low IL-13 counterparts. Delineating which patients have high IL-13 and IL-4 signatures is thought to be of value not only for disease severity but also for patient selection regarding treatment with targeted biologics against these cytokines.

Interleukin 25 and 33

Epithelial-derived cytokines, including thymic stromal lymphopoietin (TSLP), IL-25, and IL-33, are recognized for their ability to interact with lymphocytes and dendritic cells to promote type 2 inflammation.[61,62] IL-25, also known as IL-17E, is a member of the IL-17 cytokine family and has been associated with high computed tomographic (CT) scores and elevated blood eosinophil numbers in patients with CRS.[63] IL-33 is a member of the IL-1 cytokine family and is likewise a potent inducer of type 2 responses, although underlying mechanisms remain poorly defined.[64] Expression of IL-33 is elevated in CRSwNP patients with severe and recalcitrant disease.[64]

Periostin

Periostin is a secreted extracellular protein that has emerged as a marker in pathologic remodeling processes and has an important role in wound repair as well as epithelial-mesenchymal transition of cancer cells.[65] Periostin is produced mainly by epithelial cells in response to IL-4 and IL-13 and has a pivotal role in subepithelial fibrosis. Overexpression of periostin has been found in eosinophilic CRSwNP and may have roles in epithelial damage, extracellular matrix accumulation, and infiltration of inflammatory cells.[66–68] A recent study by Maxfield and colleagues[66] established that high serum levels of periostin were strongly associated with the presence of nasal polyps in patients with CRS. Zhang and colleagues[67] also found that periostin expression was elevated in active CRS, and decreased after effective treatment, suggesting that periostin could represent an indicator of disease activity and responsiveness to therapy. In addition to being a diagnostic biomarker, periostin may also be a biomarker for responsiveness to omalizumab in eosinophilic nasal polyps and has already been studied as an effective biomarker in asthma.[69]

P-Glycoprotein

P-glycoprotein is an adenosine triphosphate–dependent efflux pump that is constitutively expressed in multiple cell types.[70] It also functions as an immunomodulator capable of regulating secretion of proinflammatory cytokines from epithelial cells.[70,71] P-glycoprotein levels are elevated in all CRS subtypes, particularly those with nasal polyps, and higher levels have been associated with worse subjective and objective measures of disease severity.[70,71] The reported immunomodulatory function of P-glycoprotein coupled with its presence in sinonasal epithelium suggests that it may play an important role in CRS pathophysiology.

Cystatin

Cystatin is a type 2 cysteine protease inhibitor that plays a key role in epithelial barrier function and immunomodulatory processes and enhances eosinophil activation and recruitment. Cystatins may have mechanistic roles in both eosinophilic CRS and allergic rhinitis by interacting with type 2 cytokines, microbial antigens, and fibroblasts and by mediating inhibition of allergen-related histamine release.[72] Cystatin-1 has been described as being both transiently elevated in seasonal allergic rhinitis and overexpressed in the setting of eosinophilic CRS.[73] Similarly, recent studies have associated high cystatin-2 levels with severe and steroid-resistant asthma.[36] In a prospective study by Bleier,[71] cystatin-2 mirrored major clinical events in patients with CRSwNP with a significant reduction in levels after surgery and subsequent increases over time, suggesting that it may be closely linked to the underlying disease process.

Nitric Oxide

Nitric oxide (NO) is a ubiquitous inflammatory mediator with multiple physiologic roles. NO in the respiratory environment is a free radical that takes the form of a colorless, odorless gas. Its chemical structure is extremely reactive with a very short half-life of a few seconds and an extremely high diffusion capacity in tissue.[74] As a result of its extreme reactivity and its direct and indirect effects, NO is involved in several regulatory functions, such as vasodilatation (as a result of smooth muscle relaxation), neuronal transmission, and inhibition of platelet aggregation.[74–76] In the nasal airways, it is constitutively produced from epithelial cells lining the paranasal sinuses and contributes to local host defense via its bacteriostatic and antiviral properties and through stimulation of ciliary motility.[77] Exhaled NO is currently used as a marker of asthma control, with lower levels correlating with better disease control.[78] A frank decrease in NO has been observed in patients with nasal polyposis, potentially due to sinus ostial occlusion and failure of gaseous NO in the sinuses to reach the nasal cavities.[78,79] There is also an inverse correlation between nitric oxide levels and the severity of sinus disease as assessed by clinical and/or CT findings.[80] After surgical or medical treatment, NO levels often improve in parallel with other clinical markers, suggesting a possible role as a less invasive marker of disease status.[79,80]

Taste Receptors

Recently, genetic polymorphisms in bitter taste receptors have been recognized as potential biomarkers in CRS. Bitter taste receptors are G protein–coupled receptors expressed by upper airway ciliated cells and stimulated by gram-negative bacteria such as *P aeruginosa*.[81] When bitter taste receptors on ciliated cells are stimulated, there is a downstream antimicrobial NO response, which results in direct bacterial killing and increased ciliary beat frequency. The receptor's function is dictated by specific genetic polymorphisms with some variants resulting in decreased function, making patients more susceptible to sinonasal infections and biofilm formation.[82] Because taste receptors are expressed both on the tongue and in the upper airway, the patient's genotype can be assessed by a taste test that elicits ratings of bitter and sweet taste intensity on a continuum.[81] Patients with CRSsNP have been found to be significantly less sensitive to a broad bitter taste receptor agonist, whereas patients with CRSwNP and CRSsNP were found to be sensitive to sucrose, a sweet receptor agonist.[83] Thus, it may be possible to use bitter and sweet taste tests as biomarkers to evaluate CRS disease status.[29,84] A genotype of the bitter taste receptor TAS2R38 was also found to predict surgical outcomes in patients with CRS without nasal polyps.[85]

Adaptive Immunity

B cells are integral to humoral immunity and, along with plasma cells and T cells, are increased in nasal polyp tissue.[8] In addition to their ability to produce antibodies that contribute to disease pathogenesis, B cells can function as antigen-presenting or regulatory cells and produce a variety of cytokines and chemokines that can influence inflammation. Tissue levels of IgG_1, IgG_2, IgG_4, IgA, IgE, and IgM are all increased in nasal polyp versus healthy sinonasal tissue.[86] This increase in antibodies was only shown locally with normal levels of circulating antibodies in the peripheral blood of the same patients. This suggests that B-cell antibody production in patients with CRSwNP is not a systemic response but rather driven by a stimulus within the local sinonasal inflammatory environment. Because of this increase in local B cells and antibodies in CRSwNP, studies have evaluated whether this elevation in immunoglobulins could be due to autoreactive B cells producing antibodies against self-tissue.[87] Tan and colleagues[87] showed a statistically significant increase in autoantibodies within nasal polyp tissue compared with tissue from patients with CRSsNP as well as nondiseased tissue in patients with CRSwNP. Specifically, increases in IgG anti-dsDNA were associated with disease severity and revision surgery, indicating a possible marker for recalcitrant disease.

TREATMENT IMPLICATIONS

With different pathomechanisms underlying endotypes of CRS, a single-treatment approach is unlikely to be universally successful in all patients. Effective management of this heterogeneous disease will ultimately require a more personalized approach based on disease pathophysiology and endotypic status that can help drive medical or surgical care. For example, glucocorticoids have been found to be most effective in patients with eosinophilic nasal polyps, while being largely ineffective in patients with noneosinophilic or neutrophilic disease.[88] Conversely, long-term use of macrolide antibiotics seems to be most effective in patients with neutrophilic inflammation,[89] whereas doxycycline, which has effects on matrix metalloproteinases and IgE levels, seems to be better suited for patients with type 2 eosinophilic inflammation.[89,90] Of immediate importance, the rapid introduction of humanized monoclonal antibodies that target type 2 inflammation have hastened the need to subtype patients based on their inflammatory signature and predict treatment responses. Recent identification and characterization of inflammatory CRS endotypes has improved understanding of CRS and highlighted a need for continued research into precise mechanisms of disease. Ultimately incorporating personalized approaches that incorporate phenotypic and endotypic characteristics will likely become an essential part of clinical practice.

DISCLOSURE OF POTENTIAL CONFLICTS OF INTEREST

J.H. Turner has served as a consultant for ALK and has received grant support from the NIH/National Institute of Deafness and Communication Disorders (NIDCD) and additional support from the NIH/National Institute of Allergy and Infectious Diseases (NIAID). The remaining author has nothing to disclose.

REFERENCES

1. Smith TL, Kern RC, Palmer JN, et al. Medical therapy vs surgery for chronic rhinosinusitis: a prospective, multi-institutional study. Int Forum Allergy Rhinol 2011; 1(4):235–41.
2. Blackwell DL, Lucas JW, Clarke TC. Summary health statistics for U.S. adults: national health interview survey, 2012. Vital Health Stat 10 2014;(260):1–161.
3. Schiller JS, Lucas JW, Peregoy JA. Summary health statistics for U.S. Adults: national health interview survey, 2011. Vital Health Stat 10 2012;(256):1–218.
4. Dykewicz MS. 7. Rhinitis and sinusitis. J Allergy Clin Immunol 2003;111(2 Suppl): S520–9.
5. Bhattacharyya N. Incremental health care utilization and expenditures for chronic rhinosinusitis in the United States. Ann Otol Rhinol Laryngol 2011;120(7):423–7.
6. Bachert C, Akdis CA. Phenotypes and emerging endotypes of chronic rhinosinusitis. J Allergy Clin Immunol Pract 2016;4(4):621–8.
7. Akdis CA, Bachert C, Cingi C, et al. Endotypes and phenotypes of chronic rhinosinusitis: a PRACTALL document of the European Academy of Allergy and Clinical Immunology and the American Academy of Allergy, Asthma & Immunology. J Allergy Clin Immunol 2013;131(6):1479–90.
8. Stevens WW, Lee RJ, Schleimer RP, et al. Chronic rhinosinusitis pathogenesis. J Allergy Clin Immunol 2015;136(6):1442–53.
9. Nomura K, Obata K, Keira T, et al. Pseudomonas aeruginosa elastase causes transient disruption of tight junctions and downregulation of PAR-2 in human nasal epithelial cells. Respir Res 2014;15:21.
10. Knowles MR, Boucher RC. Mucus clearance as a primary innate defense mechanism for mammalian airways. J Clin Invest 2002;109(5):571–7.
11. Antunes MB, Cohen NA. Mucociliary clearance–a critical upper airway host defense mechanism and methods of assessment. Curr Opin Allergy Clin Immunol 2007;7(1):5–10.
12. Lee RJ, Foskett JK. Ca^{2+} signaling and fluid secretion by secretory cells of the airway epithelium. Cell Calcium 2014;55(6):325–36.
13. Mall MA, Galietta LJV. Targeting ion channels in cystic fibrosis. J Cyst Fibros 2015;14(5):561–70.
14. Wilson R, Pitt T, Taylor G, et al. Pyocyanin and 1-hydroxyphenazine produced by Pseudomonas aeruginosa inhibit the beating of human respiratory cilia in vitro. J Clin Invest 1987;79(1):221–9.
15. Zhao K-Q, Goldstein N, Yang H, et al. Inherent differences in nasal and tracheal ciliary function in response to Pseudomonas aeruginosa challenge. Am J Rhinol Allergy 2011;25(4):209–13.

16. Shen JC, Cope E, Chen B, et al. Regulation of murine sinonasal cilia function by microbial secreted factors. Int Forum Allergy Rhinol 2012;2(2):104–10.

17. Amitani R, Taylor G, Elezis EN, et al. Purification and characterization of factors produced by Aspergillus fumigatus which affect human ciliated respiratory epithelium. Infect Immun 1995;63(9):3266–71.

18. Ho J, Bailey M, Zaunders J, et al. Group 2 innate lymphoid cells (ILC2s) are increased in chronic rhinosinusitis with nasal polyps or eosinophilia. Clin Exp Allergy 2015;45(2):394–403.

19. Liao B, Cao P-P, Zeng M, et al. Interaction of thymic stromal lymphopoietin, IL-33, and their receptors in epithelial cells in eosinophilic chronic rhinosinusitis with nasal polyps. Allergy 2015;70(9):1169–80.

20. Shaw JL, Fakhri S, Citardi MJ, et al. IL-33-responsive innate lymphoid cells are an important source of IL-13 in chronic rhinosinusitis with nasal polyps. Am J Respir Crit Care Med 2013;188(4):432–9.

21. Lam EPS, Kariyawasam HH, Rana BMJ, et al. IL-25/IL-33-responsive TH2 cells characterize nasal polyps with a default TH17 signature in nasal mucosa. J Allergy Clin Immunol 2016;137(5):1514–24.

22. Wang X, Zhang N, Bo M, et al. Diversity of TH cytokine profiles in patients with chronic rhinosinusitis: a multicenter study in Europe, Asia, and Oceania. J Allergy Clin Immunol 2016;138(5):1344–53.

23. Tan BK, Klingler AI, Poposki JA, et al. Heterogeneous inflammatory patterns in chronic rhinosinusitis without nasal polyps in Chicago, Illinois. J Allergy Clin Immunol 2017;139(2):699–703.e7.

24. Zhang N, Van Zele T, Perez-Novo C, et al. Different types of T-effector cells orchestrate mucosal inflammation in chronic sinus disease. J Allergy Clin Immunol 2008;122(5):961–8.

25. Abreu NA, Nagalingam NA, Song Y, et al. Sinus microbiome diversity depletion and Corynebacterium tuberculostearicum enrichment mediates rhinosinusitis. Sci Transl Med 2012;4(151):151ra124.

26. Anderson M, Stokken J, Sanford T, et al. A systematic review of the sinonasal microbiome in chronic rhinosinusitis. Am J Rhinol Allergy 2016;30(3):161–6.

27. Boase S, Foreman A, Cleland E, et al. The microbiome of chronic rhinosinusitis: culture, molecular diagnostics and biofilm detection. BMC Infect Dis 2013; 13:210.

28. Feazel LM, Robertson CE, Ramakrishnan VR, et al. Microbiome complexity and Staphylococcus aureus in chronic rhinosinusitis. Laryngoscope 2012;122(2): 467–72.

29. Workman AD, Kohanski MA, Cohen NA. Biomarkers in chronic rhinosinusitis with nasal polyps. Immunol Allergy Clin North Am 2018;38(4):679–92.

30. Van Zele T, Claeys S, Gevaert P, et al. Differentiation of chronic sinus diseases by measurement of inflammatory mediators. Allergy 2006;61(11):1280–9.

31. Van Bruaene N, Pérez-Novo CA, Basinski TM, et al. T-cell regulation in chronic paranasal sinus disease. J Allergy Clin Immunol 2008;121(6):1435–41, 1441.e1-3.

32. Tomassen P, Vandeplas G, Van Zele T, et al. Inflammatory endotypes of chronic rhinosinusitis based on cluster analysis of biomarkers. J Allergy Clin Immunol 2016;137(5):1449–56.e4.

33. Turner JH, Chandra RK, Li P, et al. Identification of clinically relevant chronic rhinosinusitis endotypes using cluster analysis of mucus cytokines. J Allergy Clin Immunol 2018;141(5):1895–7.e7.

34. Stevens WW, Ocampo CJ, Berdnikovs S, et al. Cytokines in chronic rhinosinusitis. role in eosinophilia and aspirin-exacerbated respiratory disease. Am J Respir Crit Care Med 2015;192(6):682–94.
35. Bachert C, Zhang N, Hellings PW, et al. Endotype-driven care pathways in patients with chronic rhinosinusitis. J Allergy Clin Immunol 2018;141(5):1543–51.
36. Hinks TSC, Brown T, Lau LCK, et al. Multidimensional endotyping in patients with severe asthma reveals inflammatory heterogeneity in matrix metalloproteinases and chitinase 3-like protein 1. J Allergy Clin Immunol 2016;138(1):61–75.
37. Silkoff PE, Laviolette M, Singh D, et al. Identification of airway mucosal type 2 inflammation by using clinical biomarkers in asthmatic patients. J Allergy Clin Immunol 2017;140(3):710–9.
38. Peters MC, Mekonnen ZK, Yuan S, et al. Measures of gene expression in sputum cells can identify TH2-high and TH2-low subtypes of asthma. J Allergy Clin Immunol 2014;133(2):388–94.
39. Divekar R, Patel N, Jin J, et al. Symptom-based clustering in chronic rhinosinusitis relates to history of aspirin sensitivity and postsurgical outcomes. J Allergy Clin Immunol Pract 2015;3(6):934–40.e3.
40. Liao B, Liu J-X, Li Z-Y, et al. Multidimensional endotypes of chronic rhinosinusitis and their association with treatment outcomes. Allergy 2018;73(7):1459–69.
41. Morse JC, Shilts MH, Ely KA, et al. Patterns of olfactory dysfunction in chronic rhinosinusitis identified by hierarchical cluster analysis and machine learning algorithms. Int Forum Allergy Rhinol 2019;9(3):255–64.
42. Yancey KL, Li P, Huang L-C, et al. Longitudinal stability of chronic rhinosinusitis endotypes. Clin Exp Allergy 2019. https://doi.org/10.1111/cea.13502.
43. Newman LJ, Platts-Mills TA, Phillips CD, et al. Chronic sinusitis. Relationship of computed tomographic findings to allergy, asthma, and eosinophilia. JAMA 1994;271(5):363–7.
44. Marks SC, Shamsa F. Evaluation of prognostic factors in endoscopic sinus surgery. Am J Rhinol 1997;11(3):187–91.
45. Lavigne F, Nguyen CT, Cameron L, et al. Prognosis and prediction of response to surgery in allergic patients with chronic sinusitis. J Allergy Clin Immunol 2000; 105(4):746–51.
46. Sreeparvathi A, Kalyanikuttyamma LK, Kumar M, et al. Significance of blood eosinophil count in patients with chronic rhinosinusitis with nasal polyposis. J Clin Diagn Res 2017;11(2):MC08–11.
47. Wen W, Liu W, Zhang L, et al. Increased neutrophilia in nasal polyps reduces the response to oral corticosteroid therapy. J Allergy Clin Immunol 2012;129(6): 1522–8.e5.
48. Steinke JW, Smith AR, Carpenter DJ, et al. Lack of efficacy of symptoms and medical history in distinguishing the degree of eosinophilia in nasal polyps. J Allergy Clin Immunol Pract 2017;5(6):1582–8.e3.
49. Ikeda K, Shiozawa A, Ono N, et al. Subclassification of chronic rhinosinusitis with nasal polyp based on eosinophil and neutrophil. Laryngoscope 2013; 123(11):E1–9.
50. Kountakis SE, Arango P, Bradley D, et al. Molecular and cellular staging for the severity of chronic rhinosinusitis. Laryngoscope 2004;114(11):1895–905.
51. Soler ZM, Sauer D, Mace J, et al. Impact of mucosal eosinophilia and nasal polyposis on quality-of-life outcomes after sinus surgery. Otolaryngol Head Neck Surg 2010;142(1):64–71.
52. Sakuma Y, Ishitoya J, Komatsu M, et al. New clinical diagnostic criteria for eosinophilic chronic rhinosinusitis. Auris Nasus Larynx 2011;38(5):583–8.

53. Lou H, Zhang N, Bachert C, et al. Highlights of eosinophilic chronic rhinosinusitis with nasal polyps in definition, prognosis, and advancement. Int Forum Allergy Rhinol 2018;8(11):1218–25.
54. Calus L, Van Bruaene N, Bosteels C, et al. Twelve-year follow-up study after endoscopic sinus surgery in patients with chronic rhinosinusitis with nasal polyposis. Clin Transl Allergy 2019;9:30.
55. Bachert C, Zhang N, Holtappels G, et al. Presence of IL-5 protein and IgE antibodies to staphylococcal enterotoxins in nasal polyps is associated with comorbid asthma. J Allergy Clin Immunol 2010;126(5):962–8, 968.e1-6.
56. Gevaert P, Bachert C, Holtappels G, et al. Enhanced soluble interleukin-5 receptor alpha expression in nasal polyposis. Allergy 2003;58(5):371–9.
57. Gevaert P, Lang-Loidolt D, Lackner A, et al. Nasal IL-5 levels determine the response to anti-IL-5 treatment in patients with nasal polyps. J Allergy Clin Immunol 2006;118(5):1133–41.
58. Turner JH, Li P, Chandra RK. Mucus T helper 2 biomarkers predict chronic rhinosinusitis disease severity and prior surgical intervention. Int Forum Allergy Rhinol 2018;8(10):1175–83.
59. Riechelmann H, Deutschle T, Rozsasi A, et al. Nasal biomarker profiles in acute and chronic rhinosinusitis. Clin Exp Allergy 2005;35(9):1186–91.
60. Scavuzzo MC, Fattori B, Ruffoli R, et al. Inflammatory mediators and eosinophilia in atopic and non-atopic patients with nasal polyposis. Biomed Pharmacother 2005;59(6):323–9.
61. Soyka MB, Holzmann D, Basinski TM, et al. The induction of IL-33 in the sinus epithelium and its influence on T-helper cell responses. PLoS One 2015;10(5): e0123163.
62. Gurrola J, Borish L. Chronic rhinosinusitis: endotypes, biomarkers, and treatment response. J Allergy Clin Immunol 2017;140(6):1499–508.
63. Lam M, Hull L, McLachlan R, et al. Clinical severity and epithelial endotypes in chronic rhinosinusitis. Int Forum Allergy Rhinol 2013;3(2):121–8.
64. The role of IL-25 and IL-33 in chronic rhinosinusitis with or without nasal polyps. - PubMed - NCBI. Available at: https://www.ncbi.nlm.nih.gov/pubmed/27522661. Accessed September 24, 2019.
65. Morra L, Moch H. Periostin expression and epithelial-mesenchymal transition in cancer: a review and an update. Virchows Arch 2011;459(5):465–75.
66. Maxfield AZ, Landegger LD, Brook CD, et al. Periostin as a biomarker for nasal polyps in chronic rhinosinusitis. Otolaryngol Head Neck Surg 2018;158(1):181–6.
67. Zhang W, Hubin G, Endam LM, et al. Expression of the extracellular matrix gene periostin is increased in chronic rhinosinusitis and decreases following successful endoscopic sinus surgery. Int Forum Allergy Rhinol 2012;2(6):471–6.
68. Masuoka M, Shiraishi H, Ohta S, et al. Periostin promotes chronic allergic inflammation in response to Th2 cytokines. J Clin Invest 2012;122(7):2590–600.
69. Hanania NA, Wenzel S, Rosén K, et al. Exploring the effects of omalizumab in allergic asthma: an analysis of biomarkers in the EXTRA study. Am J Respir Crit Care Med 2013;187(8):804–11.
70. Nocera AL, Meurer AT, Miyake MM, et al. Secreted P-glycoprotein is a noninvasive biomarker of chronic rhinosinusitis. Laryngoscope 2017;127(1):E1–4.
71. Bleier BS. Regional expression of epithelial MDR1/P-glycoprotein in chronic rhinosinusitis with and without nasal polyposis. Int Forum Allergy Rhinol 2012;2(2): 122–5.

72. Yan B, Lou H, Wang Y, et al. Epithelium-derived cystatin SN enhances eosinophil activation and infiltration through IL-5 in patients with chronic rhinosinusitis with nasal polyps. J Allergy Clin Immunol 2019;144(2):455–69.

73. Kato Y, Takabayashi T, Sakashita M, et al. Expression and functional analysis of CST1 in intractable nasal polyps. Am J Respir Cell Mol Biol 2018;59(4):448–57.

74. Sahin G, Klimek L, Mullol J, et al. Nitric oxide: a promising methodological approach in airway diseases. Int Arch Allergy Immunol 2011;156(4):352–61.

75. Vaidyanathan S, Williamson P, Lipworth BJ. Comment on: nitric oxide evaluation in upper and lower respiratory tracts in nasal polyposis. Delclaux C, et al. Clin Exp Allergy 2008;38(10):1697.

76. Maniscalco M, Sofia M, Pelaia G. Nitric oxide in upper airways inflammatory diseases. Inflamm Res 2007;56(2):58–69.

77. Phillips PS, Sacks R, Marcells GN, et al. Nasal nitric oxide and sinonasal disease: a systematic review of published evidence. Otolaryngol Head Neck Surg 2011; 144(2):159–69.

78. Jeong JH, Yoo HS, Lee SH, et al. Nasal and exhaled nitric oxide in chronic rhinosinusitis with polyps. Am J Rhinol Allergy 2014;28(1):e11–6.

79. Lee JM, McKnight CL, Aves T, et al. Nasal nitric oxide as a marker of sinus mucosal health in patients with nasal polyposis. Int Forum Allergy Rhinol 2015; 5(10):894–9.

80. Colantonio D, Brouillette L, Parikh A, et al. Paradoxical low nasal nitric oxide in nasal polyposis. Clin Exp Allergy 2002;32(5):698–701.

81. Lee RJ, Kofonow JM, Rosen PL, et al. Bitter and sweet taste receptors regulate human upper respiratory innate immunity. J Clin Invest 2014;124(3):1393–405.

82. Adappa ND, Truesdale CM, Workman AD, et al. Correlation of T2R38 taste phenotype and in vitro biofilm formation from nonpolypoid chronic rhinosinusitis patients. Int Forum Allergy Rhinol 2016;6(8):783–91.

83. Workman AD, Brooks SG, Kohanski MA, et al. Bitter and sweet taste tests are reflective of disease status in chronic rhinosinusitis. J Allergy Clin Immunol Pract 2018;6(3):1078–80.

84. Yao Y, Xie S, Yang C, et al. Biomarkers in the evaluation and management of chronic rhinosinusitis with nasal polyposis. Eur Arch Otorhinolaryngol 2017; 274(10):3559–66.

85. Rowan NR, Soler ZM, Othieno F, et al. Impact of bitter taste receptor phenotype upon clinical presentation in chronic rhinosinusitis. Int Forum Allergy Rhinol 2018; 8(9):1013–20.

86. Hulse KE, Norton JE, Suh L, et al. Chronic rhinosinusitis with nasal polyps is characterized by B-cell inflammation and EBV-induced protein 2 expression. J Allergy Clin Immunol 2013;131(4):1075–83, 1083.e1-7.

87. Tan BK, Li Q-Z, Suh L, et al. Evidence for intranasal antinuclear autoantibodies in patients with chronic rhinosinusitis with nasal polyps. J Allergy Clin Immunol 2011;128(6):1198–206.e1.

88. Wang C, Lou H, Wang X, et al. Effect of budesonide transnasal nebulization in patients with eosinophilic chronic rhinosinusitis with nasal polyps. J Allergy Clin Immunol 2015;135(4):922–9.e6.

89. Peters AT, Spector S, Hsu J, et al. Diagnosis and management of rhinosinusitis: a practice parameter update. Ann Allergy Asthma Immunol 2014;113(4):347–85.

90. Van Zele T, Gevaert P, Holtappels G, et al. Oral steroids and doxycycline: two different approaches to treat nasal polyps. J Allergy Clin Immunol 2010;125(5): 1069–76.e4.

The Role of Biologics in the Treatment of Nasal Polyps

Christine B. Franzese, MD

KEYWORDS

- Nasal polyposis • Chronic rhinosinusitis • Biologic • Omalizumab • Dupilumab
- Reslizumab • Mepolizumab • Benralizumab

KEY POINTS

- Chronic sinusitis with nasal polyposis (CRSwNP) is a heterogenous disorder with multiple endotypes and various treatment options, including both surgical and medical therapies.
- CRSwNP manifests as a chronic inflammatory condition and should be viewed as a disease of exacerbations that should be controlled through intervention, rather than a disease of surgical and/or medical "failures."
- There are several biological agents that are either Food and Drug Administration–approved, completed Phase III trials with positive results, or are currently undergoing investigation for the treatment of CRSwNP.
- The role of biological agents in the treatment of CRSwNP as well as potential patient candidate characteristics for use are discussed.

INTRODUCTION

Where biological agents fit into current guidelines for the treatment of patients with chronic rhinosinusitis with nasal polyps (CRSwNP) is not as simple and straightforward as it has been with other interventions developed to treat the disease state. With the advent of any new medical or surgical intervention, when discussing where a particular treatment should fit into a therapeutic algorithm, consideration is generally given to the specific details of its usage: what its indications are, what type of patient would most benefit from it, and how to use it in actual clinical practice. Organizations (and individuals) may deliberate the further implications of where the new therapeutic option fits into currently available guidelines and its costs to the health care system, among other considerations. This scenario is complicated by the fact that chronic sinusitis with nasal polyposis [CRSwNP] is a heterogeneous disorder that is not completely understood and has different phenotypic endotypes that may or may not be associated with other systemic disorders.[1] The clinical implications of endotype designation on

Department of Otolaryngology–Head and Neck Surgery, University of Missouri-Columbia, One Hospital Drive, Suite MA314, Columbia, MO 65212, USA
E-mail address: franzesec@health.missouri.edu

Immunol Allergy Clin N Am 40 (2020) 295–302
https://doi.org/10.1016/j.iac.2019.12.006
0889-8561/20/© 2019 Elsevier Inc. All rights reserved.

immunology.theclinics.com

treatment is also not fully appreciated and options for treatment of CRSwNP include surgical and medical interventions that may vary in success, availability, and expense.[2]

Although only one biologic at present has Food and Drug Administration (FDA) approval for the treatment of CRSwNP,[3] a second has recently announced positive results from its Phase III trials,[4] and still more have ongoing Phase I, II, and III trials. Thus, it would be prudent to assume that one or more additional biologics will also receive FDA approval and to adapt current treatment parameters to accommodate these new therapeutic options for suitable patient candidates in a proactive manner. Indeed, the European Forum for Allergy and Airway Diseases published a consensus statement on the use of biologics for CRSwNP with or without asthma before any biologics receiving FDA approval for such usage.[5] Other societies, groups, and organizations either have drafted or are in the process of drafting similar statements, updates, and/or guidelines to weigh in on what is appropriate usage and to prevent misusage/overusage.

Part of the challenge is that the understanding of the different types of inflammation driving the development of CRSwNP and its various clinical presentations is continually evolving.[6] At present, 3 different types of inflammation (Type 1, Type 2, and Type 3) have been described.[6,7] Type 1 inflammation is characterized by neutrophilic inflammation, T_h1 cells, and driven by interleukin (IL)-2, interferon γ, and tumor necrosis factor alpha (TNF-α). Type 2 inflammation is characterized by eosinophilic inflammation, T_h2 cells, and driven by IL-4, IL-5, IL-10, and IL-13. Type 3 inflammation is characterized by tissue fibrosis, Th17 cells, and driven by IL-6, IL-17, IL-22, and TNF-α. Type 2 inflammation tends to be the dominant form of inflammation in CRSwNP in Western countries and the current biological therapies either approved for or under investigation for CRSwNP target aspects of Type 2 inflammation.[1,6,7] Even with specific targeted therapy, the wide-ranging effects of these agents, the scarcity of published data, and their cost make the placement of biological agents in guidelines difficult.

Indeed, use of these biological agents entails significant expanse, and due to financial factors alone, there is temptation to simply earmark biologics as a "treatment of last resort" to be used when all other measures have been exhausted or failed, and administering biologics before that is shameful overuse. However, such a designation would do a grave disservice to patients, as, unlike the question of where biologics fit into guidelines or algorithms, the role that biologics should play in the treatment of CRSwNP is more clear.

Similar to other Type 2 inflammatory disorders such as eosinophilic asthma, CRSwNP is a chronic inflammatory disease state where patients suffer from exacerbations and defining it as such can be helpful in determining the role these agents play. However, rather than episodes of wheezing, coughing, and chest tightness, patients with CRSwNP experience increased nasal congestion, polyp growth, decrease or loss of sense of smell, etc. as their exacerbations. It should not be viewed as "surgery has failed" or "medications have failed" but rather exacerbations that are either controlled with appropriate surgical and medical therapies or remain uncontrolled despite those treatments. Once the perception of CRSwNP is altered to a disease of chronic inflammation with the need to control exacerbations, the way treatment is viewed can be altered from a flow diagram type or algorithm type strategy to more of a step-wise strategy, similar to asthma. Criteria to designate asthma status as mild to severe and its control are assessed at each visit. Recommendations for controller medications then are categorized in a stepwise fashion with each particular category corresponding to one or more "steps." Each step lists appropriate medications/interventions with recommendations on additional measures for exacerbations or poor control. Treatment algorithms for CRSwNP could follow a similar fashion, establishing criteria for disease severity and accounting for different endotypes, while then designating "step" type therapy and determining on which step/disease severity biological agents should be placed.

Regardless of placement, the goal of initiating biological agents should be to improve exacerbation control in those uncontrolled patients, who would generally get further surgery or repeated high-dose and/or long-term oral corticosteroids. Oral corticosteroid use is a mainstay of therapy but has associated significant risks, particularly when used long term or at high dose.[8] In patients who have had at least one surgery for CRSwNP, the role of biologics should be to reduce or eliminate the need for additional surgical interventions and additional courses of oral corticosteroids and/or antibiotics. In patients with CRSwNP who refuse surgery or are not surgical candidates due to comorbidities, the role of biologics should be to reduce or eliminate the need for repeated additional courses of oral corticosteroids and/or antibiotics once standard treatments have been attempted and either failed or could not be tolerated.

Keeping the role of biologics in mind and given that there are multiple points in current guidelines where these agents could fit, it may instead make more sense to define or identify those characteristics that make patients suitable candidates for biological agents, as their use is not appropriate in all patients. All of the commercially available biological agents are recombinant humanized monoclonal immunoglobulins that target a specific receptor, immunoglobulin, or cytokine-producing inhibitory downstream effects on binding. **Table 1** lists the commercially available biologics approved for, have some data available for, or are under investigation for the treatment of CRSwNP, each targeting a different immunologic aspect involved in the pathogenesis of CRSwNP. Agents not currently commercially available but under investigation for CRSwNP are listed in **Table 2**. The following is a brief review of biological agents, listed by what each agent targets. Once familiar with these agents and their mechanisms, suggestions as to what types of patient characteristics make one a suitable candidate for use can be further discussed.

Target: Interleukin 4/Interleukin 13

IL-4 is responsible for inducing the differentiation of naïve T cells into Th2 cells and isotype switching of B cells into IgE-producing plasma cells, among other effects. IL-13 regulates several immune processes including IgE synthesis, mucous hypersecretion, and fibrosis.

Table 1
Commercially available biological agents under investigation for chronic rhinosinusitis with nasal polyps

Name	Target	Status for CRSwNP	Dose
Dupilumab	IL-4α subunit	FDA approved	300 mg SQ every 2 wk
Omalizumab	IgE	Phase III completed	150 mg/300 mg every 4 wk
Mepolizumab	IL-5	Phase III ongoing	100 mg SQ every 4 wk
Resilizumab	IL-5	Unknown	3 mg/kg IV infusion every 4 wk
Benralizumab	IL-5 receptor	Phase III ongoing	30 mg SQ every 4 wk X 3, then every 8 wk

Information available at clinicaltrials.gov.

Table 2			
Noncommercially available biological agents under investigation for chronic rhinosinusItis with nasal polyps			
Name	Target	Status	Dose
GB001	DP2 agonist	Phase 2a	Unknown daily dose
PF-06817024	IL-33	Phase 1	Various IV, SC doses
ACT-774312	CRTH2 receptor antagonist	Phase 2	Oral twice daily dose
Etokimab	IL-33	Phase 2a	SC dose every 4–8 wk
Fevipiprant	CRTH2 antagonist	Phase 3	Oral daily dose

Information available at clinicaltrials.gov.
Abbreviations: IV, intravenous; SC, subcutaneous.

Agent: dupilumab (Dupixent)

This antibody functions as an IL-4 receptor α-subunit antagonist.[3] Because the IL-4 receptor α-subunit is present in both Type I receptors that bind IL-4 and Type II receptors that bind IL-4 and IL-13, it modulates the effects of both cytokines. It is currently approved as an add-on maintenance treatment in adult patients with inadequately controlled CRSwNP, as well as the treatment of patients 12 years or older with moderate to severe atopic dermatitis uncontrolled by topical treatments, moderate to severe asthma with eosinophilic phenotype, and/or oral corticosteroid–dependent asthma.[3]

It has completed 2 Phase III trials, SINUS-24 and SINUS-52, both meeting their primary endpoints.[3] Dupilumab significantly improved nasal polyp score (−2.06), nasal congestion (−0.89), and SNOT-22 (−21.12) from baseline to week 24 (least square mean differences vs placebo) and reduced systemic oral corticosteroid use for nasal polyposis surgery.[3]

The dosing for dupilumab for CRSwNP is administered subcutaneously in a prefilled syringe at home or in the office. Unlike atopic dermatitis or asthma, there is no loading dose for CRNwNP. The dose is 300 mg, which is generally first given in the office, so that patient training on how to administer the medication can occur. Thereafter, it is 300 mg every 2 weeks subcutaneously given at home by the patient. Transient eosinophilia has be seen after initiation, as the inhibition of IL-4/IL-13 will cause a decrease in the migration of eosinophils into peripheral tissues faster than a decrease in the production and release of eosinophils.[3]

Target: immunoglobulin E

Immunoglobulin E is 1 of 5 classes of antibodies and is the immunoglobulin that classically participates in the pathophysiology of atopic disorders.

Agent: omalizumab (Xolair)

This antibody functions as an IgE antagonist. It binds to free-floating IgE, specifically to the Cε3 domain. The Cε3 domain is crucial to IgE binding to receptors on cell surfaces; by omalizumab complexing with this domain, it prevents serum IgE from attaching to the FcεRI high-affinity IgE receptor and the CD23 receptor.[9] This inhibits the release of inflammatory mediators and upregulates the replacement of FcεRI high-affinity IgE receptors with FcεRII low-affinity IgE receptors.[9] Omalizumab cannot bind to or displace bound IgE nor can it bind to any IgE receptors itself, thus preventing omalizumab from triggering mediator release and anaphylaxis.

Omalizumab is currently indicated for the treatment of poorly or uncontrolled moderate to severe persistent asthma despite inhaled corticosteroids in patients 6 years of age and older with a positive skin test or specific IgE reactivity to a perennial allergen and for chronic idiopathic urticaria in patients 12 years of age or older who remain symptomatic despite H1 antihistamine treatment.[10] Omalizumab can be given subcutaneously either every 2 weeks or every 4 weeks, and its dosage depends on what indication it is administered for and can be affected by weight and IgE level before initiation. It comes in a prefilled syringe or a lyophilized powder that must be reconstituted.[10] It must be administered in the office and recommendations are to monitor patient postadministration due to the risk of anaphylaxis.[10]

It has completed 2 Phase III trials, POLYP1 and POLYP2, both meeting their primary endpoints, but no published data regarding these trials are currently available.[4] For these trials, omalizumab could be given either every 2 weeks or every 4 weeks. Before this, 2 smaller clinical trials had evaluated the use of omalizumab in the treatment CRSwNP with conflicting results.[11,12]

Target: Interleukin 5

IL-5 is responsible for the regulation of eosinophil production, maturation, and survival as well as the growth and differentiation of B lymphocytes.

Agent: mepolizumab (Nucala)

This antibody functions as an IL-5 antagonist by binding to IL-5 and preventing that cytokine from binding to the IL-5 receptor α-subunit. Mepolizumab is currently indicated as add-on maintenance therapy for the treatment of patients with poorly controlled or uncontrolled severe asthma with an eosinophilic phenotype aged 6 years and older and adult patients with eosinophilic granulomatosis with polyangiitis (EGPA).[13]

The dose of mepolizumab depends on age and indication. The dose for asthma is 100 mg and the dose for EGPA is 300 mg. Regardless of indication, it is given subcutaneously every 4 weeks and comes in 3 forms: a lyophilized powder that must be reconstituted, a prefilled syringe, and a self-administered autoinjector. The prefilled syringe and the autoinjector are for patients 12 years and older and are administered at home. The reconstituted powder is administered in the office while the patient is observed for adverse reactions.

There are currently ongoing Phase III trials (SYNAPSE) involving mepolizumab in the treatment of CRSwNP.[14] No published data regarding these trials are available yet. A smaller Phase II trial demonstrated a significant reduction in polyp size with concurrent reduction in peripheral eosinophil count but did not result in symptomatic improvement.[15]

Agent: reslizumab (Cinqair)

This antibody also functions as an IL-5 antagonist by binding to IL-5 and preventing that cytokine from binding to the IL-5 receptor α-subunit. Reslizumab is currently indicated as add-on maintenance therapy for adult patients with poorly or uncontrolled severe asthma with an eosinophilic phenotype.[16] The dosage is 3 mg/kg administered by intravenous infusion over 20 to 50 minutes every 4 weeks. It must be administered in the office and recommendations are to monitor patient postadministration due to the risk of anaphylaxis.

A reduction in nasal polyp size had been shown in a small, controlled trial of 8 patients using a single dose of 1 mg/kg of reslizumab.[17] A phase III trial involving reslizumab in the treatment of CRSwNP was listed on clinicaltrails.gov but no longer seems to be available.

Agent: benralizumab (Fasenra) Although this agent does affect IL-5, it is different from the prior 2 as benralizumab actually binds to the IL-5 receptor itself. The monoclonal antibody is engineered without a fucose molecule, and thus upon binding to the IL-5 receptor, can trigger antibody-dependent cell cytotoxicity and apoptosis in eosinophils and mast cells. Benralizumab is currently indicated as add-on maintenance therapy for the treatment of patients with poorly controlled or uncontrolled severe asthma with an eosinophilic phenotype aged 12 years and older.[17] It has also been granted orphan drug status for adult patients with EGPA.[18,19]

It comes in a prefilled syringe and the dosage is 30 mg every 4 weeks for the first 12 weeks, then every 8 weeks thereafter. It must be administered in the office and recommendations are to monitor the patient postadministration.

There are currently ongoing Phase III trials (OSTRO) involving benralizumab in the treatment of CRSwNP,[20] as well as an open-label study (BITE) for the treatment of EGPA.[21] No published data regarding these trials are available yet.

BIOLOGICS: WHERE DO THEY FIT IN CLINICAL PRACTICE?

Keeping in mind the goal of using biological agents to control exacerbations without the need for additional courses of oral corticosteroids, antibiotics, or surgery in patients with CRSwNP helps with the identification of characteristics of patient candidates where these agents may be helpful. It is also important to keep in mind that no therapy is 100% successful and that many candidates do quite well after functional endoscopic sinus surgery (FESS) with continued medical management. In addition, the goals and desires of the patient should be elicited as part of shared decision-making process, so that recommendations for treatment are tailored to suit the needs of the individual.

Box 1 is the author's opinion of potential characteristics of patients who could be suitable candidates for initiation of a biological agent, given the following assumptions:

1. The patient suffers from significant symptoms consistent with the diagnosis of CRSwNP such as nasal obstruction and loss of sense of smell
2. Has endoscopic and/or computed tomographic scan findings consistent with CRSwNP and has had appropriate medical treatment[2]
3. Has had continued symptomatic polyp regrowth, despite appropriate surgical treatment and/or more than one course of high dose and/or long-term course of an oral corticosteroid in a 12-month period

---

Box 1
Some patient characteristics where a biological agent may be appropriate

Patient has symptomatic CRSwNP, despite appropriate medical/surgical therapy AND one or more of the following:
- Separately meets criteria for a second indication, such as chronic urticaria, asthma, etc.
- Has had one or more FESS with recurrence of symptomatic polyps in a short time frame (6 months or less) despite compliance with topical intranasal therapies
- Has had one or more FESS with recurrence of symptomatic polyps in a longer time frame (greater than 6 months) despite compliance with therapy but declines/refuses additional surgery
- Has contraindications or medical comorbidities such that additional courses of oral or types of corticosteroid therapy would be potentially harmful or contraindicated, such as uncontrolled or poorly controlled diabetes mellitus, osteoporosis or stress fractures, cataracts, etc.
- Declines/refuses surgery and has attempted appropriate medical management, including topical intranasal steroids, but has required more than one course of high dose and/or long-term oral corticosteroids in a 12-month period

This list is not meant to be an exhaustive enumeration of all potential characteristics, but as a guide to a starting point in the identification of possible candidates for this type of therapy.

At present, there are no Type 2 biomarkers that can definitely determine which biological treatment should be initiated or is right for the patient; however, they can serve as guides to the practitioner in selecting which one to initiate, if the patient is an appropriate candidate. The selection of which biologic to use for CRSwNP alone at this stage is a moot point, as the only FDA-approved biologic for the treatment of CRSwNP is dupilumab. If another biologic is desired for use, a separate indication for that particular agent would be required.

FUTURE CONSIDERATIONS/SUMMARY

Table 2 lists biological agents not commercially available but under investigation for nasal polyposis. Without doubt, one or more of these investigational or commercially available biologics will succeed in clinical trials and receive FDA approval for use. Adapting our practice patterns, considering appropriate patient characteristics, and using judicious caution in both the prevention of zealous overuse as well as the prevention of inappropriate restrictions will be helpful in enhancing the care and quality of life for our patients with CRSwNP. Rethinking the way CRSwNP is viewed to be more like an inflammatory condition with exacerbations that must be controlled, rather than disease of surgical or medical "failures," could be helpful in finding the right fit of treatment algorithms for these therapies. Perhaps alteration of our treatment algorithms into more of a "step-wise" paradigm would aid in designating where these agents should fit. No doubt these therapies will alter the way practitioners treat CRSwNP but exactly how practice will change remains to be seen.

DISCLOSURE

Author has the following conflicts of interest: Speaker's Bureau-ALK, GSK, AZ, Regeneron-Sanofi, Optinose; Advisory Board-ALK; Research funding-Merck, ALK, GSK, Novartis/Genetech/Roche, Optinose.

REFERENCES

1. Tomassen P, Vandeplas G, Van Zele T, et al. Inflammatory endotypes of chronic rhinosinusitis based on cluster analysis of biomarkers. J Allergy Clin Immunol 2016;137(5):1449–56.e4.

2. Orlandi RR, Kingdom TT, Hwang PH, et al. International consensus statement on allergy and rhinology: rhinosinusitis executive summary. Int Forum Allergy Rhinol 2016;6(Suppl 1):S3–21.

3. Dupilumab package insert. Available at: https://www.accessdata.fda.gov/drugsatfda_docs/label/2017/761055lbl.pdf. Accessed August 30, 2019.

4. Xolair® (omalizumab) significantly reduced nasal polyps and congestion symptoms in adults with chronic rhinosinusitis with nasal polyps in two phase III studies. Available at: https://www.biospace.com/article/releases/xolair-omalizumab-significantly-reduced-nasal-polyps-and-congestion-symptoms-in-adults-with-chronic-rhinosinusitis-with-nasal-polyps-in-two-phase-iii-studies. Accessed August 20, 2019.

5. Fokkens WJ, Lund V, Bachert C, et al. EUFOREA consensus on biologics for CRSwNP with or without asthma. Allergy 2019. https://doi.org/10.1111/all.13875.

6. Stevens WW, Peters AT, Tan BK, et al. Associations between inflammatory endo-types and clinical presentations in Chronic Rhinosinusitis. J Allergy Clin Immunol Pract 2019. https://doi.org/10.1016/j.jaip.2019.05.009.
7. Smith KA, Pulsipher A, Gabrielsen DA, et al. Biologics in chronic rhinosinusitis: an update and thoughts for future directions. Am J Rhinol Allergy 2018;32(5): 412–23.
8. Poetker DM, Reh DD. A comprehensive review of the adverse effects of systemic corticosteroids. Otolaryngol Clin North Am 2010;43(4):753–68.
9. Johansson SGO, Haahtela T, O'Byrne M. Omalizumab and the immune system: an overview of preclinical and clinical data. Ann Allergy Asthma Immunol 2002; 89:132–8.
10. Omalizumab package insert. Available at: https://www.gene.com/download/pdf/xolair_prescribing.pdf. Accessed August 30, 2019.
11. Gevaert P, Calus L, Van Zele T, et al. Omalizumab is effective in allergic and nonallergic patients with nasal polyps and asthma. J Allergy Clin Immunol 2013;131:110–6.
12. Pinto JM, Mehta N, DiTineo M, et al. A randomized, double-blind, placebo-controlled trial of anti-IgE for chronic rhinosinusitis. Rhinology 2010;48(3):318–24.
13. Mepolizumab package insert. Available at: https://gsksource.com/pharma/content/dam/GlaxoSmithKline/US/en/Prescribing_Information/Nucala/pdf/NUCALA-PI-PIL-IFU-COMBINED.PDF. Accessed August 30, 2019.
14. Effect of mepolizumab in severe bilateral nasal polyps. Available at: https://clinicaltrials.gov/ct2/show/NCT03085797. Accessed September 5, 2019.
15. Gevaert P, Van Bruaene N, Cattaert T, et al. Mepolizumab, a humanized anti-IL-5 mAb, as a treatment option for severe nasal polyposis. J Allergy Clin Immunol 2011;128(5):989–95.
16. Reslizumab package insert. Available at: https://www.cinqair.com/globalassets/cinqair/prescribinginformation.pdf. Accessed August 30, 2019.
17. Gevaert P, Lang-Loidolt D, Lackner A, et al. Nasal IL-5 levels determine the response to anti-IL-5 treatment in patients with nasal polyps. J Allergy Clin Immunol 2006;118(5):1133–41.
18. Benralizumab package insert. Available at: https://www.azpicentral.com/fasenra/fasenra.pdf#page=1. Accessed August 30, 2019.
19. FDA Grants ODD for AstraZeneca's Fasenra to Treat EGPA. Available at: https://www.pharmaceutical-technology.com/news/fda-grants-odd-for-astrazenecas-fasenra-to-treat-egpa. Accessed September 5, 2019.
20. Efficacy and Safety Study of Benralizumab for Patients With Severe Nasal Polyp-osis (OSTRO). Available at: https://clinicaltrials.gov/ct2/show/NCT03401229. Accessed September 5, 2019.
21. Benralizumab in the Treatment of Eosinophilic Granulomatosis With Polyan-giitis (EGPA) Study (BITE). Available at: https://clinicaltrials.gov/ct2/show/NCT03010436. Accessed September 5, 2019.

The Role of Macrolides and Doxycycline in Chronic Rhinosinusitis

Katherine A. Lees, MD[a], Richard R. Orlandi, MD[b],
Gretchen Oakley, MD[b], Jeremiah A. Alt, MD, PhD[b],*

KEYWORDS

- Macrolides • Doxycycline • Chronic • Sinusitis • Rhinosinusitis • Polyps
- Immunomodulation

KEY POINTS

- The role of macrolides in the management of chronic rhinosinusitis relates more to their immunomodulatory properties than their antibacterial properties. Macrolides can reduce proinflammatory cytokines, neutrophil infiltration, and oxidative damage to mucosal tissue.
- Macrolide antibiotics may be useful in the management of recalcitrant chronic rhinosinusitis without nasal polyposis, particularly in patients with low immunoglobulin E and eosinophil levels.
- Doxycycline has been effective in chronic rhinosinusitis with nasal polyposis because of its ability to inhibit matrix metalloproteinase activity.
- Macrolides have an increased risk of cardiac side effects. A review of the patient's medications and cardiac risk factors is advised before initiating therapy.

INTRODUCTION

Although antibiotics are commonly used for the treatment of acute rhinosinusitis, there is growing interest in their role for controlling upper-airway inflammation in conditions such as chronic rhinosinusitis (CRS).[1] In 1987, Kudoh and colleagues[2] reported on the use of erythromycin, a macrolide antibiotic, in patients with diffuse panbronchiolitis, resulting in improved 5-year survival from 25% to greater than 90%. This discovery led to further widespread adoption of macrolides in the management of other airway

[a] Rhinology and Anterior Skull Base Surgery, Division of Otolaryngology–Head and Neck Surgery, University of Utah, 50 North Medical Drive, #3C120, Salt Lake City, UT 84132, USA; [b] Division of Otolaryngology–Head and Neck Surgery, University of Utah, 50 North Medical Drive, #3C120, Salt Lake City, UT 84132, USA
* Corresponding author.
E-mail address: Jeremiah.Alt@hsc.utah.edu
Twitter: @TheSnotShot (K.A.L.)

Immunol Allergy Clin N Am 40 (2020) 303–315
https://doi.org/10.1016/j.iac.2019.12.005
0889-8561/20/Published by Elsevier Inc.
immunology.theclinics.com

diseases, such as cystic fibrosis, bronchiectasis, and CRS. In addition to the well-known antimicrobial properties, macrolides exhibit anti-inflammatory and immuno-modulatory effects on airway tissues, even at subtherapeutic doses. More recently, doxycycline, a tetracycline antibiotic, has been found to have similar immunomodula-tory properties in CRS.

CLINICAL APPLICATIONS
Macrolides

Macrolides, which include erythromycin, clarithromycin, azithromycin, and roxithro-mycin, exert their antimicrobial effect by reversibly binding to the 50S ribosomal sub-unit, preventing bacterial protein synthesis. These antibiotics have a propensity to accumulate in high concentrations within leukocytes and subsequently at sites of active infection or inflammation. They provide good coverage of gram-positive cocci (excluding *Enterococcus* species) as well as intracellular and atypical pathogens; however, gram-negative coverage is limited (**Table 1**). Macrolides are often used as the first-line treatment of upper-respiratory tract infections in penicillin-allergic patients.

Macrolides also affect the virulence of some bacteria without having direct antimi-crobial effects through the 50S subunit. Macrolides inhibit the production of alginate, an important component in biofilm formation, at levels below the minimal inhibitory concentration for *Pseudomonas aeruginosa* and other bacteria.[3] They also impair the motility of *Pseudomonas* by inhibiting flagellin expression, thereby preventing a mechanism of adherence to respiratory mucosa.[4,5] Finally, macrolides impair the quorum-sensing system by blocking expression of signals known as "autoinducers."[6]

Macrolides' role as immunomodulators has been used in the management of CRS, because they have been shown to have multiple anti-inflammatory properties.

Table 1 Spectrum of antimicrobial coverage of macrolides and doxycycline		
Gram positive	*S aureus*[a] Methicillin-resistant *S aureus*[c] *Streptococcus pyogenes*[a] *Streptococcus pneumoniae*[a] *Streptococcus viridens*[c] *Enterococcus*[c] *Corynebacterium diphtheria*[b] *Propionibacterium acnes* *Listeria monocytogenes*	
Gram negative	*H influenzae*[a] *Moraxella catarrhalis*[a] *Bordetella pertussis*[b] *Bacillus anthracis*[c] *Neisseria gonorrhea* *Helicobacter pylori*	*Campylobacter jejuni* *Escherichia coli*[c] *Enterobacter*[c] *Serratia*[c] *Shigella*[c] *Vibrio*[c]
Atypical	*Chlamydia* *Legionella* *Mycoplasma* *Ureaplasma* *Mycobacterium*	*Treponema pallidum* *Borrelia burgdorferi* *Rickettsia*[c] *Actinomyces*[c]

[a] Common pathogens in sinusitis.
[b] Susceptible only to macrolides.
[c] Susceptible only to doxycycline.

Macrolides promote decreased production of proinflammatory cytokines, such as interleukin-1β (IL-1β), IL-6, tumor necrosis factor-α (TNF-α), and IL-8.[7,8] IL-8 is a potent neutrophil chemoattractant but is also released by neutrophils, and in vivo studies have shown macrolide administration to reduce both IL-8 and neutrophil infiltration in nasal epithelium.[9] Macrolides have also been found to decrease the production of reactive oxygen species (ROS), thereby reducing epithelial cell damage.

The beneficial effects of macrolides on mucus production and clearance have also been described. In lower-airway diseases, such as chronic bronchitis and bronchiectasis, clarithromycin has been found to decrease sputum production by 50%.[10] Similarly, early studies of nasal secretions in CRS patients showed improved viscosity, decreased quantity,[11] and improved clearance.[12] Later studies found that mucociliary clearance, as measured objectively by saccharin transit time (STT), improved following macrolide administration.[8,13,14]

Following the encouraging results of macrolide use in the management of lower-airway diseases, several cohort studies of macrolides in CRS emerged. Moriyama and colleagues[15] retrospectively reviewed outcomes of 149 patients with CRS with nasal polyposis (CRSwNP) treated with endoscopic sinus surgery (ESS), 57 of whom received long-term low-dose erythromycin postoperatively. The erythromycin group, despite having worse disease preoperatively, had improved rhinorrhea and postnasal drainage as well as improved edema and polyps on endoscopic examination compared with the ESS-only patients. Other studies have found the symptoms most likely to respond to macrolide therapy are rhinorrhea and postnasal drainage.[11,13,16]

Several studies have investigated the role of macrolides in different CRS phenotypes. Ichimura and colleagues[17] noted that roxithromycin decreased nasal polyp size in about 50% of CRSwNP patients, but also that patients with smaller polyps were more likely to respond to macrolide therapy than those with large polyps. Patients with higher levels of IL-8 in nasal secretions have a greater response to macrolides both for CRSwNP[18] and without nasal polyposis (CRSsNP).[19] In a study of CRS patients treated with macrolides, Haruna and colleagues[20] determined the efficacy was lower in CRSwNP than CRSsNP, but increased following polypectomy, suggesting polyp burden may predict macrolide response. Patients with higher polyp eosinophil levels were more likely to be poor responders to macrolide therapy, a finding corroborated by a recent retrospective review of macrolide responders and nonresponders.[21] Finally, patients with high serum immunoglobulin E (IgE) had less symptom improvement than those with normal IgE, and both serum and nasal eosinophil counts inversely correlated with symptom improvement.[22] These studies suggest that patients with eosinophilic or Th2-dominant disease are less likely to respond to macrolide therapy.

In 2006, Wallwork and colleagues[8] published results of a randomized controlled trial (RCT) demonstrating the benefit of roxithromycin over placebo, providing the first level I evidence in support of macrolide therapy for CRSsNP. Patients reported significant symptom improvement as well as SNOT-20 scores in the roxithromycin-treated group and had improved mucociliary clearance (as measured by STT) and nasal endoscopy scores at the end of the 3-month treatment period. Furthermore, patients with low IgE levels had greater improvement in SNOT-20, nasal endoscopy scores, and STT compared with patients with high IgE. Since then, 3 RCTs have failed to convincingly demonstrate the benefit of macrolides over placebo in CRS.[23–25] However, these trials included patients both with and without nasal polyposis, and two of the studies[24,25] evaluated macrolide use specifically in the postoperative period.

Multiple RCTs in recent years have compared macrolide therapy to intranasal corticosteroid spray (INCS) for CRS.[26–31] Overall, these studies failed to demonstrate a clear benefit of macrolides over INCS for symptoms, nasal endoscopy, or computed tomographic (CT) scores. Two studies examined clarithromycin in the perioperative period for patients with CRSwNP: one administered clarithromycin for 8 weeks before ESS,[32] whereas the second randomized patients to receive clarithromycin after ESS for either 12 or 24 weeks.[28] Both studies showed improved nasal endoscopic scores in the clarithromycin-treated patients (although without significant symptomatic improvement), suggesting macrolides may prevent or postpone nasal polyp regrowth after surgery.

Because of the contradictory results from these studies, systematic reviews and metaanalyses have been performed in an attempt to draw broader conclusions from the existing literature. Shen and colleagues[33] included 7 RCTs and 4 cohort trials in their recent metaanalysis. Interestingly, when comparing Asian and non-Asian subgroups, they found that the Asian subgroup had significant improvement in SNOT scores in the macrolide-treated group compared with the control group; however, no significant difference was found for the non-Asian subgroup. This finding may be explained by findings from previous studies that Asian patients with CRS have a neutrophil predominance in nasal polyps and cytokine profiles suggestive of Th1-dominance.[34,35] Huang and Zhou[36] performed a systematic review and metaanalysis specifically of clarithromycin in CRS, which included 17 RCTs with 1738 patients. They found the addition of clarithromycin to INCS showed improvement in symptoms and endoscopic scores in the medium term (1–3 months) and long term (>3 months), but insufficient evidence to support the use of clarithromycin monotherapy when compared with INCS.

Macrolide antibiotics can be a useful adjunct in the treatment of recalcitrant CRS that has failed previous medical and surgical therapies because of its anti-inflammatory and immunomodulatory effects. It may be more effective in patients with rhinorrhea and postnasal drainage, with noneosinophilic CRS subtypes, such as CRSsNP, normal serum IgE, and low serum and nasal eosinophil levels.

Doxycycline

Doxycycline is a synthetic derivative of the tetracycline class of antibiotics, which also includes demeclocycline, minocycline, and tigecycline. Similar to macrolides' antimicrobial activity, tetracyclines inhibit protein synthesis by reversibly binding to the 30S ribosomal subunit. Doxycycline broadly covers gram-positive species, including methicillin-resistant *Staphylococcus aureus*, as well as some gram-negative bacteria (see **Table 1**).

Doxycycline has been found to have immunomodulatory effects in addition to antimicrobial properties, which has gained attention for its potential use in CRSwNP. In CRSwNP, increased levels of matrix metalloproteinase-9 (MMP-9) have been found in nasal polyps and are thought to contribute to the process of matrix remodeling, edema, and chronic inflammation.[37–39] Doxycycline exerts its anti-inflammatory effect by inhibiting MMP activity, including decreasing MMP-9 in CRSwNP.[39,40] Doxycycline administration has also been found to decrease eosinophilic cationic protein (ECP) and myeloperoxidase levels in nasal secretions, suggesting decreased activity of eosinophils and neutrophils, respectively.[39,40] Doxycycline reduces the damaging effects of ROS, decreases levels of nitric oxide synthase, and suppresses proinflammatory cytokines, including TNF-α, IL-1β, and IL-6.

To date, there have been 2 clinical trials investigating the utility of doxycycline in CRSwNP. The first RCT had 3 treatment arms: methylprednisolone taper, doxycycline, and placebo, taken for 20 days.[39] The effect on symptoms, polyp size, and inflammatory markers in nasal secretions and blood was evaluated up to 12 weeks after initiation of treatment. They found that with methylprednisolone, polyp size quickly and dramatically decreased while taking the medication, but by the end of the study period, had returned to their baseline size. In the doxycycline group, however, the decrease in polyp size was moderate by the end of the 20-day treatment period, but was maintained until the end of the trial period. When evaluating inflammatory markers, the doxycycline group had significantly decreased MMP-9, myeloperoxidase, and ECP levels in the nasal secretions, the latter two suggesting decreased neutrophil and eosinophil activity, respectively.

A second RCT evaluated the efficacy of long-term doxycycline in CRSwNP patients with persistent symptoms despite appropriate medical and surgical treatment.[41] Patients were randomized to receive a 12-week course of doxycycline plus INCS and nasal irrigations, or INCS and nasal irrigations alone. After 12 weeks, patients in the doxycycline group had significantly improved symptoms and nasal endoscopy compared with the control group. They also found that patients with aspirin-exacerbated respiratory disease, asthma, and elevated serum IgE levels were less likely to demonstrate clinically significant improvement in SNOT-20 scores, suggesting that CRSwNP with allergy or eosinophilia may be less responsive to doxycycline therapy, similar to what has been found for macrolides.

Doxycycline has been found to improve symptoms and decrease polyps specifically in the subset of patients with CRSwNP. However, this is based on a limited number of studies in small cohorts, and further research is needed in larger numbers of patients to strengthen these conclusions and determine optimal length of treatment.

DOSING AND ADMINISTRATION

For low-dose maintenance therapy for CRS with antibiotics, the general recommendation for both macrolides and doxycycline has been half the dose used to treat acute infection (**Table 2**).

Macrolides

Macrolide antibiotics demonstrate excellent penetration of sinus mucosa, partly because of their uptake by leukocytes, leading to their transportation to sites of infection and inflammation. Erythromycin was initially the most commonly used macrolide because it was the first to be discovered. However, it required 4-times-a-day dosing and was associated with high rates of gastrointestinal (GI) side effects and has now been replaced by second-generation macrolides. Clarithromycin and roxithromycin have similar half-lives and distribution, with once-daily dosing providing appropriate concentrations in nasal and sinus mucosa for CRS therapy. However, during acute CRS exacerbations, increasing to twice daily dosing is recommended for 5 to 10 days. Azithromycin is unique from the other macrolides in that it has a much longer half-life and can be detected in sinus mucosa up to 6 days following oral administration.[42] As such, it can be dosed less frequently, such as every other day, 3 days a week, or even weekly.[23]

The dose of macrolides for CRS is likely of less significance than duration of treatment. Several studies have shown increasing efficacy with prolonged use, and that clinical benefit may not become apparent until 4 to 8 weeks after initiation of treatment.[11,16,43] A trial of at least 12 weeks is recommended to determine whether a patient demonstrates responsiveness to macrolide therapy; if there is no clinical improvement after 3 months, discontinuation of macrolides and investigation into alternative treatments is appropriate. However, if the patient demonstrates improvement in symptoms and/or endoscopic examination on

Table 2
Recommended dosing and side effects of macrolides and doxycycline for use in acute exacerbation and maintenance therapy for chronic rhinosinusitis

	Dosing: Maintenance Therapy for CRS	Dosing: Acute Exacerbation CRS	Side Effects
Azithromycin	250 mg every other day	500 mg loading dose Then 250 mg daily × 4 d	GI: Nausea, vomiting, abdominal pain, diarrhea
Clarithromycin	250 mg daily Pediatric: 5 mg/kg daily	250 mg bid × 5–10 d Pediatric: 5 mg/kg bid × 5–10 d	Cardiac arrhythmias[a] Hearing loss[a]
Roxithromycin	150 mg daily Pediatric: 2.5–5 mg/kg daily	150 mg bid Pediatric: 2.5–5 mg/kg bid	*Drug interactions*: Warfarin, benzodiazepines, cyclosporine, statins (all CYP3A4 pathway)
Doxycycline	200 mg loading dose, then 100 mg daily	200 mg daily × 5–7 d OR 100 mg bid × 5–7 d	GI: Nausea, vomiting, abdominal pain, diarrhea Skin reactions: Rash, pruritus, photosensitivity Tooth discoloration, enamel hypoplasia (children <8 y)[a] Esophageal ulceration[a] Drug interactions: Calcium supplements, antacids, iron; anticonvulsants (barbiturates, carbamazepine, phenytoin); warfarin

[a] Rare side effects.

macrolide therapy, an additional 3 to 9 months of treatment may result in further improvement.[11,13,43]

For patients with creatinine clearance less than 30 mL/min, clarithromycin dosing should be reduced by half, or the dosing interval doubled; however, no adjustments are required for azithromycin.

Doxycycline

The studies on doxycycline for CRS have been remarkably consistent on the dosing, with a loading dose of 200 mg on the first day followed by 100 mg once a day thereafter (see **Table 2**). Doxycycline has rapid and very high absorption (>90%) in the duodenum, making oral dosing preferred to other methods of administration.[44] It is able to penetrate sinus mucosa and maintain therapeutic concentrations until 24 hours after administration, supporting the once-daily dosing scheduling.[45] No dosing adjustments are needed in patients with renal failure, but should be considered in patients with severe hepatic dysfunction. There is currently limited evidence as to the optimal duration therapy in CRS given the limited number of studies to date. However, patients benefited from both short-term (<3 week) and long-term (12 week) courses of doxycycline in terms of symptoms and endoscopic examinations,[39–41] suggesting there may be utility to different treatment durations in certain clinical scenarios.

SIDE EFFECTS

Macrolides and doxycycline most commonly cause adverse GI symptoms, including nausea, vomiting, diarrhea, and abdominal pain. The incidence is highest with erythromycin (15%–20%) but is reported as 5% to 10% for clarithromycin, azithromycin, and doxycycline.[46]

Development of resistance to antibiotics has been a concern for decades as multidrug-resistant bacteria have become increasingly prevalent. Bacteria have adopted 2 main strategies of resistance against macrolides and doxycycline: efflux of antibiotic out of the cell and modification of the antibiotic-binding site via ribosomal methylation.[47] Although growing rates of antibiotic resistance remain a global concern, particularly for macrolides, there has not been convincing evidence of increase in resistant strains following long-term, low-dose macrolide treatment in CRS.[8,13,23,28,31]

Both macrolides and doxycycline have unique side-effect profiles as well that deserve mention.

Macrolides

Macrolides cause prolonged QT interval, which can subsequently lead to the fatal cardiac arrhythmia, torsades de pointes. Several large observational studies have identified an increased risk of cardiovascular death in patients taking macrolides, citing 37 to 47 additional deaths per 1 million antibiotic courses.[48,49] This risk is higher in patients with an increased baseline risk of cardiovascular disease[49] and women[48]; however, 1 study found no increased risk between azithromycin and penicillin in a young and middle-aged, healthy cohort.[50] This increased cardiac risk seems limited to the period of macrolide use, with no evidence of long-term toxicity after administration.[51,52] These studies do not specify medication dose, and there are no similarly large studies on cardiac risk specifically in low-dose macrolide therapy. However, Azuma and Kudoh[53] commented on the incidence of torsades de pointes in the Japanese population taking erythromycin, in which 60% of the prescriptions are long-term, low-dose treatment. They found only 4 cases out of approximately 34,000 patients treated annually for more than 10 years, which they attributed to the subtherapeutic doses compared with other studies. Before initiation of macrolides, it is recommended to take a thorough cardiac history on patients (including family history), check for cardiac medication use, and consider a baseline electrocardiogram to evaluate for QT prolongation in high-risk patients. Macrolide use is advised against in patients with QT prolongation, ventricular arrhythmias, bradycardia, electrolyte abnormalities (eg, hypomagnesemia, hypokalemia), or other significant risk factors for cardiac events.

Hearing loss has also been reported with macrolide use, which is usually transient and more likely to occur with higher doses of medication. In a large study of 1577 patients with chronic obstructive pulmonary disease (COPD), the rate of hearing loss was significantly higher in the azithromycin group at 25% compared with the placebo group at 20%.[54]

Doxycycline

The second most common side effect of doxycycline is skin reactions, such as rash, pruritus, and photosensitivity.[55] Patients should be cautioned on the increased susceptibility to sunburn, particularly during summer months.

A side effect unique to the tetracyclines is enamel hypoplasia, causing teeth discoloration in young children.[44] Historically, the use of doxycycline has been contraindicated in children less than 8 years of age and pregnant women based on reports of yellow or brown staining of teeth following use of tetracycline specifically. However, doxycycline binds calcium significantly less than tetracycline, making this risk with doxycycline extremely low. As such, the American Academy of Pediatrics recently changed its recommendation that now children of any age can take up to a 21-day course of doxycycline.[56]

Although rare, doxycycline use has been linked to the development of esophageal ulceration, which occurs more commonly with the capsule than the tablet form of medication.[55] Patients may experience substernal burning pain and odynophagia shortly after administration, which can be avoided by taking pills with plenty of fluids while in the upright position.

DRUG INTERACTIONS
Macrolides

Erythromycin, clarithromycin, and roxithromycin are all metabolized via the cytochrome p450 pathway, specifically, through enzyme CYP3A4. Many macrolide drug interactions arise from interactions with other medications using the same CYP3A4 pathway. Of note, azithromycin is unique among the macrolides in that it is not metabolized via this pathway, so it has fewer drug interactions by comparison.

Coadministration of macrolides with warfarin can lead to slower metabolism and clearance of the warfarin, leading to potentially supratherapeutic anticoagulation. Close monitoring of international normalized ratio (INR), with warfarin dosing adjustments as needed, is recommended.

Concomitant use of benzodiazepines with macrolides can lead to increased bioavailability of the benzodiazepines; their use should be avoided or the dose decreased to avoid the potentially fatal consequences such as respiratory depression.

Cyclosporine is another drug metabolized through the CYP3A4 pathway, and taking it with macrolides can lead to elevated cyclosporine levels that can subsequently cause renal toxicity. It is important to monitor renal function (eg, serum creatinine) closely if these medications are taken together.

Finally, some studies have shown that patients taking statin medications with macrolides can develop acute renal failure, rhabdomyolysis, and increased all-cause mortality, particularly for clarithromycin and erythromycin.[57,58]

Doxycycline

Doxycycline is not metabolized by any p450 system, which decreases the potential drug interactions that it has. However, it can become bound to divalent and trivalent cations, which becomes particularly important when taking this medication orally. Doxycycline should not be taken within 1 to 2 hours of having milk, antacids, iron supplements, or other substances containing calcium, magnesium, aluminum, or iron, because these substances can bind the doxycycline and prevent its absorption from the GI tract.

Anticonvulsants, specifically barbiturates, carbamazepine, and phenytoin, can influence the metabolism of doxycycline and lead to decreased half-life. Coadministration with these medications may require alteration in the dose or frequency of doxycycline. Doxycycline can also potentiate the effects of warfarin, and close monitoring of INR is required if these medications are taken together.

FUTURE CONSIDERATIONS

The conflicting evidence on long-term, low-dose macrolide treatment in CRS derives from several RCTs with small study populations and variability in their inclusion criteria and treatment protocols. Because of this, it is difficult to draw strong conclusions as to the specific clinical scenarios in which macrolide therapy will provide the greatest benefit. A large RCT trial currently underway is the MACRO trial, which seeks to compare symptomatic improvement between clarithromycin and placebo in patients with CRS, with a goal recruitment of 600 patients.[59]

Use of macrolide antibiotics has been a primary focus of the past several decades, and only in recent years has doxycycline gained attention for use in CRS. There are very few studies by comparison investigating the use of doxycycline, all of which have been specifically in CRSwNP. However, these studies have shown encouraging results, and in combination with its favorable side-effect profile and antimicrobial coverage, further research into its role in CRS will likely continue to emerge.

Finally, there have been several in vitro studies on several macrolide derivatives that maintain the immunomodulatory effects of macrolides but without the antimicrobial properties. For instance, EM900 is an erythromycin derivative that has been shown to suppress IL-1β, TNF-α, and IL-8 production in human airway epithelial cells.[60,61] Another example is CSY0073, an azithromycin derivative. In a murine model, CSY0073 did not affect growth of *S aureus*, *Haemophilus influenzae*, or *P aeruginosa*, but did lead to decreased levels of proinflammatory cytokines and neutrophils in lung tissue and secretions similar to azithromycin.[62] These medications have great potential in long-term management of diseases such as CRS while mitigating concerns about antibiotic resistance. However, their use not yet been evaluated in human subjects and thus will not become available for several years.

SUMMARY

Macrolides and doxycycline can be useful adjuncts in the management of CRS. When administered as long-term, low-dose therapy, they exert an immunomodulatory effect on the sinuses by decreasing neutrophil infiltration, production of proinflammatory cytokines, and secretion of mucus. Macrolides, such as clarithromycin and azithromycin, are particularly effective in patients with CRSsNP with normal serum IgE and low serum and nasal eosinophil levels. Doxycycline can improve symptoms and decrease polyps in patients with CRSwNP. The most common side effect for both macrolides and doxycycline is GI symptoms, including abdominal pain, nausea, or diarrhea. Macrolides can cause prolonged QT interval, which may lead to torsades de pointes or other cardiac arrhythmias. As such, they should be used with caution in patients with increased cardiac risk.

DISCLOSURE STATEMENT

J.A. Alt is a consultant for Medtronic, Optinose, Intersect ENT, and GlycoMira Therapeutics. R.R. Orlandi is a consultant for Medtronic, Lyra Therapeutics, and BioInspire. K.A. Lees and G. Oakley have nothing to disclose.

REFERENCES

1. Soler ZM, Oyer SL, Kern RC, et al. Antimicrobials and chronic rhinosinusitis with or without polyposis in adults: an evidenced-based review with recommendations. Int Forum Allergy Rhinol 2013;3:31–47.

2. Kudoh S, Uetake T, Hagiwara K, et al. Clinical effects of low-dose long-term erythromycin chemotherapy on diffuse panbronchiolitis. Nihon Kyobu Shikkan Gakkai Zasshi 1987;25:632–42 [in Japanese].

3. Ichimiya T, Takeoka K, Hiramatsu K, et al. The influence of azithromycin on the biofilm formation of Pseudomonas aeruginosa in vitro. Chemotherapy 1996;42:186–91.

4. Yamasaki T, Ichimiya T, Hirai K, et al. Effect of antimicrobial agents on the piliation of Pseudomonas aeruginosa and adherence to mouse tracheal epithelium. J Chemother 1997;9:32–7.

5. Kawamura-Sato K, Iinuma Y, Hasegawa T, et al. Effect of subinhibitory concentrations of macrolides on expression of flagellin in Pseudomonas aeruginosa and Proteus mirabilis. Antimicrob Agents Chemother 2000;44:2869–72.

6. Sofer D, Gilboa-Garber N, Belz A, et al. 'Subinhibitory' erythromycin represses production of Pseudomonas aeruginosa lectins, autoinducer and virulence factors. Chemotherapy 1999;45:335–41.

7. Suzuki H, Shimomura A, Ikeda K, et al. Effects of long-term low-dose macrolide administration on neutrophil recruitment and IL-8 in the nasal discharge of chronic sinusitis patients. Tohoku J Exp Med 1997;182:115–24.

8. Wallwork B, Coman W, Mackay-Sim A, et al. A double-blind, randomized, placebo-controlled trial of macrolide in the treatment of chronic rhinosinusitis. Laryngoscope 2006;116:189–93.

9. Fujita K, Shimizu T, Majima Y, et al. Effects of macrolides on interleukin-8 secretion from human nasal epithelial cells. Eur Arch Otorhinolaryngol 2000;257:199–204.

10. Tamaoki J, Takeyama K, Tagaya E, et al. Effect of clarithromycin on sputum production and its rheological properties in chronic respiratory tract infections. Antimicrob Agents Chemother 1995;39:1688–90.

11. Hashiba M, Baba S. Efficacy of long-term administration of clarithromycin in the treatment of intractable chronic sinusitis. Acta Otolaryngol Suppl 1996;525:73–8.

12. Nishi K, Mizuguchi M, Tachibana H, et al. Effect of clarithromycin on symptoms and mucociliary transport in patients with sino-bronchial syndrome. Nihon Kyobu Shikkan Gakkai Zasshi 1995;33:1392–400 [in Japanese].

13. Cervin A, Kalm O, Sandkull P, et al. One-year low-dose erythromycin treatment of persistent chronic sinusitis after sinus surgery: clinical outcome and effects on mucociliary parameters and nasal nitric oxide. Otolaryngol Head Neck Surg 2002;126:481–9.

14. Ragab SM, Lund VJ, Scadding G. Evaluation of the medical and surgical treatment of chronic rhinosinusitis: a prospective, randomised, controlled trial. Laryngoscope 2004;114:923–30.

15. Moriyama H, Yanagi K, Ohtori N, et al. Evaluation of endoscopic sinus surgery for chronic sinusitis: post-operative erythromycin therapy. Rhinology 1995;33:166–70.

16. Majima Y, Kurono Y, Hirakawa K, et al. Efficacy of combined treatment with S-carboxymethylcysteine (carbocisteine) and clarithromycin in chronic rhinosinusitis patients without nasal polyp or with small nasal polyp. Auris Nasus Larynx 2012;39:38–47.

17. Ichimura K, Shimazaki Y, Ishibashi T, et al. Effect of new macrolide roxithromycin upon nasal polyps associated with chronic sinusitis. Auris Nasus Larynx 1996;23:48–56.

18. Yamada T, Fujieda S, Mori S, et al. Macrolide treatment decreased the size of nasal polyps and IL-8 levels in nasal lavage. Am J Rhinol 2000;14:143–8.

19. Luo Q, Chen F, Liu W, et al. Evaluation of long-term clarithromycin treatment in adult Chinese patients with chronic rhinosinusitis without nasal polyps. ORL J Otorhinolaryngol Relat Spec 2011;73:206–11.

20. Haruna S, Shimada C, Ozawa M, et al. A study of poor responders for long-term, low-dose macrolide administration for chronic sinusitis. Rhinology 2009;47: 66–71.

21. Oakley GM, Christensen JM, Sacks R, et al. Characteristics of macrolide responders in persistent post-surgical rhinosinusitis. Rhinology 2018;56:111–7.

22. Suzuki H, Ikeda K, Honma R, et al. Prognostic factors of chronic rhinosinusitis under long-term low-dose macrolide therapy. ORL J Otorhinolaryngol Relat Spec 2000;62:121–7.

23. Videler WJ, Badia L, Harvey RJ, et al. Lack of efficacy of long-term, low-dose azithromycin in chronic rhinosinusitis: a randomized controlled trial. Allergy 2011;66: 1457–68.

24. Haxel BR, Clemens M, Karaiskaki N, et al. Controlled trial for long-term low-dose erythromycin after sinus surgery for chronic rhinosinusitis. Laryngoscope 2015; 125:1048–55.

25. Amali A, Saedi B, Rahavi-Ezabadi S, et al. Long-term postoperative azithromycin in patients with chronic rhinosinusitis: a randomized clinical trial. Am J Rhinol Allergy 2015;29:421–4.

26. Zeng M, Long XB, Cui YH, et al. Comparison of efficacy of mometasone furoate versus clarithromycin in the treatment of chronic rhinosinusitis without nasal polyps in Chinese adults. Am J Rhinol Allergy 2011;25:e203–7.

27. Korkmaz H, Ocal B, Tatar EC, et al. Biofilms in chronic rhinosinusitis with polyps: is eradication possible? Eur Arch Otorhinolaryngol 2014;271:2695–702.

28. Varvyanskaya A, Lopatin A. Efficacy of long-term low-dose macrolide therapy in preventing early recurrence of nasal polyps after endoscopic sinus surgery. Int Forum Allergy Rhinol 2014;4:533–41.

29. Deng J, Chen F, Lai Y, et al. Lack of additional effects of long-term, low-dose clarithromycin combined treatment compared with topical steroids alone for chronic rhinosinusitis in China: a randomized, controlled trial. Int Forum Allergy Rhinol 2018;8:8–14.

30. Zeng M, Wang H, Liao B, et al. Comparison of efficacy of fluticasone propionate versus clarithromycin for postoperative treatment of different phenotypic chronic rhinosinusitis: a randomized controlled trial. Rhinology 2019;57:101–9.

31. Wu SH, Hsu SH, Liang KL, et al. The effects of erythromycin towards the treatment of persistent rhinosinusitis after functional endoscopic sinus surgery: a randomized, active comparator-controlled study. J Chin Med Assoc 2019;82:322–7.

32. Peric A, Baletic N, Milojevic M, et al. Effects of preoperative clarithromycin administration in patients with nasal polyposis. West Indian Med J 2014;63:721–7.

33. Shen S, Lou H, Wang C, et al. Macrolide antibiotics in the treatment of chronic rhinosinusitis: evidence from a meta-analysis. J Thorac Dis 2018;10:5913–23.

34. Zhang N, Van Zele T, Perez-Novo C, et al. Different types of T-effector cells orchestrate mucosal inflammation in chronic sinus disease. J Allergy Clin Immunol 2008;122:961–8.

35. Cao PP, Li HB, Wang BF, et al. Distinct immunopathologic characteristics of various types of chronic rhinosinusitis in adult Chinese. J Allergy Clin Immunol 2009;124:478–84, 84.e1-2.

36. Huang Z, Zhou B. Clarithromycin for the treatment of adult chronic rhinosinusitis: a systematic review and meta-analysis. Int Forum Allergy Rhinol 2019;9:545–55.

37. Watelet JB, Bachert C, Claeys C, et al. Matrix metalloproteinases MMP-7, MMP-9 and their tissue inhibitor TIMP-1: expression in chronic sinusitis vs nasal polyposis. Allergy 2004;59:54–60.
38. Kostamo K, Tervahartiala T, Sorsa T, et al. Metalloproteinase function in chronic rhinosinusitis with nasal polyposis. Laryngoscope 2007;117:638–43.
39. Van Zele T, Gevaert P, Holtappels G, et al. Oral steroids and doxycycline: two different approaches to treat nasal polyps. J Allergy Clin Immunol 2010;125: 1069–76.e4.
40. De Schryver E, Derycke L, Calus L, et al. The effect of systemic treatments on periostin expression reflects their interference with the eosinophilic inflammation in chronic rhinosinusitis with nasal polyps. Rhinology 2017;55:152–60.
41. Pinto Bezerra Soter AC, Bezerra TF, Pezato R, et al. Prospective open-label evaluation of long-term low-dose doxycycline for difficult-to-treat chronic rhinosinusitis with nasal polyps. Rhinology 2017;55:175–80.
42. Fang AF, Palmer JN, Chiu AG, et al. Pharmacokinetics of azithromycin in plasma and sinus mucosal tissue following administration of extended-release or immediate-release formulations in adult patients with chronic rhinosinusitis. Int J Antimicrob Agents 2009;34:67–71.
43. Nakamura Y, Suzuki M, Yokota M, et al. Optimal duration of macrolide treatment for chronic sinusitis after endoscopic sinus surgery. Auris Nasus Larynx 2013;40: 366–72.
44. Joshi N, Miller DQ. Doxycycline revisited. Arch Intern Med 1997;157:1421–8.
45. Sundberg L, Eden T, Ernstson S. Penetration of doxycycline in respiratory mucosa. Acta Otolaryngol 1983;96:501–8.
46. Hansen MP, Scott AM, McCullough A, et al. Adverse events in people taking macrolide antibiotics versus placebo for any indication. Cochrane Database Syst Rev 2019;(1):CD011825.
47. Richter SS, Heilmann KP, Beekmann SE, et al. Macrolide-resistant Streptococcus pyogenes in the United States, 2002-2003. Clin Infect Dis 2005;41:599–608.
48. Svanstrom H, Pasternak B, Hviid A. Use of clarithromycin and roxithromycin and risk of cardiac death: cohort study. BMJ 2014;349:g4930.
49. Ray WA, Murray KT, Hall K, et al. Azithromycin and the risk of cardiovascular death. N Engl J Med 2012;366:1881–90.
50. Svanstrom H, Pasternak B, Hviid A. Use of azithromycin and death from cardiovascular causes. N Engl J Med 2013;368:1704–12.
51. Schembri S, Williamson PA, Short PM, et al. Cardiovascular events after clarithromycin use in lower respiratory tract infections: analysis of two prospective cohort studies. BMJ 2013;346:f1235.
52. Inghammar M, Nibell O, Pasternak B, et al. Long-term risk of cardiovascular death with use of clarithromycin and roxithromycin: a nationwide cohort study. Am J Epidemiol 2018;187:777–85.
53. Azuma A, Kudoh S. Securing the safety and efficacy of macrolide therapy for chronic small airway diseases. Intern Med 2005;44:167–8.
54. Albert RK, Connett J, Bailey WC, et al. Azithromycin for prevention of exacerbations of COPD. N Engl J Med 2011;365:689–98.
55. Smith K, Leyden JJ. Safety of doxycycline and minocycline: a systematic review. Clin Ther 2005;27:1329–42.
56. Stultz JS, Eiland LS. Doxycycline and tooth discoloration in children: changing of recommendations based on evidence of safety. Ann Pharmacother 2019;53(11): 1162–6.

57. Patel AM, Shariff S, Bailey DG, et al. Statin toxicity from macrolide antibiotic co-prescription: a population-based cohort study. Ann Intern Med 2013;158:869–76.
58. Lund M, Svanstrom H, Pasternak B, et al. Concomitant use of statins and macrolide antibiotics and risk of serious renal events: a nationwide cohort study. Int J Cardiol 2018;269:310–6.
59. Philpott C, le Conte S, Beard D, et al. Clarithromycin and endoscopic sinus surgery for adults with chronic rhinosinusitis with and without nasal polyps: study protocol for the MACRO randomised controlled trial. Trials 2019;20:246.
60. Otsu K, Ishinaga H, Suzuki S, et al. Effects of a novel nonantibiotic macrolide, EM900, on cytokine and mucin gene expression in a human airway epithelial cell line. Pharmacology 2011;88:327–32.
61. Tojima I, Shimizu S, Ogawa T, et al. Anti-inflammatory effects of a novel non-antibiotic macrolide, EM900, on mucus secretion of airway epithelium. Auris Nasus Larynx 2015;42:332–6.
62. Balloy V, Deveaux A, Lebeaux D, et al. Azithromycin analogue CSY0073 attenuates lung inflammation induced by LPS challenge. Br J Pharmacol 2014;171:1783–94.

Topical Irrigations for Chronic Rhinosinusitis

Victoria S. Lee, MD

KEYWORDS

- Topical therapies • Irrigations • Chronic rhinosinusitis • Saline • Topical steroids
- Topical antibiotics • Topical antifungals • Manuka honey

KEY POINTS

- Saline irrigations and topical corticosteroid sprays are recommended in the treatment of chronic rhinosinusitis.
- Topical corticosteroid irrigations are recommended as an option particularly in the postoperative setting. Further research on their effect on the hypothalamic-pituitary-adrenal axis is needed.
- Topical antibiotics are not recommended in the treatment of routine chronic rhinosinusitis but may have a role in recalcitrant cases.
- Topical antifungals are not recommended, but their effect in the allergic fungal subtype is unclear and warrants further investigation.
- Investigations are underway on a variety of topical alternative therapies, with additional ones, such as topical probiotics, on the horizon.

INTRODUCTION

The sinonasal cavity is easily accessible and therefore particularly amenable to topical therapy. Topical therapy offers multiple advantages over systemic therapy. It is administered directly onto the affected tissue, has the potential to be delivered at higher local concentrations, and minimizes systemic absorption, thereby reducing the potential for adverse systemic effects.[1] The existing data support optimal sinus delivery using a high-volume irrigation device, and in surgically opened sinuses and the head down and forward position.[2–6]

Saline irrigations are the oldest and most widely used of the topical therapies. As the understanding of the primary cause of chronic rhinosinusitis (CRS) has shifted away from infection toward inflammation, topical corticosteroid sprays have also become a mainstay of treatment with irrigations an option in the postoperative setting. The

Department of Otolaryngology–Head and Neck Surgery, University of Illinois at Chicago, 1855 West Taylor Street, MC 648, Room 3.87, Chicago, IL 60611, USA
E-mail address: vlee39@uic.edu

Immunol Allergy Clin N Am 40 (2020) 317–328
https://doi.org/10.1016/j.iac.2019.12.014
0889-8561/20/© 2019 Elsevier Inc. All rights reserved.
immunology.theclinics.com

popularity of topical antibiotics has subsequently waned with their use reserved for recalcitrant cases, and the use of topical antifungals is now defunct in the treatment of routine CRS. In recent years with the growing concern over the role of biofilms in CRS, topical alternative therapies that target biofilms, such as surfactants and manuka honey, have also gained increasing recognition. This article summarizes the existing literature on the various topical therapies that have been studied, also highlighting exciting new avenues of research, such as topical probiotics.[5]

SALINE IRRIGATIONS
Indications

The proposed physiologic benefits of nasal saline irrigations include improved mucociliary clearance and disruption and removal of mucus, blood, and environmental allergens.[7,8] Nasal saline irrigations are indicated as an adjunct to other medical therapies for CRS. A 2007 systematic review with metanalysis by Harvey and colleagues[9] included eight randomized controlled trials (RCTs) with a variety of study designs, comparing saline with no treatment, placebo, or as an adjunct to other treatments. The study concluded that the benefits of saline outweigh the drawbacks and that saline may be used as an adjunctive treatment of CRS, because it seemed to improve symptoms as a sole treatment modality but was less effective compared with intranasal corticosteroid (INCS) therapy.[9] The 2013 evidence-based reviews by Rudmik and colleagues[1] and Wei and colleagues[10] reached similar conclusions, as did the 2016 International Consensus Statement on Allergy and Rhinology: Rhinosinusitis.[5]

Saline irrigations may also be useful in the immediate postoperative period for patients that have undergone endoscopic sinus surgery (ESS). An RCT by Liang and colleagues[11] found that saline irrigations combined with postoperative debridement improved symptoms and endoscopic appearance compared with debridement alone in the mild CRS group, although not in the moderate-severe CRS group. In another RCT, Freeman and colleagues[12] noted improved endoscopic appearance and mucociliary function at 3 weeks with saline irrigations, but these improvements were not sustained at 3 months. The study, however, used a suboptimal low-volume delivery protocol, and it is difficult to determine the extent to which this may have contributed to the lack of sustained improvement. The 2016 International Consensus Statement on Allergy and Rhinology: Rhinosinusitis has recommended nasal saline irrigations for postoperative care.[5]

Volume, Formulations, and Cost

Studies support the superiority of high-volume irrigations over low-volume sprays and nebulizers. In an RCT by Pynnonen and colleagues,[13] patients with chronic sinus and nasal symptoms that received high-volume irrigations achieved lower Sino-Nasal Outcome Test (SNOT)-20 scores compared with patients that received nasal spray over an 8-week period. The use of high-volume nasal saline irrigations, defined as greater than 200 mL, is recommended over low-volume methods.[5] The cost of high-volume irrigation devices is also favorably low, estimated at approximately $0.24 per day.[5]

In addition to determining optimal volume, studies have focused on evaluating which saline formulation, isotonic versus hypertonic, is most effective. Studies comparing isotonic and hypertonic saline irrigations have shown that both improved symptoms but there were no significant differences between the groups.[14,15] Overall, the data do not support a difference in effectiveness between isotonic and hypertonic formulations.[1,9]

Safety Profile

Saline irrigations are generally well-tolerated.[5] The most frequently reported adverse effects are nasal burning, local irritation, and nausea. Headaches, epistaxis, postnasal drainage, and ear pain/congestion have also been reported.[5,8] These side effects may occur more frequently with hypertonic solutions.[5]

Although extremely rare, there have been deaths from amebic meningoencephalitis believed to be related to sinus irrigations with contaminated water. As a result, it is recommended to use a clean water source for irrigations, avoiding well/tap water, until this is better elucidated.[16] Bacterial colonization of irrigation bottles is also well-known, but it does not seem to be associated with increased clinical infections in CRS.[7] Nevertheless, it is suggested that patients regularly clean their nasal irrigation devices. Microwave decontamination has been suggested as a possible cleaning strategy.[17]

TOPICAL CORTICOSTEROIDS
Mechanism

Corticosteroids suppress inflammation via a variety of mechanisms. They reduce circulating leukocytes and inhibit proinflammatory transcription factors, arachidonic acid metabolites, histamine and leukotriene release from basophils, neuropeptide-induced inflammation, and lysozyme release. Corticosteroids also decrease vascular permeability, and inhibit glycoprotein release from submucosal glands, thinning mucus secretions.[18]

Indications

Standard delivery (sprays)

Standard INCS refers to metered-dose topical corticosteroid solutions that are approved by the Food and Drug Administration for nasal use. In patients with CRC without nasal polyposis (CRSsNP), systematic reviews with meta-analyses by Kalish and colleagues[19] and Snidvongs and colleagues[20] have been performed evaluating standard INCS. Kalish and colleagues[19] combined results from five RCTs and concluded there was no significant benefit with INCS, although there was significant heterogeneity between studies. Total symptom scores were reported in three of the trials; however, with a standardized mean difference favoring INCS, suggesting a symptom benefit.[19] Snidvongs and colleagues[20] pooled symptom scores for five RCTs and found a significant improvement with INCS, with no significant heterogeneity between studies noted.

In patients with CRS with nasal polyposis (CRSwNP), systematic reviews with meta-analyses by Joe and colleagues,[21] Rudmik and colleagues,[22] and Snidvongs and colleagues[20] have been performed evaluating standard INCS. Pooled data demonstrated significant reduction in polyp size and significant symptom and nasal peak inspiratory flow improvement. A 2016 systematic review by Chong and colleagues[23] included 18 RCTs, 14 studies including patients with CRSwNP and 4 studies including patients with CRSsNP. The study concluded that there seemed to be an improvement for all symptoms.[23] Overall, standard delivery of topical corticosteroids is well-supported in the literature, and its use is recommended in CRSsNP and CRSwNP.[5]

Nonstandard delivery (irrigations)

Standard INCS, however, has limited distribution beyond the nasal cavities, especially in patients that have not undergone ESS.[3] Nonstandard INCS refers to off-label therapies, such as high-volume topical corticosteroid irrigations, which are designed to deliver a higher volume and concentration of corticosteroid.[5] Despite the widespread use of these irrigations in clinical practice, there is a paucity of high-quality data.

Rotenberg and colleagues[24] in 2011 published an RCT evaluating the effect of budesonide irrigations in patients with Samter triad who had undergone ESS. Patients were randomized into three arms: (1) saline irrigation alone, (2) saline irrigation plus separate budesonide nasal spray, and (3) saline irrigation mixed with budesonide nasal spray. Outcome measures were symptom, radiographic, and endoscopic scores. All groups showed improvement in outcomes, but there were no significant differences among the groups.[24]

Tait and colleagues[25] in 2018 published the only other RCT evaluating the effectiveness of high-volume budesonide irrigations in patients with CRS. Patients with and without polyps were enrolled. Sixty-one patients were included in the per-protocol analysis, 29 randomized to perform budesonide irrigations and 32 randomized to perform saline irrigations for 1 month. The budesonide group showed greater mean improvement in SNOT-22 and endoscopic scores compared with the saline group, although there were no significant differences between the groups. It is worth noting, however, that the budesonide group exceeded the minimal clinically important difference for the SNOT-22, whereas the saline group did not, suggesting that budesonide may have clinically meaningful benefits beyond saline alone.[25]

Several less scientifically rigorous studies have also demonstrated significant improvements in outcomes with topical corticosteroid irrigations.[26] Given the conflicting results and overall lack of high-quality data, evidence-based reviews and consensus statements have found it challenging to provide a recommendation for or against the use of topical corticosteroid irrigations. They are currently recommended as an option in the treatment of CRSsNP and CRSwNP, especially in the postoperative setting.[1,5]

Formulations and Cost

Standard sprays come in a variety of formulations.[1] Second-generation sprays have less than 2% systemic bioavailability compared with 10% to 50% for first-generation sprays.[27] There is insufficient evidence to recommend one spray formulation over another.[28] The most widely studied formulation of nonstandard high-volume topical corticosteroid irrigations is budesonide. Common formulations are listed in **Table 1**. The spray formulations are low in cost. The cost of the irrigations, however,

Table 1 Common formulations for topical corticosteroids		
Class		**Generic Name (Brand Name)**
Standard (sprays)	1st generation	Beclomethasone (Beconase AQ, Qnasl)
		Budesonide (Rhinocort Aqua[b])
		Triamcinolone (Nasacort AQ[a,b])
	2nd generation	Ciclesonide (Omnaris, Zetonna)
		Fluticasone (Veramyst[a], Flonase[b])
		Mometasone (Nasonex[a])
Nonstandard (irrigations)		Budesonide (0.25–2 mg/2 mL in 240 mL saline)
		Mometasone

[a] Indicates approved for age 2 and older.
[b] Indicates available over-the-counter.
Adapted from Lee VS, Lin SY. Allergy and the Pediatric Otolaryngologist. Otolaryngol Clin North Am 2019;52(5):870; with permission.

is prohibitive for some patients because they are frequently not covered by insurance given their off-label usage. The increasing availability of special compounding pharmacies has helped to lower out-of-pocket costs.

Safety Profile

Given that the dosing of budesonide used in concentrated irrigations is much higher than in spray formulations, there is concern for unwanted systemic absorption that could lead to hypothalamic-pituitary-adrenal (HPA) axis suppression and/or increased intraocular pressure. Small studies looking at short-term use of budesonide irrigations, at least 6 to 8 weeks in duration, found no evidence of HPA axis suppression or increased intraocular pressure.[29,30]

More recently, two studies have evaluated more long-term use of budesonide irrigations. Smith and colleagues[31] completed a cross-sectional cohort study of 35 post-ESS patients with CRS who performed budesonide irrigations for at least 12 months. They concluded that there was no detectable HPA axis suppression. Soudry and colleagues[32] evaluated 48 post-ESS patients with CRS who were treated with budesonide irrigations for at least 6 months. Of note, 32 of the 48 patients were also using other topical steroid formulations. Intraocular pressure was normal in all patients. Eleven of the 48 patients, however, had abnormally low stimulated cortisol levels on corticotropin stimulation testing, although they were not symptomatic. Four repeated the testing after stopping the budesonide irrigation for 30 days, and three had increased stimulated cortisol levels.[32]

The current literature suggests that high-volume budesonide irrigations do not affect intraocular pressure but that there may be a low risk of HPA axis suppression with long-term use. Further research is needed to evaluate the true impact of long-term topical steroid irrigations on the HPA axis, especially in the setting of concomitant use of other topical steroid formulations. Determining this along with their clinical effectiveness will help to shape recommendations regarding their use in the future.

TOPICAL ANTI-INFECTIVES
Topical Antibiotics

CRS was once thought to be primarily the result of bacterial infection, fueling interest in topical antibiotic therapies. Over time, however, there has been a paradigm shift away from an infectious cause of CRS and toward an inflammatory one.[8] Several RCTs and systematic reviews have examined topical antibiotics in CRS, primarily in the post-ESS setting, failing to show any benefit and recommending against their use because of lack of evidence.[1,7,10,33–39]

Mupirocin irrigations have perhaps the strongest data supporting their use of any topical antibiotic. Jervis-Bardy and colleagues[40,41] published an RCT studying the use of mupirocin irrigations to target Staphylococcus aureus. Twenty-two patients were included in the per-protocol analysis, 13 randomized to perform mupirocin irrigations and 9 randomized to perform saline irrigations for 1 month. The study demonstrated significant improvement in positive culture rates, although a high long-term microbiologic failure rate was reported in a follow-up study. Additionally, there were no significant improvements in symptom or endoscopic outcomes.[40,41]

In summary, topical antibiotics are not recommended in the treatment of routine CRS. Some case series have reported benefit in recalcitrant cases, indicating that there may be a role for topical antibiotics in challenging cases ideally in a culture-directed fashion.[5]

Topical Antifungals

Since the 1990s, fungal elements have been known to be present in the sinonasal cavity in patients with CRS, and it was hypothesized that they were contributing to the inflammation in CRS. In 2002, a pilot study examining topical amphotericin B in patients with CRS showed promising improvements in symptom and endoscopic measures, driving a subsequent flurry of RCTs and metanalyses that have overall failed to show any benefit.[1,42–47]

Allergic fungal rhinosinusitis (AFRS) represents a unique subtype of patients with CRS, and fungi may play a greater role in its pathophysiology. Unfortunately, there are minimal data evaluating topical antifungal therapy in patients with AFRS specifically. Pilot data suggest that there may be some benefit, although the studies suffered from serious methodologic issues.[44,48] In summary, topical antifungal therapy is not recommended in the treatment of CRSsNP or CRSwNP. Further research is needed to determine if it has any beneficial effects in AFRS specifically.

Formulations and Cost

Formulations of topical antibiotic therapy are directed toward the presumed pathogen. The most frequently implicated pathogenic bacteria in CRS are S aureus, targeted most commonly with mupirocin irrigations, and Pseudomonas aeruginosa, targeted most commonly with tobramycin irrigations. The most widely studied formulation of topical antifungal therapy is amphotericin B. Like topical corticosteroid irrigations, the cost for topical anti-infective irrigations is high and is often not covered by insurance. Special compounding pharmacies can lower out-of-pocket costs.

Safety Profile

Topical anti-infective therapy is generally well-tolerated. Adverse effects are similar to other topical therapies and include irritation, dryness, burning, itching, epistaxis, postnasal drainage, ear pain, and sore throat. There is a theoretic risk of ototoxicity and nephrotoxicity with topical aminoglycosides, although this has not been documented with irrigations. Resistance development is also a concern.[5] In the mupirocin RCT by Jervis Bardy and Wormald,[41] there was a documented case of mupirocin-resistant S aureus. Exacerbation of respiratory symptoms, such as asthma, has been reported with topical antifungal therapy.[1]

TOPICAL ALTERNATIVE THERAPIES
Inhibitors of Biofilm Formation

Although the cause of CRS is now believed to be primarily inflammatory, infection may potentially still play a role in recalcitrant disease. The ability of pathogenic bacteria in CRS, particularly S aureus and P aeruginosa, to form biofilms, well-organized structures of bacterial communities encased in a self-produced polymeric matrix tightly adhered to the sinonasal mucosa, has been proposed to contribute to their recalcitrance.[49,50] Several topical alternative therapies have emerged targeting these biofilms.

Surfactants

Surfactants are compounds that are hydrophobic and hydrophilic. In the orthopedic literature, chemical surfactants, such as those found in shampoos, have been shown to inhibit biofilm formation. Naturally occurring surfactants in the respiratory system also decrease the surface tension and viscosity of mucus.[5] Given these properties, the effect of baby shampoo irrigations has been studied in the setting of CRS. Despite favorable initial pilot studies, an RCT comparing 1% baby shampoo and hypertonic saline irrigations showed no significant differences in symptom scores between the two groups, and the baby shampoo group had a higher rate of discontinued use because of side effects, most commonly nasal irritation.[51] Baby shampoo has also been shown to increase mucociliary clearance time.[52] There is currently not enough evidence to provide recommendations regarding surfactant irrigations in CRS.[5]

Manuka honey

Manuka honey has long been used in the treatment of wounds, which are prone to bacterial biofilm formation. The mechanisms behind its ability to inhibit biofilm formation are postulated to be related to multiple properties, including its high sugar content and therefore osmolarity; its acidity; its hydrogen peroxide activity; and the presence of unique phytochemical compounds, such as methylglyoxal (MGO).[53–56] Manuka honey is also effective against a broad range of bacteria, including most relevantly S aureus and P aeruginosa.[57]

Two RCTs have been performed examining manuka honey irrigations in CRS, both in the post-ESS setting on a particularly recalcitrant subset of patients. In the study by Lee and colleagues,[58] 42 patients were included in the per-protocol analysis, 20 randomized to perform manuka honey irrigations and 22 randomized to perform saline irrigations for 1 month. Both groups achieved clinically meaningful improvement in SNOT-22 scores. SNOT-22 scores, endoscopic scores, and post-treatment culture negativity rates were better in the manuka honey group compared with the saline group, but these differences were not significant. A limitation of this study was that adjunctive systemic therapies were offered at the clinician's discretion. In a subgroup analysis of patients who did not receive any adjunctive treatment, the manuka honey group achieved significantly better culture negativity rates than the saline group, suggesting that manuka honey may have microbiologic benefit and that the relative importance of systemic therapy may be higher in patients receiving saline irrigation alone.[58] In the study by Ooi and colleagues,[59] 25 patients were included in the per-protocol analysis, 15 randomized to receive manuka honey irrigations with an MGO additive and 10 randomized to receive saline and culture-directed oral antibiotics. Saline and culture-directed oral antibiotics seemed to be superior to manuka honey only in eradication of infection on culture. There were no significant differences in symptom or endoscopic scores between the groups. The study was intended as a phase 1 safety and tolerability study, and as a result, the authors state it was likely underpowered. Smell function was assessed by Ooi and colleagues[59] and unchanged with the manuka honey irrigations. The irrigations were well-tolerated, and no serious adverse effects were reported in either study.[58,59] At higher concentrations of MGO than used in the study by Ooi and colleagues, it does become ciliotoxic.[54,60]

In summary, these studies focused on the recalcitrant post-ESS subset of CRS suggest that manuka honey irrigations may have the greatest effect on microbiologic outcomes. There is no evidence of a symptomatic or endoscopic benefit compared with saline. These data, however, are limited with only two RCTs, one of which is underpowered. Larger prospective studies are needed to make recommendations regarding the use of these irrigations in CRS.[5]

Xylitol

Xylitol enhances the activity of innate immune factors present in respiratory secretions, eliciting a downstream bactericidal effect. There is only one small RCT with substantial participant dropout, which demonstrated a significant symptomatic benefit with xylitol irrigations.[61] Further research is needed to make a recommendation regarding their use in CRS.[5]

Table 2
Summary of topical therapies in chronic rhinosinusitis

Type	Recommended?	Formulation	Cost	Specific Safety Concerns
Saline irrigation	Yes, routine Yes, postoperative	High-volume (>200 mL)	Low ($0.24/d)	None
Corticosteroid sprays	Yes, routine Yes, postoperative	Metered-dose solutions	Low	None
Corticosteroid irrigations	Option, mainly postoperative	Variable (eg, budesonide)	Higher (lower with compounding pharmacies)	Possible HPA axis suppression
Antibiotic irrigations	No, routine May have role in recalcitrant cases Ideally culture-directed	Highly variable	Higher (lower with compounding pharmacies)	Resistance development Ototoxicity/ nephrotoxicity (aminoglycosides)
Antifungal irrigations	No Further research needed for allergic fungal subtype	Variable (eg, amphotericin B)	Higher (lower with compounding pharmacies)	Exacerbation of respiratory conditions
Alternative therapies (surfactants, manuka honey, xylitol)	Insufficient evidence	Highly variable	Highly variable	None specifically

Probiotics: The New Frontier

In recent years, there has been an increasing focus on the commensal sinonasal microbiome and its role in the development of a functional immune system. It has been theorized that infections in CRS may be related to a decrease in diversity of the commensal microbiome and an increase in pathogenic bacteria. The concept behind the therapeutic potential of topical probiotics is that they outcompete pathogenic bacteria via a variety of mechanisms, including creating suboptimal environmental conditions, competing for cell surface receptors and thus limiting pathogen adherence, and producing antibacterial metabolites. In doing so, topical probiotics restore the commensal microbiome.

Recent research has focused on determining what constitutes this microbiome, which has proved to be a difficult task. A goal of these efforts is to better inform the selection of topical probiotics to restore it. There are little data evaluating topical probiotics in the treatment of CRS, but the data examining topical probiotics in otitis media and recurrent tonsillitis are promising and demonstrate an excellent safety profile. The therapeutic potential of topical probiotics in CRS is still in its infancy, but it is an exciting new area of research.[62]

SUMMARY

Topical therapies allow for delivery at higher local concentrations and minimize systemic absorption, providing attractive treatment options given the accessibility of the sinonasal cavity (**Table 2**). Saline irrigations and topical corticosteroid sprays are recommended in the treatment of CRS. Further research on the effect of topical corticosteroid irrigations and possible HPA axis suppression is needed to make a recommendation regarding their use, which is currently an option primarily in the postoperative setting. Topical antibiotics and antifungals are not recommended in the treatment of routine CRS but may have a role in recalcitrant CRS and AFRS, respectively. Investigations are currently underway on a variety of topical alternative therapies, with additional ones, such as topical probiotics, on the horizon.

DISCLOSURE

The author has nothing to disclose.

REFERENCES

1. Rudmik L, Hoy M, Schlosser RJ, et al. Topical therapies in the management of chronic rhinosinusitis: an evidence-based review with recommendations. Int Forum Allergy Rhinol 2013;3(4):281–98.
2. Grobler A, Weitzel EK, Buele A, et al. Pre- and postoperative sinus penetration of nasal irrigation. Laryngoscope 2008;118(11):2078–81.
3. Thomas WW 3rd, Harvey RJ, Rudmik L, et al. Distribution of topical agents to the paranasal sinuses: an evidence-based review with recommendations. Int Forum Allergy Rhinol 2013;3(9):691–703.
4. Habib AR, Thamboo A, Manji J, et al. The effect of head position on the distribution of topical nasal medication using the mucosal atomization device: a cadaver study. Int Forum Allergy Rhinol 2013;3(12):958–62.
5. Orlandi RR, Kingdom TT, Hwang PH, et al. International consensus statement on allergy and rhinology: rhinosinusitis. Int Forum Allergy Rhinol 2016;6(Suppl 1): S22–209.
6. Orlandi RR, Smith TL, Marple BF, et al. Update on evidence-based reviews with recommendations in adult chronic rhinosinusitis. Int Forum Allergy Rhinol 2014; 4(Suppl 1):S1–15.
7. Huang A, Govindaraj S. Topical therapy in the management of chronic rhinosinusitis. Curr Opin Otolaryngol Head Neck Surg 2013;21(1):31–8.
8. Luk LJ, DelGaudio JM. Topical drug therapies for chronic rhinosinusitis. Otolaryngol Clin North Am 2017;50(3):533–43.
9. Harvey R, Hannan SA, Badia L, et al. Nasal saline irrigations for the symptoms of chronic rhinosinusitis. Cochrane Database Syst Rev 2007;(3):CD006394.
10. Wei CC, Adappa ND, Cohen NA. Use of topical nasal therapies in the management of chronic rhinosinusitis. Laryngoscope 2013;123(10):2347–59.
11. Liang KL, Su MC, Tseng HC, et al. Impact of pulsatile nasal irrigation on the prognosis of functional endoscopic sinus surgery. J Otolaryngol Head Neck Surg 2008;37(2):148–53.
12. Freeman SR, Sivayoham ES, Jepson K, et al. A preliminary randomised controlled trial evaluating the efficacy of saline douching following endoscopic sinus surgery. Clin Otolaryngol 2008;33(5):462–5.
13. Pynnonen MA, Mukerji SS, Kim HM, et al. Nasal saline for chronic sinonasal symptoms: a randomized controlled trial. Arch Otolaryngol Head Neck Surg 2007;133(11):1115–20.
14. Bachmann G, Hommel G, Michel O. Effect of irrigation of the nose with isotonic salt solution on adult patients with chronic paranasal sinus disease. Eur Arch Otorhinolaryngol 2000;257(10):537–41.

15. Hauptman G, Ryan MW. The effect of saline solutions on nasal patency and mucociliary clearance in rhinosinusitis patients. Otolaryngol Head Neck Surg 2007; 137(5):815–21.

16. Sowerby LJ, Wright ED. Tap water or "sterile" water for sinus irrigations: what are our patients using? Int Forum Allergy Rhinol 2012;2(4):300–2.

17. Shargorodsky J, Lane AP. What is the best modality to minimize bacterial contamination of nasal saline irrigation bottles? Laryngoscope 2015;125(7):1515–6.

18. Rudmik L, Soler ZM. Medical therapies for adult chronic sinusitis: a systematic review. JAMA 2015;314(9):926–39.

19. Kalish LH, Arendts G, Sacks R, et al. Topical steroids in chronic rhinosinusitis without polyps: a systematic review and meta-analysis. Otolaryngol Head Neck Surg 2009;141(6):674–83.

20. Snidvongs K, Kalish L, Sacks R, et al. Topical steroid for chronic rhinosinusitis without polyps. Cochrane Database Syst Rev 2011;(8):CD009274.

21. Joe SA, Thambi R, Huang J. A systematic review of the use of intranasal steroids in the treatment of chronic rhinosinusitis. Otolaryngol Head Neck Surg 2008; 139(3):340–7.

22. Rudmik L, Schlosser RJ, Smith TL, et al. Impact of topical nasal steroid therapy on symptoms of nasal polyposis: a meta-analysis. Laryngoscope 2012;122(7): 1431–7.

23. Chong LY, Head K, Hopkins C, et al. Intranasal steroids versus placebo or no intervention for chronic rhinosinusitis. Cochrane Database Syst Rev 2016;(4):CD011996.

24. Rotenberg BW, Zhang I, Arra I, et al. Postoperative care for Samter's triad patients undergoing endoscopic sinus surgery: a double-blinded, randomized controlled trial. Laryngoscope 2011;121(12):2702–5.

25. Tait S, Kallogjeri D, Suko J, et al. Effect of budesonide added to large-volume, low-pressure saline sinus irrigation for chronic rhinosinusitis: a randomized clinical trial. JAMA Otolaryngol Head Neck Surg 2018;144(7):605–12.

26. Huang ZZ, Chen XZ, Huang JC, et al. Budesonide nasal irrigation improved Lund-Kennedy endoscopic score of chronic rhinosinusitis patients after endoscopic sinus surgery. Eur Arch Otorhinolaryngol 2019;276(5):1397–403.

27. Lee VS, Lin SY. Allergy and the pediatric otolaryngologist. Otolaryngol Clin North Am 2019;52(5):863–73.

28. Chong LY, Head K, Hopkins C, et al. Different types of intranasal steroids for chronic rhinosinusitis. Cochrane Database Syst Rev 2016;(4):CD011993.

29. Bhalla RK, Payton K, Wright ED. Safety of budesonide in saline sinonasal irrigations in the management of chronic rhinosinusitis with polyposis: lack of significant adrenal suppression. J Otolaryngol Head Neck Surg 2008;37(6):821–5.

30. Welch KC, Thaler ER, Doghramji LL, et al. The effects of serum and urinary cortisol levels of topical intranasal irrigations with budesonide added to saline in patients with recurrent polyposis after endoscopic sinus surgery. Am J Rhinol Allergy 2010;24(1):26–8.

31. Smith KA, French G, Mechor B, et al. Safety of long-term high-volume sinonasal budesonide irrigations for chronic rhinosinusitis. Int Forum Allergy Rhinol 2016; 6(3):228–32.

32. Soudry E, Wang J, Vaezeafshar R, et al. Safety analysis of long-term budesonide nasal irrigations in patients with chronic rhinosinusitis post endoscopic sinus surgery. Int Forum Allergy Rhinol 2016;6(6):568–72.

33. Soler ZM, Oyer SL, Kern RC, et al. Antimicrobials and chronic rhinosinusitis with or without polyposis in adults: an evidenced-based review with recommendations. Int Forum Allergy Rhinol 2013;3(1):31–47.
34. Sykes DA, Wilson R, Chan KL, et al. Relative importance of antibiotic and improved clearance in topical treatment of chronic mucopurulent rhinosinusitis. A controlled study. Lancet 1986;2(8503):359–60.
35. Videler WJ, van Drunen CM, Reitsma JB, et al. Nebulized bacitracin/colimycin: a treatment option in recalcitrant chronic rhinosinusitis with *Staphylococcus aureus*? A double-blind, randomized, placebo-controlled, cross-over pilot study. Rhinology 2008;46(2):92–8.
36. Desrosiers MY, Salas-Prato M. Treatment of chronic rhinosinusitis refractory to other treatments with topical antibiotic therapy delivered by means of a large-particle nebulizer: results of a controlled trial. Otolaryngol Head Neck Surg 2001;125(3):265–9.
37. Lee JT, Chiu AG. Topical anti-infective sinonasal irrigations: update and literature review. Am J Rhinol Allergy 2014;28(1):29–38.
38. Lim M, Citardi MJ, Leong JL. Topical antimicrobials in the management of chronic rhinosinusitis: a systematic review. Am J Rhinol 2008;22(4):381–9.
39. Woodhouse BM, Cleveland KW. Nebulized antibiotics for the treatment of refractory bacterial chronic rhinosinusitis. Ann Pharmacother 2011;45(6):798–802.
40. Jervis-Bardy J, Boase S, Psaltis A, et al. A randomized trial of mupirocin sinonasal rinses versus saline in surgically recalcitrant staphylococcal chronic rhinosinusitis. Laryngoscope 2012;122(10):2148–53.
41. Jervis-Bardy J, Wormald PJ. Microbiological outcomes following mupirocin nasal washes for symptomatic, *Staphylococcus aureus*-positive chronic rhinosinusitis following endoscopic sinus surgery. Int Forum Allergy Rhinol 2012;2(2):111–5.
42. Ebbens FA, Scadding GK, Badia L, et al. Amphotericin B nasal lavages: not a solution for patients with chronic rhinosinusitis. J Allergy Clin Immunol 2006;118(5):1149–56.
43. Gerlinger I, Fittler A, Fonai F, et al. Postoperative application of amphotericin B nasal spray in chronic rhinosinusitis with nasal polyposis, with a review of the antifungal therapy. Eur Arch Otorhinolaryngol 2009;266(6):847–55.
44. Khalil Y, Tharwat A, Abdou AG, et al. The role of antifungal therapy in the prevention of recurrent allergic fungal rhinosinusitis after functional endoscopic sinus surgery: a randomized, controlled study. Ear Nose Throat J 2011;90(8):E1–7.
45. Liang KL, Su MC, Shiao JY, et al. Amphotericin B irrigation for the treatment of chronic rhinosinusitis without nasal polyps: a randomized, placebo-controlled, double-blind study. Am J Rhinol 2008;22(1):52–8.
46. Ponikau JU, Sherris DA, Weaver A, et al. Treatment of chronic rhinosinusitis with intranasal amphotericin B: a randomized, placebo-controlled, double-blind pilot trial. J Allergy Clin Immunol 2005;115(1):125–31.
47. Sacks PL, Harvey RJ, Rimmer J, et al. Topical and systemic antifungal therapy for the symptomatic treatment of chronic rhinosinusitis. Cochrane Database Syst Rev 2011;(8):CD008263.
48. Jen A, Kacker A, Huang C, et al. Fluconazole nasal spray in the treatment of allergic fungal sinusitis: a pilot study. Ear Nose Throat J 2004;83(10):692, 694–5.
49. Fokkens WJ, Lund VJ, Mullol J, et al. European position paper on rhinosinusitis and nasal polyps 2012. Rhinol Suppl 2012;23. 3 p preceding table of contents, 1-298.
50. Ramadan HH, Sanclement JA, Thomas JG. Chronic rhinosinusitis and biofilms. Otolaryngol Head Neck Surg 2005;132(3):414–7.

51. Farag AA, Deal AM, McKinney KA, et al. Single-blind randomized controlled trial of surfactant vs hypertonic saline irrigation following endoscopic endonasal surgery. Int Forum Allergy Rhinol 2013;3(4):276–80.
52. Isaacs S, Fakhri S, Luong A, et al. The effect of dilute baby shampoo on nasal mucociliary clearance in healthy subjects. Am J Rhinol Allergy 2011;25(1):e27–9.
53. Cooper RA, Molan PC, Harding KG. The sensitivity to honey of gram-positive cocci of clinical significance isolated from wounds. J Appl Microbiol 2002; 93(5):857–63.
54. Jervis-Bardy J, Foreman A, Bray S, et al. Methylglyoxal-infused honey mimics the anti-*Staphylococcus aureus* biofilm activity of manuka honey: potential implication in chronic rhinosinusitis. Laryngoscope 2011;121(5):1104–7.
55. Kilty SJ, Duval M, Chan FT, et al. Methylglyoxal: (active agent of manuka honey) in vitro activity against bacterial biofilms. Int Forum Allergy Rhinol 2011;1(5): 348–50.
56. Lu J, Turnbull L, Burke CM, et al. Manuka-type honeys can eradicate biofilms produced by *Staphylococcus aureus* strains with different biofilm-forming abilities. PeerJ 2014;2:e326.
57. Lusby PE, Coombes AL, Wilkinson JM. Bactericidal activity of different honeys against pathogenic bacteria. Arch Med Res 2005;36(5):464–7.
58. Lee VS, Humphreys IM, Purcell PL, et al. Manuka honey sinus irrigation for the treatment of chronic rhinosinusitis: a randomized controlled trial. Int Forum Allergy Rhinol 2017;7(4):365–72.
59. Ooi ML, Jothin A, Bennett C, et al. Manuka honey sinus irrigations in recalcitrant chronic rhinosinusitis: phase 1 randomized, single-blinded, placebo-controlled trial. Int Forum Allergy Rhinol 2019;9(12):1470–7.
60. Paramasivan S, Drilling AJ, Jardeleza C, et al. Methylglyoxal-augmented manuka honey as a topical anti-*Staphylococcus aureus* biofilm agent: safety and efficacy in an in vivo model. Int Forum Allergy Rhinol 2014;4(3):187–95.
61. Weissman JD, Fernandez F, Hwang PH. Xylitol nasal irrigation in the management of chronic rhinosinusitis: a pilot study. Laryngoscope 2011;121(11):2468–72.
62. Cervin AU. The potential for topical probiotic treatment of chronic rhinosinusitis, a personal perspective. Front Cell Infect Microbiol 2018;7:530.

Nasal Polyposis and Aspirin-Exacerbated Respiratory Disease

Kathleen Luskin, MD[a,b,*], Hiral Thakrar, MD[a,b],
Andrew White, MD[a,b]

KEYWORDS

• Nasal • Polyp • AERD • Aspirin • Exacerbated • Respiratory • disease

KEY POINTS

• Aspirin-exacerbated respiratory disease (AERD) is characterized by persistent and difficult-to-treat nasal polyposis, eosinophilic chronic sinusitis, asthma, and nonsteroidal anti-inflammatory drug reactions and is often accompanied by alcohol sensitivity.

• The underlying pathophysiology of AERD seems to involve dysregulated arachidonic acid metabolism and receptor signaling, along with eosinophil and mast cell byproducts, including increased leukotriene E4 and prostaglandin D2 and decreased prostaglandin E2.

• There are a variety of therapies available for AERD, including those that interfere with leukotriene production or signaling, topical and systemic corticosteroids, biologics, dietary modification, and aspirin.

• Aspirin challenge is the gold standard for AERD diagnosis, and desensitization provides a unique and effective therapeutic alternative; the decision about procedure timing and location must be individualized based on patient factors.

• Aspirin therapy is generally well tolerated, although side effects and lack of response or maintenance of desensitization can occur in a minority of patients.

INTRODUCTION

Aspirin-exacerbated respiratory disease (AERD) is seen in a subset of patients with nasal polyposis who have comorbid asthma and acute upper and lower respiratory tract reactions with exposure to aspirin (acetylsalicylic acid) or other cyclooxygenase-1 (COX-1)-inhibiting nonsteroidal anti-inflammatory drugs (NSAIDs).

[a] Allergy-Immunology, Scripps Health, San Diego, CA, USA; [b] Scripps Clinic Carmel Valley, 3811 Valley Centre Drive, San Diego, CA 92130, USA
* Corresponding author. Scripps Clinic Carmel Valley, 3811 Valley Centre Drive, San Diego, CA 92130.
E-mail address: luskin.kathleen@scrippshealth.org

Immunol Allergy Clin N Am 40 (2020) 329–343
https://doi.org/10.1016/j.iac.2019.12.002
0889-8561/20/© 2019 Elsevier Inc. All rights reserved.

immunology.theclinics.com

AERD is usually diagnosed in the third or fourth decades of life, with approximately 50% of patients reporting a viral syndrome at initiation. Reactions to aspirin/NSAIDs depend on inhibition of the COX-1 enzyme inhibition rather than being immunoglobulin E (IgE) mediated. NSAID tolerance before the development of NSAID reactions is typical. Although NSAID hypersensitivity can precede respiratory disease, most patients develop asthma and chronic rhinosinusitis with nasal polyposis (CRSwNP) first, with NSAID reactions occurring later in the disease. NSAID reactions occur typically between 30 minutes and 3 hours after ingestion, and severity may be dose-related.[1] Typical reactions include nasal congestion, rhinorrhea, ocular pruritis with erythema, and bronchospasm.[2] Less commonly, cutaneous (rash and flushing) or gastrointestinal symptoms (abdominal pain, diarrhea, vomiting) can be the predominant findings.[3]

ASPIRIN-EXACERBATED RESPIRATORY DISEASE BURDEN

Approximately 7.9% of the US population has asthma, and among adult asthmatic patients, about 7% have AERD, with the prevalence increasing to 30% in patients with asthma and nasal polyps.[4–6] There are significant financial, physical, and emotional costs in AERD, in part due to the severity and persistence of their sinus and airway disease.[7]

In 2013, it was estimated that the total cost of asthma in the United States was $81.9 billion.[8] Poor asthma control was associated with a greater prevalence of sleep problems, depression, functional impairment, and negative impact on work and regular activities.[9] Although patients with AERD comprise a small portion of all patients with asthma, they tend to have more severe and poorly-controlled disease requiring aggressive therapy. Compared with non-AERD asthmatics, patients with AERD had higher rates of intubation and high-dose inhaled corticosteroid use and lower mean post-bronchodilator forced expiratory volume at 1 second (FEV1).[10] In addition to asthma, patients with AERD have severe sinus disease, with 10 times as many functional endoscopic sinus surgeries (FESS) and higher rates of polyp recurrence than non-AERD patients.[11] Patients with AERD likely comprise a significant portion of the $3.4 to 5 billion annual cost of CRS.[12] Chronic nasal symptoms, anosmia, and inability to enjoy eating contribute to poor quality of life in AERD.[13]

Although CRSwNP and asthma have significant disease-associated financial costs and morbidity, the AERD subgroup bears a disproportionate burden of disease and medical utilization. Given the high burden of disease, it is imperative to identify impactful, cost-effective therapies.

Alcohol Reactivity in Aspirin-Exacerbated Respiratory Disease

Alcohol sensitivity was first described in 1986, when asthmatic patients developed alcohol-induced respiratory reactions after ingestion of red wine.[14,15] NSAID intolerance was identified in 17% of patients with alcohol-induced nasal symptoms.[16] One study demonstrated the prevalence of alcohol-induced reactions were significantly higher in patients with AERD (75%) compared with aspirin-tolerant asthmatics (33%), CRS (30%), and healthy controls (14%).[17] Similar prevalence was reported in a survey, where 77% of the 190 AERD respondents reported alcohol reactivity.[13]

The mechanism for alcohol reactivity is unknown, although it is suspected that cysteinyl leukotrienes (CysLTs) or other mast cell mediators play a key role in these reactions.[17] Alcohol sensitivity as a manifestation of the underlying inflammatory milieu of AERD is supported by the finding that the severity of aspirin-induced reactions positively correlated with the severity of alcohol-induced reactions.[17] Moreover, aspirin desensitization has been shown to improve alcohol-induced respiratory reactions in AERD.[18]

Inflammatory Basis of Aspirin-Exacerbated Respiratory Disease

Since AERD was originally identified, there has been an increased understanding of disease pathophysiology. Mechanisms underlying AERD are thought to involve abnormal arachidonic acid metabolism, overproduction of CysLTs and pro-inflammatory prostaglandins, and underproduction of the anti-inflammatory prostaglandin PGE2.[3]

The role of CysLTs is evidenced by studies that have demonstrated improvement in anosmia, polyp size, and FEV1 that corresponded to a decrease in urine LTE4 (uLTE4) seen with leukotriene modifier drugs.[19] Patients with AERD have increased CysLT burden and responsiveness in AERD, with an increase in CysLT1 receptors and heightened airway sensitivity to LTE4 compared with aspirin-tolerant patients.[20,21] Aspirin reactions are characterized by increased uLTE4, and those with more severe reactions have higher baseline and larger increase in uLTE4.[3,22,23]

It is not known whether LTE4 causes bronchoconstriction directly or whether it acts through prostaglandin production, especially prostaglandin D2 (PGD2). PGD2 is found in high levels in mast cells and promotes vasodilation, bronchoconstriction, and eosinophil and basophil chemotaxis. Mast cell functionality in AERD is supported by the increase in tryptase with aspirin reactions and the observation that cromolyn improves nasal symptoms and FEV1 at baseline and with aspirin challenge.[24–26] Leukotrienes result in mast cell PGD2 production, either directly through LTE4 binding to CysLT1 receptor or indirectly via binding epithelial GPR99 receptors that subsequently cause mast cell activation.[27–29] Although PGD2 is a primary mast cell mediator, in AERD eosinophils have high hematopoetic prostaglandin D synthase expression and can be stimulated by aspirin to produce PGD2.[30] In addition, eosinophils demonstrate production of and response to interferon gamma (IFN-γ), which may augment the pro-inflammatory state in AERD.[31] The balance of pro- to anti-inflammatory molecules is important, and PGE2 seems to be protective. Lower PDG2:PGE2 ratio, less peripheral eosinophilia, and attenuated increase in uLTE4 was found in post-polypectomy AERD patients who underwent re-challenge and did not react compared with those who reacted.[32] Moreover, polyps seem to be physiologically active inflammatory tissue as evidenced by a decrease in aspirin challenge reaction rate and severity; increase in plasma lipoxin A; and decrease in baseline uLTE4, PGD2 metabolite, and FeNO in post- versus pre-surgery AERD subjects.[32]

Several other discoveries shed light on unique inflammatory pathways involved in AERD. Adherent platelets on leukocytes can form a unit that augments the production of cysLTs in AERD.[33] Type 2 innate lymphocytes (ILC2) traffic to the sinuses during aspirin-induced reactions and may contribute to inflammation in AERD.[34] In addition to the different cell recruitment and function, signaling may be abnormal in AERD. Aberrant LTE4 signaling through recently described receptors, GPR99 and P2Y12, in addition to CysLT1/2 are avenues for further study.[35–37] Although the underlying phenotype of nasal polyposis, eosinophilia, and asthma may be indistinguishable across the spectrum, the pathophysiology of AERD is distinct and has unique inflammatory characteristics.

MEDICAL MANAGEMENT OF ASPIRIN-EXACERBATED RESPIRATORY DISEASE

Given the overproduction of the CysLTs in AERD, medications mitigating the effects of these molecules are cornerstones of the AERD therapeutic regimen and improve safety in aspirin desensitization.[38,39] There are 2 identified leukotriene receptor antagonists (LTRA), montelukast and zafirlukast, which block the CysLT1 receptor but have minimal effects on leukotriene B4 (LTB4) and LTE4 signaling. Zileuton is a 5-lipoxygenase (5-LO) inhibitor that blocks the synthesis of both CysLTs and LTB4. Montelukast improves lung function, reduces bronchodilator use and asthma exacerbations, improves quality of life, decreases nasal polyp eosinophilia, and improves nasal symptom scores.[40,41] Zileuton improves pulmonary function and nasal inspiratory flow, increases sense of smell, and decreases rhinorrhea in patients with AERD.[19] Zileuton, which may be more potent than LTRA, may be underused in AERD.[13,42]

Corticosteroids are important components of AERD treatment. Intranasal glucocorticoids may be helpful in preventing polyp regrowth after sinus surgery in AERD, but not all studies demonstrate efficacy, and polyp recurrence continues to be problematic.[43–45] Fluticasone propionate is available in a new Food and Drug Administration–approved delivery device (Xhance) and decreased nasal polyp size and improved quality-of-life and symptoms in CRSwNP but was not specifically studied in AERD.[46] Nasal rinses with budesonide respules are also used for the reduction of nasal polyps and are effective in reducing sinus computed tomographic scores, symptoms, and anosmia in those with chronic eosinophilic sinusitis.[47] Budesonide rinses have not been specifically studied in AERD.

Other therapies for patients with AERD are being studied. This includes platelet-targeted therapies, including a P2Y12-receptor antagonist and a thromboxane receptor (TP) antagonist. Although a treatment effect was not seen in AERD overall, a P2Y12 inhibitor was effective in inhibiting aspirin-induced symptoms in a subgroup of patients who had greater baseline platelet activation and milder upper respiratory symptoms.[48] Ifetroban, an oral TP-receptor antagonist, is undergoing investigation currently in patients with AERD (NCT03028350).

There is potential to modify a dysregulated arachidonic acid pathway through dietary intervention. Two prospective crossover trials on low salicylate diets demonstrated improvement in nasal symptoms and endoscopy scores, with one trial demonstrating improvement in asthma symptoms.[49,50] Effects of fatty acid (FA) ingestion include inhibition of cellular 5-LO pathways and decreased uLTE4,[51,52] whereas omega-6 FA interferes with the anti-inflammatory effects of omega-3 FA.[53] One study showed that low omega-6, high omega-3 FA diet decreased uLTE4, PGD metabolites, and nasal and asthma symptoms.[54]

BIOLOGICS

Although there are no biological therapies specifically approved for AERD, there are medications with indications for both asthma and nasal polyposis. This allows for on-label use of all 5 biological therapies on the market for high-T2 airway disease. Omalizumab is a recombinant antibody that binds to free IgE, thereby decreasing IgE density on mast cells and basophils. Omalizumab was initially approved for treatment of asthma, has demonstrated efficacy in AERD by decreasing symptoms during aspirin challenges.[55–57] This effect may be related to the downregulation of high-affinity receptors on mast cells, resulting in decreased mast cell activation and mediator production, with lower uLTE4 and PGD2 metabolite levels.[58] A recent phase 3 study evaluating the effectiveness of omalizumab in CRSwNP has been completed, but results are not yet available (NCT03280537).

Mepolizumab is a humanized monoclonal antibody that binds free interleukin 5 (IL-5), preventing it from binding to its receptor on the surface of eosinophils. Mepolizumab has shown efficacy in patients with eosinophilic asthma[59,60] and CRSwNP.[61] Patients with AERD treated with mepolizumab for greater than 3 months showed improvement in nasal congestion, anosmia, and asthma control.[62] No comparator studies have been done with mepolizumab in AERD.

Reslizumab, which acts similarly to mepolizumab, is also approved for severe eosinophilic asthma. Treatment effect in patients with CRSwNP was evaluated in a post-hoc analysis of 2 asthma clinical trials. Patients with a history consistent with AERD had an 84% reduction in asthma exacerbations; sinus outcomes were not evaluated.[63]

Benralizumab is a monoclonal antibody against the IL-5 receptor with a fucosylated modification that attracts natural killer cells to accelerate apoptosis. After administration, there is a dramatic decline in tissue eosinophils with nearly undetectable peripheral eosinophils.[64] Currently, benralizumab is approved for use in severe asthma with an eosinophilic phenotype but has not been specifically studied in AERD.

Dupilumab, a human monoclonal antibody that binds the alpha subunit of the IL-4 receptor, thereby blocking signaling of the Th2 cytokines IL-4 and IL-13, has been extensively studied in eosinophilic asthma, nasal polyposis, and atopic dermatitis.[65,66] Approved for nasal polyposis in 2019, dupilumab has not been studied specifically in AERD. However, in a subgroup analysis of patients with AERD, improvement in polyp outcome was equivalent to all those with CRSwNP.[67]

Biological therapies will likely be of enormous benefit to patients with AERD. Given the disease severity and highly eosinophilic nature of the disease, many patients with AERD qualify for biologic therapy. Whether a given biologic is superior or whether the magnitude of effect in AERD is similar to non-AERD patients merits further study.

UNIQUE EFFECTS OF ASPIRIN IN ASPIRIN-EXACERBATED RESPIRATORY DISEASE

Aspirin is an effective treatment in AERD, but the exact mechanism of action related to this benefit is poorly understood. It is thought that NSAID reactions arise in part from a shunting of arachidonic acid down the leukotriene pathway, with COX-1 inhibition, leading to excess CysLT production and PGE2 depletion.

The Mechanism of Aspirin Benefit in Aspirin-Exacerbated Respiratory Disease

Aspirin desensitization is characterized by diminished airway LTE4 responsiveness and nasal mucosal CysLT1 receptor expression.[20,21] This is likely secondary to a decrease in receptor-mediated signaling, as LTE4 is still produced at significant levels in patients with AERD on chronic aspirin therapy.[3,68] The beneficial effects of aspirin desensitization may, in part, be mediated by IL-4 and STAT6, as aspirin and ketorolac can decrease IL-4 induced STAT6 expression.[69] Desensitization is characterized by a decrease in prostanoid metabolites (thromboxane, PGE2, and PGD2), which is consistent with the effects of aspirin COX-1 antagonism.[3] There are increases in serum eosinophils and basophils with desensitization, possibly mediated by the chemokine receptor homologous molecule expressed on Th2 lymphocytes/D prostanoid 2 receptor (CRTH2/DP2) that causes PDG2-induced vasodilation and chemotaxis.[3,70–72] Aspirin-induced decrease in PDG2 CRTH2/DP2 stimulation may play a role in the changes seen in desensitization, with decreased tissue recruitment of eosinophils and thereby increased peripheral eosinophils, as is seen in aspirin reactions and chronic therapy.[3]

CLINICAL TRIALS OF ASPIRIN THERAPY IN ASPIRIN-EXACERBATED RESPIRATORY DISEASE

Aspirin therapy after desensitization (ATAD) is an effective treatment of upper and lower airway manifestations of AERD, with noticeable improvement as soon as 4 weeks after aspirin initiation[73,74] **(Table 1)**. After 6 months of treatment, a decrease

Table 1
Comparison of oral aspirin therapy after desensitization trials

	Stevenson et al,[81] 1984	Swierczynska-Krepa et al,[82] 2014	Esmaeilzadeh et al,[83] 2015	Fruth et al,[84] 2013
Study Type	Double-Blind Crossover	RDBPCT	RDBPCT	RCBPCT
Population	25 ATA	20 AIA, 14 ATA	34 CRSwNP, asthma, aspirin hypersensitivity	70 nasal polyps and CRS after sinus surgery, analgesic intolerance test >0.7
Duration	Two 3 month arms, 1 month washout	6 months	7 months	36 months
Aspirin dose	325 mg QD, 325 mg QID, 650 mg QID	624 mg QD	650 mg BID for 1 mo → 325 mg BID	100 mg QD
Definition of positive challenge	FEV1 decrease ≥25% compared with baseline	FEV1 decrease ≥20% compared with baseline	FEV1 decrease ≥20% compared with baseline or FEV1 decrease 15%–19% with nasoocular reaction/urticaria/angioedema	Not specified
Upper airway findings: aspirin vs placebo	• Decrease in nasal congestion and sinus pain • Trend but NS decrease in anosmia	• Decrease in SNOT-20, anosmia, sneeze, nasal blockade, and increase in peak nasal inspiratory flow • No change in sinus CT Lund-Mackay score	• Decrease in SNOT-22 • Decrease in sinus CT Lund-Mackay score	• Tendency but NS decrease in polyp relapse, anosmia • Later and less frequent polyp relapse on Kaplan-Meier curve • Improved nasal and paranasal quality of life and symptoms (nasal obstruction, postnasal drip, cephalgia, cough, sneeze, subjective olfaction)
Lower airway findings: aspirin vs placebo	• NS change in chest tightness, wheeze, cough, shortness of breath, chest congestion • 48% had decrease in asthma symptoms	• Decrease ACQ • No change in FEV1, PEF	• Increase in FEV1	Not measured

Effects on medication use: aspirin vs placebo	• Decrease in nasal beclomethasone; no change in prednisone dose	• No change in asthma rescue medication use; • Decrease in ICS dose	• Trend but NS improvement in doctor-rated medication scores (significantly better in aspirin group after treatment compared with baseline)	• Not measured
Other results	• Tendency but NS improvement in upper and lower airway symptoms with increased aspirin dose	• Effects only seen in those with AIA on aspirin, not ATA on aspirin or placebo nor AIA on placebo • Higher baseline uLTE4 AIA vs ATA, increase only seen with aspirin challenge in AIA; no change with prolonged aspirin therapy • Increase in baseline 9α,11β-PGF2 AIA vs ATA, no change with aspirin challenge or prolonged therapy	• Placebo group had less severe disease (significantly lower SNOT-22 and Lund-Mackay scores) vs active group • NS change in eosinophils, IL-10, IFN-γ, and TGF-β in active vs placebo group after treatment	• 55.7% drop out rate (none due to medication side effects), no intention to treat analysis • Improved general health quality of life in aspirin group

Abbreviations: ACQ, asthma control; AIA, aspirin-intolerant asthma; ATA, aspirin-tolerant asthma; BID, twice daily; ICS, inhaled corticosteroid; NS, non-significant; PEF, peak expiratory flow; PGF2, prostaglandin F2; QD, daily; QID, four times daily; RDBPCT, randomized double-blind placebo-controlled trial; SNOT, Sino-nasal Outcome Test.

in the number of sinus infections, sinus/nasal and asthma symptoms and courses of oral steroids was observed, with sustained improvement seen at 1 year in one study.[75] In patients with AERD who are on aspirin treatment for greater than 1 year, there was a decrease in hospitalizations, upper respiratory infections, sinus surgeries, use of systemic and inhaled steroids, and nasal endoscopy scores along with an improved sense of smell and increased nasal inspiratory flow.[76–78] In a group of 172 patients, 87% of those who were able to continue therapy for 1 year experienced improvement.[75] Re-operation is needed about every 3 years in AERD patients before desensitization, but aspirin therapy can decrease this to once every 10 years.[76,77] Long-term studies have demonstrated no additional sinus surgeries in AERD patients on aspirin during follow-up periods ranging from 24 to 30 months post-desensitization, compared with 80% of non-desensitized AERD patients needing revision surgery at 24 months in one study.[78–80] Desensitization has also been shown to improve alcohol tolerance in AERD.[18]

ASPIRIN-EXACERBATED RESPIRATORY DISEASE DIAGNOSIS

Aspirin challenge is the gold standard for AERD diagnosis, as there are no validated in vitro tests. uLTE4 is a promising AERD biomarker, but currently is not standardized for diagnostic purposes.[3] Obtaining a history of either NSAID hypersensitivity or tolerance is not sufficient to diagnose AERD; in one study, 15% of asthmatics became aware of aspirin sensitivity only following challenge.[85] As NSAID sensitivity is acquired over time, history of symptoms with NSAID ingestion may not be present, especially in those who have avoided these medications. Alternatively, symptoms may be attributed to a flare in the underlying disease or to the condition that prompted ingestion (respiratory infection, menses) rather than the NSAID itself. Moreover, tolerance of low-dose aspirin does not exclude NSAID sensitivity, as demonstrated in a case series where 6 subjects on 81 mg aspirin daily had positive challenges after stopping aspirin for 10 days, with 5 of those subjects reacting to 81 mg or less.[86]

Challenges are optimally performed before polypectomy to maximize diagnostic sensitivity, as 43% of patients who had pre-operative positive challenges were asymptomatic (silent challenge) with post-surgical challenge.[1,32] Conversely, desensitizations are optimally performed 2 to 4 weeks post-polypectomy. There are several different desensitization protocols that have been published; the benefits and drawbacks to these various protocols have been outlined elsewhere.[87]

DESENSITIZATION AND ASPIRIN MAINTENANCE THERAPY

Desensitization is often necessary, as non-aspirin therapies are often suboptimally effective, especially for preventing polyp regrowth and reducing symptoms and medication burden in AERD.[45,78,88] It provides an alternative to NSAID avoidance and decreases the medication burden while improving symptoms compared with AERD patients not taking aspirin.[76]

Maintenance of desensitization is accomplished via daily aspirin or other COX-1–blocking NSAID, but only aspirin has demonstrated efficacy in decreasing polyp regrowth and improving asthma and sinus symptoms. Re-sensitization occurs over a period of days after NSAIDs are discontinued, with partial (2–5 days) or complete (>5 days) repeat desensitization indicated depending on time from last dose.[89] Cross-desensitization to other NSAIDs is accomplished with at least 325 mg daily of aspirin or an equivalent dose of a COX-1 inhibitor, with perioperative ibuprofen bridging being done without adverse events or loss of desensitization.[89–91]

The lowest dose of maintenance aspirin required for symptom improvement is not well-defined. In a series of 137 patients, about 50% were able to decrease their maintenance dose from 650 to 325 mg aspirin twice daily without recurrence of symptoms.[92] Most patients have an increase in nasal congestion when the dose is less than 325 mg aspirin twice daily, although some studies have demonstrated efficacy when using 300 to 325 mg daily; lower doses (100 mg) may improve quality of life but do not decrease polyp regrowth.[79,81,84,91,92]

ASPIRIN SIDE EFFECTS AND COMPLICATIONS OF THERAPY

In patients with AERD who are on adequate aspirin doses, a lack of response to desensitization and maintenance therapy indicates either misdiagnosis or nonresponse. Symptom improvement was seen in 78% after excluding those who stopped aspirin; of those patients who did not improve, most had uncontrolled comorbidities.[75] There are patients without identified comorbidities who still fail to demonstrate improvement. Ethnicity may play a role in aspirin response, as all those who failed to complete desensitization or improve in one study were African American or Latino.[93] Differences in underlying inflammation may also be contributing to a lack of response to aspirin therapy. The arachidonic acid metabolite 15-Hydroxyeicosatetraenoic acid was significantly higher at baseline and after 4 weeks of treatment in AERD patients who had improvement in asthma symptoms and FEV1 compared with patients who worsened with ATAD.[32,93]

Failure to maintain desensitization, with NSAID-induced reactions occurring after an initial period of aspirin tolerance, is rare but has been reported.[94,95] The mechanism has not been fully elucidated but may be similar to those patients who are not able to tolerate the desensitization process, with increased baseline PGD2 and thromboxane levels and a larger increase in PDG2 during desensitization.[3]

Side effects occurred in about 23.3% of patients in one study, and the rate of discontinuation is reported to be 3.5% to 14%.[75,80,92] Gastrointestinal side effects are the most common, namely dyspepsia, gastrointestinal bleeding, and ulcers, although pancreatitis both during desensitization and maintenance therapy has been reported.[92,96,97]

SUMMARY

AERD is an important phenotype of nasal polyposis. Given the paucity of pharmacologic studies on this condition, AERD seems to be still underappreciated. Patients with AERD have the highest rates of polyp recurrence, have more difficult-to-control asthma, and likely account for a disproportionate share of health care costs compared with their aspirin-tolerant peers. The role of ATAD merits ongoing study, and the future potential of biological therapy offers promise. Further mechanistic insights into the cause and propagation of this intensely type 2–mediated disease will continue to inform our understanding of nasal polyposis and severe asthma.

DISCLOSURE

Drs K. Luskin and H. Thakrar have nothing to disclose. Dr A. White has served on the speakers bureau for Regeneron/Sanofi and AstraZeneca; the advisory board for Optinose and ALK; the board of directors for WSAAI; and a primary investigator for Cumberland Therapeutics.

REFERENCES

1. Woessner KM, White AA. Evidence-based approach to aspirin desensitization in aspirin-exacerbated respiratory disease. J Allergy Clin Immunol 2014;133(1): 286–7.e1-9.
2. Berges-Gimeno MP, Simon RA, Stevenson DD. The natural history and clinical characteristics of aspirin-exacerbated respiratory disease. Ann Allergy Asthma Immunol 2002;89(5):474–8.
3. Cahill KN, Bensko JC, Boyce JA, et al. Prostaglandin D2: A dominant mediator of aspirin exacerbated respiratory disease. J Allergy Clin Immunol 2015;135(1): 245–52.
4. U.S. Department of Health & Human Services. Most recent asthma data. Centers for Disease Control and Prevention. <cdc.gov/asthma/most_recent_data.htm>
5. Rajan JP, Wineinger NE, Stevenson DD, et al. Prevalence of aspirin-exacerbated respiratory disease among asthmatic patients: A meta-analysis of the literature. J Allergy Clin Immunol 2015;135(3):676–81.e1.
6. Li KL, Lee AY, Abuzeid WM. Aspirin exacerbated respiratory disease: epidemiology, pathophysiology, and management. Med Sci (Basel) 2019;7(3) [pii:E45].
7. Chang JE, White A, Simon RA, et al. Aspirin-exacerbated respiratory disease: burden of disease. Allergy Asthma Proc 2012;33(2):117–21.
8. Nurmagambetov T, Kuwahara R, Garbe P. The economic burden of asthma in the United States, 2008-2013. Ann Am Thorac Soc 2018;15(3):348–56.
9. Wertz DA, Pollack M, Rodgers K, et al. Impact of asthma control on sleep, attendance at work, normal activities, and disease burden. Ann Allergy Asthma Immunol 2010;105(2):118–23.
10. Lee JH, Haselkorn T, Borish L, et al. Risk factors associated with persistent airflow limitation in severe or difficult-to-treat asthma: insights from the TENOR study. Chest 2007;132(6):1882–9.
11. Kim JE, Kountakis SE. The prevalence of Samter's triad in patients undergoing functional endoscopic sinus surgery. Ear Nose Throat J 2007;86(7):396–9.
12. Pleis JR, Lucas JW, Ward BW. Summary health statistics for U.S. adults: National Health Interview Survey, 2008. Vital Health Stat 10 2009;(242):1–157.
13. Ta V, White AA. Survey-defined patient experiences with aspirin-exacerbated respiratory disease. J Allergy Clin Immunol Pract 2015;3(5):711–8.
14. Vally H, de Klerk N, Thompson PJ. Alcoholic drinks: important triggers for asthma. J Allergy Clin Immunol 2000;105(3):462–7.
15. Dahl R, Henriksen JM, Harving H. Red wine asthma: a controlled challenge study. J Allergy Clin Immunol 1986;78(6):1126–9.
16. Nihlen U, Greiff LJ, Nyberg P, et al. Alcohol-induced upper airway symptoms: prevalence and co-morbidity. Respir Med 2005;99(6):762–9.
17. Cardet JC, White AA, Barrett NA, et al. Alcohol-induced respiratory symptoms are common in patients with aspirin exacerbated respiratory disease. J Allergy Clin Immunol Pract 2014;2(2):208–13.
18. Glicksman JT, Parasher AK, Doghramji L, et al. Alcohol-induced respiratory symptoms improve after aspirin desensitization in patients with aspirin-exacerbated respiratory disease. Int Forum Allergy Rhinol 2018;8(10):1093–7.
19. Dahlén B, Nizankowska E, Szczeklik A, et al. Benefits from adding the 5-lipoxygenase inhibitor zileuton to conventional therapy in aspirin-intolerant asthmatics. Am J Respir Crit Care Med 1998;157(4 Pt 1):1187–94.

20. Sousa AR, Parikh A, Scadding G, et al. Leukotriene-receptor expression on nasal mucosal inflammatory cells in aspirin-sensitive rhinosinusitis. N Engl J Med 2002; 347(19):1493–9.
21. Arm JP, O'Hickey SP, Spur BW, et al. Airway responsiveness to histamine and leukotriene E4 in subjects with aspirin-induced asthma. Am Rev Respir Dis 1989;140(1):148–53.
22. Nizankowska E, Bestynska-Krypel A, Cmiel A, et al. Oral and bronchial provocation tests with aspirin for diagnosis of aspirin-induced asthma. Eur Respir J 2000; 15(5):863–9.
23. Daffern PJ, Muilenburg D, Hugli TE, et al. Association of urinary leukotriene E4 excretion during aspirin challenges with severity of respiratory responses. J Allergy Clin Immunol 1999;104(3 Pt 1):559–64.
24. Yoshida S, Amayasu H, Sakamoto H, et al. Cromolyn sodium prevents broncho-constriction and urinary LTE4 excretion in aspirin-induced asthma. Ann Allergy Asthma Immunol 1998;80(2):171–6.
25. Imokawa S, Sato A, Taniguchi M, et al. Sodium cromoglycate nebulized solution has an acute bronchodilative effect in patients with aspirin-intolerant asthma (AIA). Arerugi 1992;41(10):1515–20.
26. Cahill KN, Murphy K, Singer J, et al. Plasma tryptase elevation during aspirin-induced reactions in aspirin-exacerbated respiratory disease. J Allergy Clin Immunol 2019;143(2):799–803.e2.
27. Bankova LG, Lai J, Yoshimoto E, et al. Leukotriene E4 elicits respiratory epithelial cell mucin release through the G-protein-coupled receptor, GPR99. Proc Natl Acad Sci U S A 2016;113(22):6242–7.
28. Bankova LG, Boyce JA. A new spin on mast cells and cysteinyl leukotrienes: Leukotriene E4 activates mast cells in vivo. J Allergy Clin Immunol 2018;142(4): 1056–7.
29. Lazarinis N, Bood J, Gomez C, et al. Leukotriene E4 induces airflow obstruction and mast cell activation through the cysteinyl leukotriene type 1 receptor. J Allergy Clin Immunol 2018;142(4):1080–9.
30. Feng X, Ramsden MK, Negri J, et al. Eosinophil production of prostaglandin D2 in patients with aspirin-exacerbated respiratory disease. J Allergy Clin Immunol 2016;138(4):1089–97.e3.
31. Steinke JW, Liu L, Huyett P, et al. Prominent role of IFN-gamma in patients with aspirin-exacerbated respiratory disease. J Allergy Clin Immunol 2013;132(4): 856–65.e1-3.
32. Jerschow E, Edin ML, Chi Y, et al. Sinus surgery is associated with a decrease in aspirin-induced reaction severity in patients with aspirin exacerbated respiratory disease. J Allergy Clin Immunol Pract 2019;7(5):1580–8.
33. Laidlaw TM, Kidder MS, Bhattacharyya N, et al. Cysteinyl leukotriene overproduction in aspirin-exacerbated respiratory disease is driven by platelet-adherent leukocytes. Blood 2012;119(16):3790–8.
34. Eastman JJ, Cavagnero KJ, Deconde AS, et al. Group 2 innate lymphoid cells are recruited to the nasal mucosa in patients with aspirin-exacerbated respiratory disease. J Allergy Clin Immunol 2017;140(1):101–8.e3.
35. Kanaoka Y, Maekawa A, Austen KF. Identification of GPR99 protein as a potential third cysteinyl leukotriene receptor with a preference for leukotriene E4 ligand. J Biol Chem 2013;288(16):10967–72.
36. Sarau HM, Ames RS, Chambers J, et al. Identification, molecular cloning, expression, and characterization of a cysteinyl leukotriene receptor. Mol Pharmacol 1999;56(3):657–63.

37. Steinke JW, Wilson JM. Aspirin-exacerbated respiratory disease: pathophysiological insights and clinical advances. J Asthma Allergy 2016;9:37–43.
38. White AA, Stevenson DD, Simon RA. The blocking effect of essential controller medications during aspirin challenges in patients with aspirin-exacerbated respiratory disease. Ann Allergy Asthma Immunol 2005;95(4):330–5.
39. Berges-Gimeno MP, Simon RA, Stevenson DD. The effect of leukotriene-modifier drugs on aspirin-induced asthma and rhinitis reactions. Clin Exp Allergy 2002; 32(10):1491–6.
40. Dahlén SE, Malmström K, Nizankowska E, et al. Improvement of aspirin-intolerant asthma by montelukast, a leukotriene antagonist: a randomized, double-blind, placebo-controlled trial. Am J Respir Crit Care Med 2002;165(1):9–14.
41. Lee DK, Haggart K, Robb FM, et al. Montelukast protects against nasal lysine-aspirin challenge in patients with aspirin-induced asthma. Eur Respir J 2004; 24(2):226–30.
42. White AA, Laidlaw TM, Woessner K. Anaphylaxis and hypersensitivity reactions. In: Castells MC, editor. Anaphylaxis and hypersensitivity reactions. New York: Humana Press; 2019. p. 116.
43. Small CB, Hernandez J, Reyes A, et al. Efficacy and safety of mometasone furoate nasal spray in nasal polyposis. J Allergy Clin Immunol 2005;116(6):1275–81.
44. Stjärne P, Olsson P, Alenius M. Use of mometasone furoate to prevent polyp relapse after endoscopic sinus surgery. Arch Otolaryngol Head Neck Surg 2009;135(3):296–302.
45. Rotenberg BW, Zhang I, Arra I, et al. Postoperative care for Samter's triad patients undergoing endoscopic sinus surgery: a double-blinded, randomized controlled trial. Laryngoscope 2011;121(12):2702–5.
46. Leopold DA, Elkayam D, Messina JC, et al. NAVIGATE II: randomized, double-blind trial of the exhalation delivery system with fluticasone for nasal polyposis. J Allergy Clin Immunol 2019;143(1):126–34.e5.
47. Steinke JW, Payne SC, Tessier ME, et al. Pilot study of budesonide inhalant suspension irrigations for chronic eosinophilic sinusitis. J Allergy Clin Immunol 2009; 124(6):1352–4.e7.
48. Laidlaw TM, Cahill KN, Cardet JC, et al. A trial of type 12 purinergic (P2Y12) receptor inhibition with prasugrel identifies a potentially distinct endotype of patients with aspirin-exacerbated respiratory disease. J Allergy Clin Immunol 2019;143(1):316–24.e7.
49. Sommer DD, Hoffbauer S, Au M, et al. Treatment of aspirin exacerbated respiratory disease with a low salicylate diet: a pilot crossover study. Otolaryngol Head Neck Surg 2015;152(1):42–7.
50. Sommer DD, Rotenberg BW, Sowerby LJ, et al. A novel treatment adjunct for aspirin exacerbated respiratory disease: the low-salicylate diet: a multicenter randomized control crossover trial. Int Forum Allergy Rhinol 2016;6(4):385–91.
51. von Schacky C, Kiefl R, Jendraschak E, et al. n-3 fatty acids and cysteinyl-leukotriene formation in humans in vitro, ex vivo, and in vivo. J Lab Clin Med 1993;121(2):302–9.
52. Lee TH, Hoover RL, Williams JD, et al. Effect of dietary enrichment with eicosapentaenoic and docosahexaenoic acids on in vitro neutrophil and monocyte leukotriene generation and neutrophil function. N Engl J Med 1985;312(19): 1217–24.
53. Innes JK, Calder PC. Omega-6 fatty acids and inflammation. Prostaglandins Leukot Essent Fatty Acids 2018;132:41–8.

54. Schneider TR, Johns CB, Palumbo ML, et al. Dietary fatty acid modification for the treatment of aspirin-exacerbated respiratory disease: a prospective pilot trial. J Allergy Clin Immunol Pract 2018;6(3):825–31.
55. Bobolea I, Barranco P, Fiandor A, et al. Omalizumab: a potential new therapeutic approach for aspirin-exacerbated respiratory disease. J Investig Allergol Clin Immunol 2010;20(5):448–9.
56. Bergmann KC, Zuberbier T, Church MK. Omalizumab in the treatment of aspirin-exacerbated respiratory disease. J Allergy Clin Immunol Pract 2015;3(3):459–60.
57. Lang DM, Aronica MA, Maierson ES, et al. Omalizumab can inhibit respiratory reaction during aspirin desensitization. Ann Allergy Asthma Immunol 2018;121(1): 98–104.
58. Hayashi H, Mitsui C, Nakatani E, et al. Omalizumab reduces cysteinyl leukotriene and 9α,11β-prostaglandin F2 overproduction in aspirin-exacerbated respiratory disease. J Allergy Clin Immunol 2016;137(5):1585–7.e4.
59. Bel EH, Wenzel SE, Thompson PJ, et al. Oral glucocorticoid-sparing effect of mepolizumab in eosinophilic asthma. N Engl J Med 2014;371(13):1189–97.
60. Ortega HG, Liu MC, Pavord ID, et al. Mepolizumab treatment in patients with severe eosinophilic asthma. N Engl J Med 2014;371(13):1198–207.
61. Gevaert P, Van Bruaene N, Cattaert T, et al. Mepolizumab, a humanized anti-IL-5 mAb, as a treatment option for severe nasal polyposis. J Allergy Clin Immunol 2011;128(5):989–95.e1-8.
62. Tuttle KL, Buchheit KM, Laidlaw TM, et al. A retrospective analysis of mepolizumab in subjects with aspirin-exacerbated respiratory disease. J Allergy Clin Immunol Pract 2018;6(3):1045–7.
63. Katial RH F, Germinaria M, McDonald M. Efficacy of reslizumab in asthma patients with aspirin sensitivity and elevated blood eosinophils. J Allergy Clin Immunol 2017;139(2):AB8.
64. Pelaia C, Calabrese C, Vatrella A, et al. Benralizumab: from the basic mechanism of action to the potential use in the biological therapy of severe eosinophilic asthma. Biomed Res Int 2018;2018:4839230.
65. Wenzel S, Ford L, Pearlman D, et al. Dupilumab in persistent asthma with elevated eosinophil levels. N Engl J Med 2013;368(26):2455–66.
66. Beck LA, Thaçi D, Hamilton JD, et al. Dupilumab treatment in adults with moderate-to-severe atopic dermatitis. N Engl J Med 2014;371(2):130–9.
67. Laidlaw TM, Mullol J, Fan C, et al. Dupilumab improves nasal polyp burden and asthma control in patients with CRSwNP and AERD. J Allergy Clin Immunol Pract 2019;7(7):2462–5.e1.
68. Nasser SM, Patel M, Bell GS, et al. The effect of aspirin desensitization on urinary leukotriene E4 concentrations in aspirin-sensitive asthma. Am J Respir Crit Care Med 1995;151(5):1326–30.
69. Steinke JW, Culp JA, Kropf E, et al. Modulation by aspirin of nuclear phosphosignal transducer and activator of transcription 6 expression: Possible role in therapeutic benefit associated with aspirin desensitization. J Allergy Clin Immunol 2009;124(4):724–30.e4.
70. Kupczyk M, Kurmanowska Z, Kuprys-Lipinska I, et al. Mediators of inflammation in nasal lavage from aspirin intolerant patients after aspirin challenge. Respir Med 2010;104(10):1404–9.
71. Hirai H, Tanaka K, Yoshie O, et al. Prostaglandin D2 selectively induces chemotaxis in T helper type 2 cells, eosinophils, and basophils via seven-transmembrane receptor CRTH2. J Exp Med 2001;193(2):255–61.

72. Xue L, Salimi M, Panse I, et al. Prostaglandin D2 activates group 2 innate lymphoid cells through chemoattractant receptor-homologous molecule expressed on TH2 cells. J Allergy Clin Immunol 2014;133(4):1184–94.

73. Berges-Gimeno MP, Simon RA, Stevenson DD. Early effects of aspirin desensitization treatment in asthmatic patients with aspirin-exacerbated respiratory disease. Ann Allergy Asthma Immunol 2003;90(3):338–41.

74. Williams AN, Woessner KM. The clinical effectiveness of aspirin desensitization in chronic rhinosinusitis. Curr Allergy Asthma Rep 2008;8(3):245–52.

75. Berges-Gimeno MP, Simon RA, Stevenson DD. Long-term treatment with aspirin desensitization in asthmatic patients with aspirin-exacerbated respiratory disease. J Allergy Clin Immunol 2003;111(1):180–6.

76. Sweet JM, Stevenson DD, Simon RA, et al. Long-term effects of aspirin desensitization–treatment for aspirin-sensitive rhinosinusitis-asthma. J Allergy Clin Immunol 1990;85(1 Pt 1):59–65.

77. Stevenson DD, Hankammer MA, Mathison DA, et al. Aspirin desensitization treatment of aspirin-sensitive patients with rhinosinusitis-asthma: long-term outcomes. J Allergy Clin Immunol 1996;98(4):751–8.

78. McMains KC, Kountakis SE. Medical and surgical considerations in patients with Samter's triad. Am J Rhinol 2006;20(6):573–6.

79. Rozsasi A, Polzehl D, Deutschle T, et al. Long-term treatment with aspirin desensitization: a prospective clinical trial comparing 100 and 300 mg aspirin daily. Allergy 2008;63(9):1228–34.

80. Cho KS, Soudry E, Psaltis AJ, et al. Long-term sinonasal outcomes of aspirin desensitization in aspirin exacerbated respiratory disease. Otolaryngol Head Neck Surg 2014;151(4):575–81.

81. Stevenson DD, Pleskow WW, Simon RA, et al. Aspirin-sensitive rhinosinusitis asthma: a double-blind crossover study of treatment with aspirin. J Allergy Clin Immunol 1984;73(4):500–7.

82. Swierczynska-Krepa M, Sanak M, Bochenek G, et al. Aspirin desensitization in patients with aspirin-induced and aspirin-tolerant asthma: a double-blind study. J Allergy Clin Immunol 2014;134(4):883–90.

83. Esmaeilzadeh H, Nabavi M, Aryan Z, et al. Aspirin desensitization for patients with aspirin-exacerbated respiratory disease: A randomized double-blind placebo-controlled trial. Clin Immunol 2015;160(2):349–57.

84. Fruth K, Pogorzelski B, Schmidtmann I, et al. Low-dose aspirin desensitization in individuals with aspirin-exacerbated respiratory disease. Allergy 2013;68(5):659–65.

85. Szczeklik A, Nizankowska E, Duplaga M. Natural history of aspirin-induced asthma. AIANE Investigators. European Network on Aspirin-Induced Asthma. Eur Respir J 2000;16(3):432–6.

86. Lee-Sarwar K, Johns C, Laidlaw TM, et al. Tolerance of chronic low-dose aspirin does not preclude aspirin exacerbated respiratory disease. J Allergy Clin Immunol Pract 2015;3(3):449–51.

87. White AA, Stevenson DD. Aspirin desensitization: faster protocols for busy patients. J Allergy Clin Immunol Pract 2019;7(4):1181–3.

88. Havel M, Ertl L, Braunschweig F, et al. Sinonasal outcome under aspirin desensitization following functional endoscopic sinus surgery in patients with aspirin triad. Eur Arch Otorhinolaryngol 2013;270(2):571–8.

89. Lee RU, Stevenson DD. Aspirin-exacerbated respiratory disease: evaluation and management. Allergy Asthma Immunol Res 2011;3(1):3–10.

90. Stevenson DD. Aspirin sensitivity and desensitization for asthma and sinusitis. Curr Allergy Asthma Rep 2009;9(2):155–63.
91. Do TT, Ishmael FT, Craig T. Long-term follow-up of patients with aspirin-exacerbated respiratory disease status post-desensitization. J Allergy Clin Immunol 2018;141(2):AB215.
92. Lee JY, Simon RA, Stevenson DD. Selection of aspirin dosages for aspirin desensitization treatment in patients with aspirin-exacerbated respiratory disease. J Allergy Clin Immunol 2007;119(1):157–64.
93. Jerschow E, Edin ML, Pelletier T, et al. Plasma 15-hydroxyeicosatetraenoic acid predicts treatment outcomes in aspirin-exacerbated respiratory disease. J Allergy Clin Immunol Pract 2017;5(4):998–1007.e2.
94. Rothe T, Achermann R, Hug J, et al. Incomplete aspirin desensitization in an aspirin-sensitive asthmatic. Int Arch Allergy Immunol 1996;109(3):298–300.
95. White AA, Hope AP, Stevenson DD. Failure to maintain an aspirin-desensitized state in a patient with aspirin-exacerbated respiratory disease. Ann Allergy Asthma Immunol 2006;97(4):446–8.
96. Hoyte FC, Weber RW, Katial RK. Pancreatitis as a novel complication of aspirin therapy in patients with aspirin-exacerbated respiratory disease. J Allergy Clin Immunol 2012;129:1684–6.
97. Durrani SR, Kelly JT. Pancreatitis as a complication of aspirin desensitization for aspirin-exacerbated respiratory disease. J Allergy Clin Immunol 2013;131(1):244–6.

Current Concepts in the Management of Allergic Fungal Rhinosinusitis

Matthew A. Tyler, MD[a], Amber U. Luong, MD, PhD[b,c],*

KEYWORDS

- Allergic fungal rhinosinusitis • Chronic rhinosinusitis • Nasal polyps
- Type 2 inflammation • Allergic sinusitis • Fungal sinusitis • Fungal allergy
- Eosinophilic mucin rhinosinusitis

KEY POINTS

- The Bent and Kuhn diagnostic criteria serve as the framework for diagnosis of allergic fungal rhinosinusitis (AFRS).
- The pathophysiology of AFRS is hypothesized to result from a combination of defective mucosal barrier function, altered innate immune signaling, and fungal overgrowth, which culminate in a localized, hyperallergic type 2 immune response.
- Standard therapy for AFRS includes complete surgery in combination with systemic and topical steroids.
- Adjunctive treatments like immunotherapy, antifungal therapy, and biologic therapy may have some benefit in recalcitrant cases of AFRS.

INTRODUCTION

Katzenstein and colleagues[1,2] were among the first to describe a unique type of fungal sinusitis in 7 patients, characterized by the presence of thick, mucinous material with impacted fungal elements and termed it, "allergic *Aspergillus* sinusitis." The investigators noted a striking similarity with allergic bronchopulmonary

[a] Department of Otolaryngology–Head and Neck Surgery, University of Minnesota Medical School, 516 Delaware Street Southeast, # 8A, Minneapolis, MN 55455, USA; [b] Department of Otorhinolaryngology–Head & Neck Surgery, McGovern Medical School at the University of Texas Health Science Center, Texas Sinus Institute, 6431 Fannin Street, MSB 5.036, Houston, TX 77030, USA; [c] Center for Immunology and Autoimmune Diseases, Institute of Molecular Medicine, McGovern Medical School at the University of Texas Health Science Center, Houston, TX, USA
* Corresponding author. Department of Otorhinolaryngology–Head & Neck Surgery, McGovern Medical School at the University of Texas Health Science Center, Texas Sinus Institute, 6431 Fannin Street, MSB 5.036, Houston, TX 77030.
E-mail address: amber.u.luong@uth.tmc.edu

Immunol Allergy Clin N Am 40 (2020) 345–359
https://doi.org/10.1016/j.iac.2019.12.001
0889-8561/20/© 2019 Elsevier Inc. All rights reserved.
immunology.theclinics.com

aspergillosis, where thick concretions of mucin lead to lower airway obstruction in the lung. Allergic fungal rhinosinusitis (AFRS) initially was conceptualized by many to represent a subtype of fungal sinusitis along with invasive fungal sinusitis and sinus fungus ball; now, it is instead thought to be a subtype of chronic rhinosinusitis (CRS). Subsequent investigations showed that a variety of fungal species could be associated with an identical clinical presentation, so the more encompassing term, *allergic fungal rhinosinusitis*, was adopted. In 1993, Bent and Kuhn[3] established criteria for diagnosis of AFRS based on their prospective review of 15 patients. These 5 diagnostic criteria are

1. Type I hypersensitivity to fungi
2. Characteristic areas of hyperattenuation on computed tomography (CT)
3. Eosinophilic mucin
4. Nasal polyps
5. Presence of noninvasive fungus within sinus mucin[3]

EPIDEMIOLOGY AND RISK FACTORS IN ALLERGIC FUNGAL RHINOSINUSITIS

AFRS demonstrates a higher prevalence in South Central and Southeastern United States, where it is believed that higher mold counts lead to greater disease burden in these territories.[4] It remains unclear, however, if mold counts truly correlate with the rate of AFRS in these regions. AFRS is more common in men and presents at a mean age range of 21 years to 33 years.[5–9] Certain studies have identified patients with lower socioeconomic status as more prone to advanced presentation, including bone erosion and orbitocranial complications; however, these studies have been disputed by other investigators showing that socioeconomic status has no association with disease severity.[7,10–12] Where early descriptions of AFRS cited a high rate of comorbid asthma, recent studies have found that the prevalence of asthma is approximately half that of patients with non-AFRS CRS with nasal polyps (CRSwNP), suggesting a unique underlying pathophysiology in AFRS.[9,13–15]

DIAGNOSIS OF ALLERGIC FUNGAL RHINOSINUSITIS

Among otolaryngologists, the Bent and Kuhn diagnostic criteria still serve as the framework for diagnosis of AFRS. Sometimes, advanced presentation on physical examination is heralded by the presence of proptosis or extensive polyposis. The radiographic findings in patients with AFRS is remarkable; some investigators propose that these features are among the most clinically differentiating characteristics of AFRS (**Fig. 1**).[16] The classic CT radiographic appearance includes unilateral diseased sinuses, bony expansion/erosion of the sinus walls, and areas of hyperattenuation. Imaging in AFRS may mimic that in inverted papilloma or, more worrisome, malignancy. AFRS typically, however, is an expansile process and does not exhibit features of bony or soft tissue invasion. Peripheral eosinophilia may not always be present; however, serum IgE levels often are elevated, many times more than 1000 U/mL. Fungal-specific hypersensitivity, by itself, is not specific for AFRS, because fungal-specific IgE and IgG are present in both non-AFRS CRS and AFRS.[17–19] Similarly, positive fungal cultures can be recovered from both non-AFRS CRS and healthy controls.[20,21] Intraoperatively, the thick, tenacious mucin should further alert a surgeon to the possibility of AFRS, and, along with the presence of noninvasive fungal elements on pathologic analysis, the diagnosis is more likely. The challenge of making a diagnosis of AFRS arises in cases of revision surgery, when polyposis and thick mucinous debris may not be as apparent as in the primary surgery.

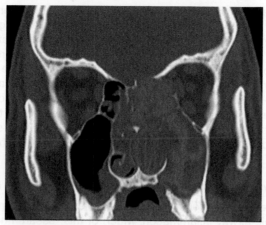

Fig. 1. Imaging features characteristic of AFRS. This coronal image demonstrates predominately unilateral disease with expansion of the ethmoid cavity. There is demineralization of the lamina papyracea and ethmoid roof. Central hyperattenuation suggests the presence of inspissated, eosinophilic mucin with fungal elements.

PATHOPHYSIOLOGY OF ALLERGIC FUNGAL RHINOSINUSITIS
Alterations in Innate Immunity and Barrier Function

The sinonasal mucosa, its epithelium, and a diverse milieu of proteins and peptides make up a constitutive line of defense in the prevention of pathogen infiltration and immune stimulation in the sinonasal cavity. The immune barrier hypothesis in CRS hypothesizes that alterations in mucosal barrier function lead to chronic inflammation by (1) permitting over-colonization of sinonasal mucosa with pathogenic microbiota, which (2) acts as a source of antigenic stimulation and inflammation in the sinuses.[22] Preliminary studies have indicated that defective barrier function may be a source of fungal over-colonization and overactive adaptive immune stimulation in AFRS. For example, in vitro studies have shown that AFRS epithelial resistance is lowered compared with controls, which may be the result of increased expression of type 2 inflammatory cytokines, like interleukin (IL)-4 and IL-13.[23,24] Studies in AFRS also have shown reduced expression of antimicrobial peptides, including surfactant protein D, lactoferrin, and histatins.[13,25,26]

Type 2 Inflammation and Adaptive Immunity

More recently, an emphasis has been placed on type 2 inflammation and eosinophilia in categorizing subtypes, or endotypes, of CRS, because this often is a marker of recalcitrant sinus inflammation in CRS. Certainly, AFRS represents an exaggerated type 2 inflammatory response characterized by allergic-type, eosinophilic inflammation. Underlying this profound type 2 inflammatory response seems to be an alteration in the local, sinonasal adaptive immune response. For instance, patients with AFRS demonstrates altered frequencies in HLA major histocompatibility complex class II (MHC II) DQB1*03 allelic variants.[27] Separate investigations have shown that local and circulating dendritic cells are elevated in AFRS, although this also has been observed in CRSwNP.[28,29] Furthermore, Pant and Macardle[30] have shown that patients with AFRS exhibit defective CD8$^+$ T-cell response to fungi, suggesting that this alteration may permit local fungal accumulation in these patients, and the resultant inflammatory response can be exacerbated by the presence of fungal/allergic hypersensitivity. In a recent study performed by Tyler and colleagues,[13] whole-genome analysis was performed using inflamed sinus mucosal specimen from AFRS and CRSwNP, in which approximately 3000 unique gene expression variations were identified in AFRS that differentiated it from CRSwNP. Many of these unique gene expression variations were associated with alterations in gene expression pathways associated with adaptive immunity, including antigen-sensing pathways, costimulatory signaling, and T-cell receptor signaling. Additional studies are needed to better understand the mechanisms leading to this profound over-activation of the adaptive immune system in AFRS; however, this appears to be a distinct feature that separates this subtype from other subtypes of CRS.

The Role of Fungus in the Immunopathogenesis of Allergic Fungal Rhinosinusitis

Mechanistic studies have demonstrated a direct role of fungal elements in the pathogenesis of allergic airway inflammation. Much of this research has been proliferated in the field of asthma and allergy. These studies have provided insight in regard to fungal immunopathogenesis in AFRS. Important proinflammatory fungal molecules, either secreted or present in the cell wall, include β-glucan, chitin, glycosidases, and fungal proteases. Fungal proteases are among the most studied disease mediators in allergy, asthma and AFRS. Proteases from *Aspergillus* species have been shown to induce classic molecular signatures of type 2 inflammation, including IL-4, IL-5, and IL-13 production; eosinophilia; and airway goblet hyperplasia.[31–33] This has been shown to be mediated partially by cleavage of fibrinogen, which signals through pattern recognition receptors, such as Toll-like receptor 4 (TLR4), to induce antifungal and allergic airway inflammation.[32] Fungal elements also promote innate immune cells to secrete cytokines that promote type 2 inflammation. Patel and colleagues[34] have shown that fungal extracts promote solitary chemosensory cells isolated from AFRS patient polyps to expand and increase secretion of the innate inflammatory mediator, IL-25. Other studies have demonstrated that fungal extracts promote the release of innate inflammatory mediators, like IL-33, a potent effector of type 2 helper T cell (T_H2) polarization and type 2 inflammation, from airway epithelial cells.[35] Increasing emphasis also has been placed on the importance of the group 2 innate lymphoid cells in fungal-mediated allergic airway inflammation.[36] This relatively recently described population of cells is responsive to IL-25 and IL-33 and represents an important effector cell type responsible for T_H2 polarization in response to fungal stimulation.[36–38]

To summarize, the observed phenotype in AFRS may be the result of innate barrier dysfunction and a dysfunctional antifungal response. As a result, fungal conidia accumulate in the sinuses, germinating to fungal hyphae, and promote the over-activation of local innate and adaptive type 2 immune responses. A diagram summarizing proposed mechanisms of the pathophysiology in AFRS is presented in **Fig. 2**.

TREATMENT OF ALLERGIC FUNGAL RHINOSINUSITIS
Surgery

Endoscopic sinus surgery (ESS) represents a standard of care in the management of AFRS. Complete evacuation of fungus and eosinophilic mucin from involved sinuses is of paramount importance. Leaving residual fungi and eosinophilic debris can lead to a rapid recurrence in fungal colonization, inflammation, and patient symptoms. Infrequently, erosion and expansion of the bony walls of the sinuses occur to the extent

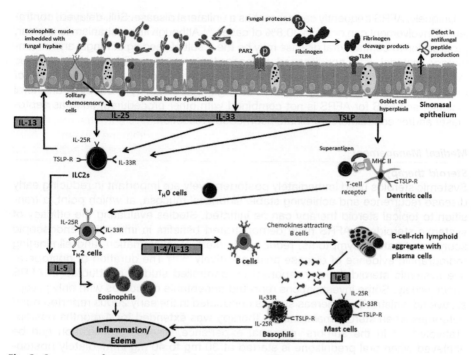

Fig. 2. Summary of proposed pathophysiology in AFRS. There are several mechanisms that may contribute to the overactive type 2 inflammatory response observed in AFRS. Loss of antifungal peptides, changes in epithelial permeability, fungal proteases, and other fungal elements together contribute to production of innate inflammatory cytokines, including IL-25, IL-33, and thymic stromal lymphopoietin (TSLP). Innate lymphoid cells, which are IL-25 responsive and IL-33 responsive, are capable of producing IL-5, which promotes eosinophil recruitment and activation. Dendritic cells respond to the presence of innate inflammatory mediators, like TSLP, and antigenic stimulation by fungal (and other) microbiota, which then promotes T_H2 cell development. In addition, T-cell activation can be activated further by superantigens. T_H2 activation affects B-cell isotype switching and differentiation to IgE-producing and IgG-producing plasma cells, further promoting a hyperallergic inflammation within the sinuses. TSLP-R, thymic stromal lymphopoietin receptor; ILC2, type 2 innate lymphoid cell.

that there is a risk of orbital and/or cranial complications.[39,40] These complications can occur in severe cases that are left untreated. Despite a significant expansion of the sinus boundaries causing cranial compression, dural invasion and CSF fistulae usually are not present. Not only can surgery be undertaken to prevent, and many times reverse, complication but also a thorough and complete evacuation of inflammatory mucin and fungal elements can be performed in the same setting, such that staging of surgery is not necessary. Given that distortion of normal anatomic landmarks is commonplace in AFRS, computerized image guidance is an indispensable tool in these endeavors.

The expansion of the sinuses often makes complete evacuation of fungal elements and inflammatory mucin challenging. The authors have found specialized instrumentation, including the Hydrodebrider (Medtronic, Minneapolis, Minnesota), a valuable tool that allows for complete removal of inflammatory debris and fungus. This powered irrigation system includes a flexible and rotatable instrument tip that aids with clearing of tenacious inflammatory debris residing within deep recesses of expanded sinuses.

Uniquely, AFRS frequently can present as a unilateral disease. Still, delayed, contralateral involvement can occur in 30.8% of cases.[41] Although its mechanism is unclear, progression to contralateral disease may be the result of seeding of fungal and inflammatory material into nondiseased mucosa that is susceptible to hyperallergic inflammatory response. For this reason, in the authors' practice, instrumentation of the contralateral side typically is limited during primary surgery in cases of unilateral disease; and ESS for AFRS is not combined with other procedures, such as septoplasty and/or contralateral turbinate submucous resection.

Medical Management

Steroid therapy

Systemic steroids used immediately postoperatively are important in reducing early disease recurrence and achieving stable sinonasal mucosa, at which point, a transition to topical steroid therapy can be initiated. Studies evaluating the efficacy of systemic steroids in AFRS have demonstrated benefits in improving endoscopic scores and patient symptoms, reducing markers of inflammation, and eliminating radiographic evidence of disease postoperatively.[42–45] The duration of postoperative systemic steroid therapy reported by controlled studies conducted in AFRS varies widely. Some investigations reported acceptable outcomes with only preoperative administration, whereas studies conducted in the early 2000s reported good outcomes when steroid maintenance therapy was extended for 4 months postoperatively.[42–45] In the authors' personal experience, disease stabilization can be achieved when oral prednisone is started at 30 mg to 40 mg immediately postoperatively and tapered 7 days to 14 days after surgery, when topical steroid therapy can be initiated.

Like systemic steroids, topical nasal steroids are a mainstay in the management of AFRS. Regular topical nasal steroids delivered via standard spray device have demonstrated efficacy in reducing symptoms and polyp size in the setting of CRSwNP.[46–48] There have been limited studies conducted in the context of AFRS; however, expert opinion indicates that the use of long-term topical nasal steroids is indicated in AFRS. In the authors' personal experience, the use of nonstandard, or off-label, topical nasal steroids, like high-volume budesonide irrigations (0.25-mg/2 mL or 0.5-mg/2 mL respules in 240 mL of nasal saline solution), is effective in reducing inflammation in the sinonasal cavity early postoperatively, especially in cases of severe disease. When indicated, high-volume steroid irrigations can be continued long term, because studies have demonstrated that use for 1 year or longer can be safe. Regular testing of cortisol levels to ensure no HPA axis suppression occurs, however, may be necessary.[49,50]

Antifungal therapy

The use of antifungal therapy typically is limited to the azole class of antifungals (ie, posaconazole, itraconazole, and others), because this drug class targets the genus of fungi commonly associated with AFRS. There currently is a paucity of high-quality evidence that supports the use of oral antifungals in the setting of AFRS; however, the available studies performed in AFRS suggest that there may be some benefit. Rojita and colleagues[51] conducted a prospective randomized clinical trial in 60 patients with AFRS diagnosed by the Bent and Kuhn criteria, in which they compared systemic steroids (given for 1 month postoperatively) plus nasal steroid spray versus oral itraconazole (100 mg twice a day, given for 6 months postoperatively). The study found no difference between the 2 groups using mean 20-item Sino-Nasal Outcome Test (SNOT-20), serum IgE level, and eosinophil count as outcomes. The investigators conclude that itraconazole used postoperatively may be a safe and effective alternative to systemic steroid therapy in AFRS patients.

A handful of retrospective studies have evaluated the efficacy of systemic antifungal therapies in AFRS. The largest was performed by Rains and Mineck,[52] including 139 patients diagnosed with AFRS using the Bent and Kuhn criteria. The investigators describe a regimen of high-dose itraconazole (400 mg/d for 1 month, 300 mg/d for 1 month, 200 mg/d for 1 month, or until clear by endoscopy) along with routine steroid taper and topical nasal steroid postoperatively. They reported a recurrence rate of 50.3% and reoperation rate of 20.5% during an average follow-up of 31.4 months. The use of itraconazole also has been studied in cases of recalcitrant disease, when standard therapy fails. Chan and colleagues[53] performed a pilot study in 32 patients with AFRS who had disease refractory to prednisone, nasal steroids, and amphotericin B nasal sprays. The investigators treated with oral itraconazole for a minimum of 3 months. They found endoscopic improvement in 12 cases and no improvement or worse endoscopic appearance in 20 patients; 56% of patients reported moderate to significant symptom improvement, whereas 44% reported little or no change in symptoms. Seiberling and Wormald[54] also performed a retrospective chart review in 23 patients with AFRS and nonallergic eosinophilic fungal rhinosinusitis who failed maximal medical and surgical therapy. All patients were treated with oral itraconazole (100 mg twice a day) for 6 months when recurrence developed after surgery. The investigators found that 19 patients had a decrease in symptoms and endoscopic scores. Sixteen patients required a decreased amount of oral steroids, and a significant portion of the patients remained disease-free at a mean of 15.7 months of follow-up.

Although the cumulative evidence does not strongly support the use of antifungals for AFRS, they may be considered an option in cases of disease recurrence when standard maximum medical therapy and/or surgery has failed. Serious toxicities have not been reported in the available published studies; however, transaminitis has been reported to occur in 4% to 19% of patients, so liver function should be monitored closely.[53,54] A summary of these selected studies evaluating oral antifungal therapy in AFRS is presented in **Table 1**.

Immunotherapy

Several studies have demonstrated that immunotherapy (IT) is a safe adjunct in the management of AFRS; however, because of limitations in study design, limited conclusions can be made regarding its efficacy. Mabry and colleagues[55–58] reported results from case series following AFRS patients receiving IT for 3 years, which demonstrated improved endoscopic examinations and reduced need for corticosteroids; however, these observational studies were limited by lack of a defined control group. Bassichis and colleagues[59] and Folker and colleagues[60] have conducted case-control studies in patients with AFRS and compared outcomes in those receiving IT with those not receiving IT. Together, these studies demonstrated improved endoscopic examinations and symptom scores and reduced need for systemic steroids and revision surgery when IT was used. Taken together, the available evidence indicates that IT for AFRS is a safe adjunct with unclear benefit (given few studies with design limitations); however, it remains an option in the management of AFRS.[61]

Biologic therapy

Biologic therapy includes antibody-based therapies that target mediators of type 2 inflammation. A majority of biologic therapies investigated in CRS were developed

Table 1
Summary of selected studies evaluating oral antifungal therapy in allergic fungal rhinosinusitis

Study, Year	Design (n)	Intervention Group	Control Group	Outcomes	Results
Rojita et al,[51] 2017	Prospective, randomized (60 pts)	Oral itraconazole, 100 mg bid for 6 mo	Oral prednisolone for 1 mo, then topical nasal steroids for 6 mo postoperatively	SNOT-20; Kupferberg endoscopic staging; AEC; total serum IgE	No significant difference in outcomes between groups
Seiberling & Wormald,[54] 2009	Retrospective chart review in recalcitrant AFRS and nonallergic eosinophilic fungal sinusitis (23 pts)	Oral itraconazole, 100 mg bid for 6 mo	None	Time to recurrence; endoscopic examination; oral steroid use; liver function tests	19 pts with clinical response 16 pts with decrease in oral steroid use 11 pts disease-free at mean 15.7 mo 3 pts stopped tx for elevated liver enzymes
Chan et al,[53] 2008	Prospective, pilot study in recalcitrant AFRS (32 pts)	Oral itraconazole for minimum of 3 mo	None	Endoscopic score; serum IgE; RSOM-31; liver function testing	Endoscopic improvement: 12 cases No improvement/worse on endoscopy: 20 patients Mean increase in serum IgE post-treatment (581 → 766 μg/L) Moderate–significant symptom improvement: 56% Little or no change in symptoms: 44%

| Rains & Mineck,[52] 2003 | Retrospective (139 pts) | Postoperative regimen Itraconazole: 400 mg/d for 1 mo, 300 mg/d for 1 mo, 200 mg/d for 1 mo, or until clear by endoscopy. PLUS postoperative steroid taper and nasal steroid spray | None | Recurrence: 50.3% Revision: 20.5% No serious adverse events |

Abbreviations: AEC, absolute eosinophil count; pts, patients; RSOM-31, 31-item rhinosinusitis outcome measure; tx, treatment.

for the management of asthma and other atopic diseases.[62] Recently, the Food and Drug Administration (FDA) approved the use of dupilumab—an antibody that binds the IL-4Rα subunit of the IL-4 and IL-13 receptors and prevents IL-4–mediated and IL-13–mediated signaling—for use in patients with nasal polyposis. The approval came after 2 phase 3 studies (24-week outcomes [Liberty NP SINUS-24], and 52-week outcomes [Liberty NP SINUS-52]) enrolling a total of 724 subjects were completed. Collectively, the studies found that patients previously treated with surgery and systemic corticosteroids receiving dupilumab (300 mg, every 2 weeks for the first 24 weeks, and then every 4 weeks for the subsequent 28 weeks) had significant improvements in olfaction (measured by University of Pennsylvania Smell Identification Test), nasal polyp score, CT Lund-Mackay score, and 22-item SNOT (SNOT-22) and reduced the need for systemic corticosteroid and surgery. Additionally, patients with comorbid asthma (59.6% of cohort) had improved lung function (forced expiratory volume in the first second of expiration) and asthma control (Asthma Control Questionnaire 6).[63,64] These studies, however, specifically excluded AFRS patients despite the shared type 2 immune response with other CRSwNP subtypes.

Other biologic therapies that target type 2 inflammation in CRS include mepolizumab and reslizumab, monoclonal antibodies that bind IL-5; benralizumab, a monoclonal antibody directed against the IL-5 α-chain receptor; and omalizumab, an antibody that binds free and membrane-bound IgE. None of these biologic therapies is FDA approved for use in CRS; however, they have demonstrated some utility in studies performed in patients with CRSwNP. Bachert and colleagues[65] conducted a randomized, double-blind, placebo-controlled clinical trial in 105 patients with CRSwNP, testing the efficacy of mepolizumab. This study found patients receiving mepolizumab (n = 54) had reduced need for surgery and demonstrated a significant improvement in nasal polyp score and SNOT-22 symptoms scores compared with a placebo group. Rivero completed a meta-analysis of 5 studies that evaluated the efficacy of biologics (mepolizumab, reslizumab, and omalizumab) for the treatment of CRSwNP and found a significant improvement in patients' nasal polyp scores.[66] Bidder and colleagues[67] prospectively evaluated the efficacy of omalizumab in patients with allergic asthma who also had comorbid CRSwNP. The investigators found a similar improvement in SNOT-22 scores in patients receiving omalizumab (n = 13) without surgery compared with a control group of patients (n = 24) with asthma/CRSwNP undergoing surgery.

Although these studies do not specify the subtype of CRSwNP included and in some cases excluded AFRS disease in their patient cohort, it seems that given the profound local type 2 inflammation observed in AFRS, biologic therapy may have a role in AFRS patients who fail standard therapy.

Prognosis After Treatment

Patients with AFRS undergoing ESS have significant improvements in quality of life after surgery.[68,69] Like patients with CRSwNP, the recurrence and revision rate for AFRS can be high. Younis and Ahmed[70] conducted a retrospective study in 117 patients with AFRS and eosinophilic mucin CRS, and they found that 22% of patients required a revision surgery an average of 2.6 years after the initial surgery. Data from the CRS epidemiology study performed in the United Kingdom reported a median interval to revision surgery of 2 years in patients with AFRS.[71] Reasons for disease recurrence and need for revision surgery likely are multifactorial and difficult to identify in these studies; however, these observations highlight the challenge in controlling inflammation in AFRS.

SUMMARY AND FUTURE CONSIDERATIONS

AFRS is a subtype of CRS characterized by an exaggerated, localized, type 2 inflammatory response within the paranasal sinuses and a characteristic clinical presentation. When good surgical techniques are combined with adequate steroid therapy, AFRS patients often obtain durable disease control with overall improvements in their quality of life. Certainly, the challenge lies in cases of recalcitrant disease. Future clinical studies will need to address the efficacy of antifungals, biologics, and IT in AFRS, especially those with difficult-to-treat disease. From a basic science viewpoint, a greater understanding of the molecular signatures that differentiate AFRS from other subtypes of CRS (altered barrier function, overactive adaptive immune signaling, and defective antifungal immunity) has been arrived at; however, a better understanding of the mechanisms that lead up to these stages of diseases is greatly needed. These studies would identify new disease targets for the development of novel therapies.

DISCLOSURE

A.U. Luong serves as a consultant for Aerin Medical (Sunnyvale, California), Arrinex (Redwood City, California), Lyra Therapeutics (Watertown, Massachusetts), and Stryker (Kalamazoo, Michigan). She is on the advisory board for ENTvantage (Austin, Texas), Sanofi (Paris, France), and Novartis (Basel, Switzerland).

REFERENCES

1. Katzenstein AL, Sale SR, Greenberger PA. Allergic Aspergillus sinusitis: a newly recognized form of sinusitis. J Allergy Clin Immunol 1983;72:89–93.
2. Katzenstein AL, Sale SR, Greenberger PA. Pathologic findings in allergic aspergillus sinusitis. A newly recognized form of sinusitis. Am J Surg Pathol 1983;7: 439–43.
3. Bent JP 3rd, Kuhn FA. Diagnosis of allergic fungal sinusitis. Otolaryngol Head Neck Surg 1994;111:580–8.
4. Ferguson BJ, Barnes L, Bernstein JM, et al. Geographic variation in allergic fungal rhinosinusitis. Otolaryngol Clin North Am 2000;33:441–9.
5. Wise SK, Venkatraman G, Wise JC, et al. Ethnic and gender differences in bone erosion in allergic fungal sinusitis. Am J Rhinol 2004;18:397–404.
6. Ghegan MD, Lee FS, Schlosser RJ. Incidence of skull base and orbital erosion in allergic fungal rhinosinusitis (AFRS) and non-AFRS. Otolaryngol Head Neck Surg 2006;134:592–5.
7. Ghegan MD, Wise SK, Gorham E, et al. Socioeconomic factors in allergic fungal rhinosinusitis with bone erosion. Am J Rhinol 2007;21:560–3.
8. Thahim K, Jawaid MA, Marfani MS. Presentation and management of allergic fungal sinusitis. J Coll Physicians Surg Pak 2007;17:23–7.
9. Tyler MA, Russell CB, Smith DE, et al. Large-scale gene expression profiling reveals distinct type 2 inflammatory patterns in chronic rhinosinusitis subtypes. J Allergy Clin Immunol 2017;139:1061–1064 e1064.
10. Wise SK, Ghegan MD, Gorham E, et al. Socioeconomic factors in the diagnosis of allergic fungal rhinosinusitis. Otolaryngol Head Neck Surg 2008;138:38–42.
11. Miller JD, Deal AM, McKinney KA, et al. Markers of disease severity and socioeconomic factors in allergic fungal rhinosinusitis. Int Forum Allergy Rhinol 2014; 4:272–9.

12. Lu-Myers Y, Deal AM, Miller JD, et al. Comparison of socioeconomic and demographic factors in patients with chronic rhinosinusitis and allergic fungal rhinosinusitis. Otolaryngol Head Neck Surg 2015;153:137–43.

13. Tyler MA, Padro Dietz CJ, Russell CB, et al. Distinguishing molecular features of allergic fungal rhinosinusitis. Otolaryngol Head Neck Surg 2018;159(1):185–93.

14. Clark DW, Wenaas A, Luong A, et al. Staphylococcus aureus prevalence in allergic fungal rhinosinusitis vs other subsets of chronic rhinosinusitis with nasal polyps. Int Forum Allergy Rhinol 2013;3:89–93.

15. Promsopa C, Kansara S, Citardi MJ, et al. Prevalence of confirmed asthma varies in chronic rhinosinusitis subtypes. Int Forum Allergy Rhinol 2016;6:373–7.

16. Fokkens WJ, Lund VJ. Mullol Jet al. EPOS 2012: European position paper on rhinosinusitis and nasal polyps 2012. A summary for otorhinolaryngologists. Rhinology 2012;50:1–12.

17. Pant H, Kette FE, Smith WB, et al. Fungal-specific humoral response in eosinophilic mucus chronic rhinosinusitis. Laryngoscope 2005;115:601–6.

18. Pant H, Kette FE, Smith WB, et al. Eosinophilic mucus chronic rhinosinusitis: clinical subgroups or a homogeneous pathogenic entity? Laryngoscope 2006;116:1241–7.

19. Pant H, Beroukas D, Kette FE, et al. Nasal polyp cell populations and fungal-specific peripheral blood lymphocyte proliferation in allergic fungal sinusitis. Am J Rhinol Allergy 2009;23:453–60.

20. Ponikau JU, Sherris DA, Kern EB, et al. The diagnosis and incidence of allergic fungal sinusitis. Mayo Clin Proc 1999;74:877–84.

21. Collins M, Nair S, Smith W, et al. Role of local immunoglobulin E production in the pathophysiology of noninvasive fungal sinusitis. Laryngoscope 2004;l114:1242–6.

22. Tieu DD, Kern RC, Schleimer RP. Alterations in epithelial barrier function and host defense responses in chronic rhinosinusitis. J Allergy Clin Immunol 2009;124:37–42.

23. Den Beste KA, Hoddeson EK, Parkos CA, et al. Epithelial permeability alterations in an in vitro air-liquid interface model of allergic fungal rhinosinusitis. Int Forum Allergy Rhinol 2013;3:19–25.

24. Wise SK, Laury AM, Katz EH, et al. Interleukin-4 and interleukin-13 compromise the sinonasal epithelial barrier and perturb intercellular junction protein expression. Int Forum Allergy Rhinol 2014;4:361–70.

25. Ooi EH, Wormald PJ, Carney AS, et al. Surfactant protein d expression in chronic rhinosinusitis patients and immune responses in vitro to Aspergillus and alternaria in a nasal explant model. Laryngoscope 2007;117:51–7.

26. Psaltis AJ, Bruhn MA, Ooi EH, et al. Nasal mucosa expression of lactoferrin in patients with chronic rhinosinusitis. Laryngoscope 2007;117:2030–5.

27. Schubert MS, Hutcheson PS, Graff RJ, et al. HLA-DQB1 *03 in allergic fungal sinusitis and other chronic hypertrophic rhinosinusitis disorders. J Allergy Clin Immunol 2004;114:1376–83.

28. Ayers CM, Schlosser RJ, O'Connell BP, et al. Increased presence of dendritic cells and dendritic cell chemokines in the sinus mucosa of chronic rhinosinusitis with nasal polyps and allergic fungal rhinosinusitis. Int Forum Allergy Rhinol 2011;1:296–302.

29. Mulligan JK, Bleier BS, O'Connell B, et al. Vitamin D3 correlates inversely with systemic dendritic cell numbers and bone erosion in chronic rhinosinusitis with nasal polyps and allergic fungal rhinosinusitis. Clin Exp Immunol 2011;164:312–20.

30. Pant H, Macardle P. CD8(+) T cells implicated in the pathogenesis of allergic fungal rhinosinusitis. Allergy Rhinol (Providence) 2014;5:146–56.

31. Kim JH, Yi JS, Gong CH, et al. Development of Aspergillus protease with ovalbumin-induced allergic chronic rhinosinusitis model in the mouse. Am J Rhinol Allergy 2014;28:465–70.

32. Millien VO, Lu W, Shaw J, et al. Cleavage of fibrinogen by proteinases elicits allergic responses through Toll-like receptor 4. Science 2013;341:792–6.

33. Porter P, Susarla SC, Polikepahad S, et al. Link between allergic asthma and airway mucosal infection suggested by proteinase-secreting household fungi. Mucosal Immunol 2009;2:504–17.

34. Patel NN, Triantafillou V, Maina IW, et al. Fungal extracts stimulate solitary chemosensory cell expansion in noninvasive fungal rhinosinusitis. Int Forum Allergy Rhinol 2019;9:730–7.

35. Shaw JL, Fakhri S, Citardi MJ, et al. IL-33-responsive innate lymphoid cells are an important source of IL-13 in chronic rhinosinusitis with nasal polyps. Am J Respir Crit Care Med 2013;188:432–9.

36. Bartemes KR, Kita H. Innate and adaptive immune responses to fungi in the airway. J Allergy Clin Immunol 2018;142:353–63.

37. Doherty TA, Khorram N, Chang JE, et al. STAT6 regulates natural helper cell proliferation during lung inflammation initiated by Alternaria. Am J Physiol Lung Cell Mol Physiol 2012;303:L577–88.

38. Bartemes KR, Iijima K, Kobayashi T, et al. IL-33-responsive lineage- CD25+ CD44(hi) lymphoid cells mediate innate type 2 immunity and allergic inflammation in the lungs. J Immunol 2012;188:1503–13.

39. Illing EA, Dunlap Q, Woodworth BA. Outcomes of pressure-induced cranial neuropathies from allergic fungal rhinosinusitis. Otolaryngol Head Neck Surg 2015; 152:541–5.

40. Bobart SA, Dimov V, Sider D, et al. Proptosis and vision loss as grave complications of allergic fungal sinusitis and polyposis. Ann Allergy Asthma Immunol 2017;118:728–9.

41. AlQahtani A, Alshaikh N, Alzarei A, et al. Contralateral sinus involvement of surgically treated unilateral allergic fungal rhinosinusitis. Eur Arch Otorhinolaryngol 2017;274:3097–101.

42. Kupferberg SB, Bent JP 3rd, Kuhn FA. Prognosis for allergic fungal sinusitis. Otolaryngol Head Neck Surg 1997;117:35–41.

43. Kuhn FA, Javer AR. Allergic fungal sinusitis: a four-year follow-up. Am J Rhinol 2000;14:149–56.

44. Woodworth BA, Joseph K, Kaplan AP, et al. Alterations in eotaxin, monocyte chemoattractant protein-4, interleukin-5, and interleukin-13 after systemic steroid treatment for nasal polyps. Otolaryngol Head Neck Surg 2004;131:585–9.

45. Landsberg R, Segev Y, DeRowe A, et al. Systemic corticosteroids for allergic fungal rhinosinusitis and chronic rhinosinusitis with nasal polyposis: a comparative study. Otolaryngol Head Neck Surg 2007;136:252–7.

46. Joe SA, Thambi R, Huang J. A systematic review of the use of intranasal steroids in the treatment of chronic rhinosinusitis. Otolaryngol Head Neck Surg 2008;139: 340–7.

47. Kalish LH, Arendts G, Sacks R, et al. Topical steroids in chronic rhinosinusitis without polyps: a systematic review and meta-analysis. Otolaryngol Head Neck Surg 2009;141:674–83.

48. Rudmik L, Schlosser RJ, Smith TL, et al. Impact of topical nasal steroid therapy on symptoms of nasal polyposis: a meta-analysis. Laryngoscope 2012;122: 1431–7.

49. Soudry E, Wang J, Vaezeafshar R, et al. Safety analysis of long-term budesonide nasal irrigations in patients with chronic rhinosinusitis post endoscopic sinus surgery. Int Forum Allergy Rhinol 2016;6:568–72.

50. Smith KA, French G, Mechor B, et al. Safety of long-term high-volume sinonasal budesonide irrigations for chronic rhinosinusitis. Int Forum Allergy Rhinol 2016;6: 228–32.

51. Rojita M, Samal S, Pradhan P, et al. Comparison of steroid and itraconazole for prevention of recurrence in allergic fungal rhinosinusitis: a randomized controlled trial. J Clin Diagn Res 2017;11:MC01–3.

52. Rains BM 3rd, Mineck CW. Treatment of allergic fungal sinusitis with high-dose itraconazole. Am J Rhinol 2003;17:1–8.

53. Chan KO, Genoway KA, Javer AR. Effectiveness of itraconazole in the management of refractory allergic fungal rhinosinusitis. J Otolaryngol Head Neck Surg 2008;37:870–4.

54. Seiberling K, Wormald PJ. The role of itraconazole in recalcitrant fungal sinusitis. Am J Rhinol Allergy 2009;23:303–6.

55. Mabry RL, Marple BF, Mabry CS. Outcomes after discontinuing immunotherapy for allergic fungal sinusitis. Otolaryngol Head Neck Surg 2000;122:104–6.

56. Mabry RL, Marple BF, Folker RJ, et al. Immunotherapy for allergic fungal sinusitis: three years' experience. Otolaryngol Head Neck Surg 1998;119:648–51.

57. Mabry RL, Mabry CS. Allergic fungal sinusitis: the role of immunotherapy. Otolaryngol Clin North Am 2000;33:433–40.

58. Mabry RL, Mabry CS. Immunotherapy for allergic fungal sinusitis: the second year. Otolaryngol Head Neck Surg 1997;117:367–71.

59. Bassichis BA, Marple BF, Mabry RL, et al. Use of immunotherapy in previously treated patients with allergic fungal sinusitis. Otolaryngol Head Neck Surg 2001;125:487–90.

60. Folker RJ, Marple BF, Mabry RL, et al. Treatment of allergic fungal sinusitis: a comparison trial of postoperative immunotherapy with specific fungal antigens. Laryngoscope 1998;108:1623–7.

61. Gan EC, Thamboo A, Rudmik L, et al. Medical management of allergic fungal rhinosinusitis following endoscopic sinus surgery: an evidence-based review and recommendations. Int Forum Allergy Rhinol 2014;4:702–15.

62. Gauthier M, Ray A, Wenzel SE. Evolving concepts of asthma. Am J Respir Crit Care Med 2015;192:660–8.

63. Han JK, Bachert C, Desrosiers M, et al. Efficacy and Safety of Dupilumab in Patients with Chronic Rhinosinusitis with Nasal Polyps: Results from the Randomized Phase 3 Sinus-24 Study. J Allergy Clin Immunol 2019;143:AB422.

64. Bachert C, Desrosiers M, Mullol J, et al. A Randomized Phase 3 Study, Sinus-52, Evaluating the Efficacy and Safety of Dupilumab in Patients with Severe Chronic Rhinosinusitis with Nasal Polyps. J Allergy Clin Immunol 2019;143:AB433.

65. Bachert C, Sousa AR, Lund VJ, et al. Reduced need for surgery in severe nasal polyposis with mepolizumab: Randomized trial. J Allergy Clin Immunol 2017;140: 1024–1031 e1014.

66. Rivero A, Liang J. Anti-IgE and anti-IL5 biologic therapy in the treatment of nasal polyposis: a systematic review and meta-analysis. Ann Otol Rhinol Laryngol 2017;126:739–47.

67. Bidder T, Sahota J, Rennie C, et al. Omalizumab treats chronic rhinosinusitis with nasal polyps and asthma together-a real life study. Rhinology 2018;56:42–5.
68. Champagne JP, Antisdel JL, Woodard TD, et al. Epidemiologic factors affect surgical outcomes in allergic fungal sinusitis. Laryngoscope 2010;120:2322–4.
69. Masterson L, Egro FM, Bewick J, et al. Quality-of-life outcomes after sinus surgery in allergic fungal rhinosinusitis versus nonfungal chronic rhinosinusitis. Am J Rhinol Allergy 2016;30:e30–5.
70. Younis RT, Ahmed J. Predicting revision sinus surgery in allergic fungal and eosinophilic mucin chronic rhinosinusitis. Laryngoscope 2017;127:59–63.
71. Philpott C, Hopkins C, Erskine S, et al. The burden of revision sinonasal surgery in the UK-data from the Chronic Rhinosinusitis Epidemiology Study (CRES): a cross-sectional study. BMJ Open 2015;5:e006680.

Odontogenic Sinusitis
Current Concepts in Diagnosis and Treatment

Hillary A. Newsome, MD[a,b], David M. Poetker, MD[a,b],*

KEYWORDS

- Odontogenic sinusitis • Unilateral maxillary sinusitis • Dental origin
- Periapical abscess • Implant

KEY POINTS

- Odontogenic sinusitis is most commonly caused by iatrogenic injury to the Schneiderian membrane from dentoalveolar procedures followed by periapical abscesses.
- Although radiographic findings such as periodontal disease, oroantral fistula, and periapical abscesses are often present, they may not be mentioned as a source of sinusitis in imaging reports.
- A combination of medical therapy, dental procedures, and endoscopic sinus surgery is used to treat odontogenic sinusitis.
- The microbial population differs from that of chronic sinusitis, with a higher incidence of polymicrobial infections and anaerobes.

INTRODUCTION

The overall health cost burden of adult chronic sinusitis has been estimated to be upward of US$22 billion.[1] Maxillary sinusitis of dental origin (MSDO), also termed odontogenic sinusitis (OS), is a unique cause of sinusitis that requires special attention. Although the mainstays of chronic sinusitis treatments, such as endoscopic sinus surgery (ESS) and medical therapy, are often used to treat OS, treatment failure can occur, highlighting the nuances of this disorder.[2,3] Care for these patients often falls to both the otolaryngologist and dental professional to determine an appropriate treatment plan when it comes to diagnosis, timing of surgery, decision to treat the oral cavity source, and type of antibiotics.

[a] Rhinology and Skull Base Division, Department of Otolaryngology & Communication Sciences, Medical College of Wisconsin, 9200 West Wisconsin Avenue, Milwaukee, WI 53226, USA; [b] Zablocki VAMC, Milwaukee, WI, USA
* Corresponding author. Rhinology and Skull Base Division, Department of Otolaryngology & Communication Sciences, Medical College of Wisconsin, 9200 West Wisconsin Avenue, Milwaukee, WI 53226.
E-mail address: dpoetker@mcw.edu

Immunol Allergy Clin N Am 40 (2020) 361–369
https://doi.org/10.1016/j.iac.2019.12.012
0889-8561/20/© 2019 Elsevier Inc. All rights reserved.

RELEVANT ANATOMY AND PATHOGENESIS

The description of MSDO has largely been credited to Bauer in 1943 who, through a series of microscopic cadaveric dissections, helped clarify possible routes of pathogenesis for this disorder.[4] The maxillary sinus and maxillary molar roots are intimately related. The floor of the maxillary sinus ranges in thickness and can be interrupted with exposed tooth roots in patients with bone loss or be up to 12 mm thick.[5] Even in a normal maxilla, the periodontal membrane of the tooth roots can be in direct contact with the respiratory epithelium (also known as the Schneiderian membrane) of the maxillary sinus, providing a potential source of contamination.[4,5] One of the most critical points from Bauer's work was the finding that in cases of a thick bony floor, a network of blood vessels and lymphatics connect the periodontal membrane to the bone marrow of the maxilla. The resulting inflammatory reaction leads to fibrous tissue that decreases the efficiency of the sinus cilia.[4] Later studies have gone on to confirm the posterior maxillary teeth, specifically the first and second molars, as the most commonly offending teeth.[6,7] Single or multiple tooth roots can be involved, and the palatal root of the first molar, followed by the mesiobuccal root of the second molar, were most frequently associated with OS in a study reviewing cone-beam computed tomography (CBCT) images of cases with unilateral or bilateral sinusitis.[6] It should come as no surprise that sinusitis of dental origin can also be implicated in cases of sinusitis beyond the maxillary sinus, considering that obstruction of the maxillary sinus ostium can cause blockage of the osteomeatal complex and lead to anterior ethmoidal and frontal sinusitis (**Fig. 1**).[8] In fact, in 2014 Saibene and colleagues[9] found that upward of 40% of OS patients had more extensive sinus involvement than the maxillary sinus alone, and in 2019 Whyte and Boeddinghaus[10] noted more than 60% of cases involving multiple sinuses.

Additionally, trauma to the epithelial cells of the respiratory epithelium, which typically have gap junctions in between them to form a physical barrier, allows oral cavity pathogens into the maxillary sinus.[5] Natural causes of trauma to the membrane come in the form of dental disorder such as periapical infections or inflammation (**Fig. 2**), periodontal and endodontal disease, and dentigerous cysts; multiple studies have gone on to cite periapical abscess as a natural leading cause of OS.[2,8,11–14] The

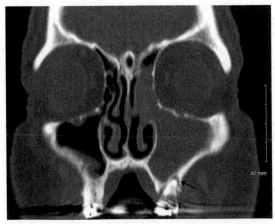

Fig. 1. Typical appearance of odontogenic sinusitis on coronal computed tomography scan. This patient has left unilateral sinusitis (maxillary sinusitis with involvement of ethmoids) as a result of a periapical abscess (denoted by *black arrow*).

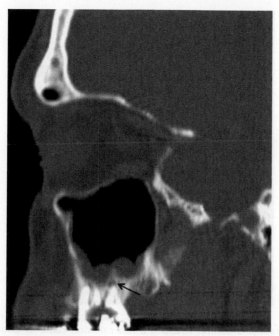

Fig. 2. Periapical disease can be seen on this computed tomography scan as radiolucency at the end of the tooth root (denoted by *black arrow*). A resulting thickening of the sinus mucosa can occur. Periapical abscess is a common cause of odontogenic sinusitis.

term "endo-antral syndrome" was coined by Selden several decades ago to describe the passage of infection from periapical and antral tissues.[15,16] The iatrogenic causes of OS are many and include fractures from dental implants, foreign bodies in the sinus, sinus augmentation procedures, and postoperative oroantral fistulas **(Fig. 3)**.[5,11,13] Regardless of the cause, MSDO is a problem of increasing clinical significance.

EPIDEMIOLOGY

In most literature regarding OS, the incidence of maxillary sinusitis related to an odontogenic source is quoted at between 10% and 12%.[2,3,5–9,12,14,17–24] This has historically been the teaching since a 1968 paper by Maloney and Doku; however, more recent studies within the past decade have called this number into question for multiple reasons.[17] A 2011 case series by Longhini and Ferguson[25] included an indepth review of the literature on the incidence of OS. Of note, the investigators found that the oft quoted 1968 study is actually a secondary source, and the primary sources of these numbers do not contain any data to support their incidence claims.[17,25] Longhini and Ferguson go on to say that the real incidence of OS is unknown but is likely higher than previously thought. In the mid 1980s, Melen and colleagues[26] found that in a cohort of patients with refractory chronic sinusitis, nearly 40% of patients actually had an odontogenic source of their disease. When specifically considering unilateral maxillary sinusitis, the incidence of odontogenic origin jumps up to greater than 70% as seen in several studies.[5,13,20] The real incidence of this disease is likely unknown because diagnostic and inclusion criteria vary between studies (e.g., chronic versus acute sinusitis patients, unilateral versus bilateral maxillary sinus opacification patients), and imaging technology (panoramic X-ray versus computed tomography [CT] scans) has greatly improved from early investigations.

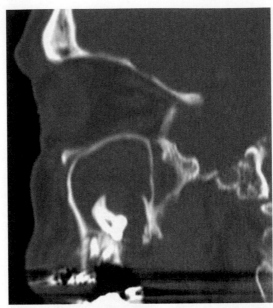

Fig. 3. Oroantral fistula with maxillary sinus opacification demonstrated by sagittal computed tomography. Oroantral fistula is a less common cause of odontogenic sinusitis than periapical disease.

There may be a slight propensity for OS to affect women over men, as several larger-scale studies have shown.[3,9,11,27] OS usually presents in middle-aged patients with both case series and reviews giving average patient ages in the 40s to 50s.[8,11,19,20] One potential cause of this fairly consistent age of presentation is that patients at this age have had sufficient time for periodontal disease and maxillary bone loss to occur. Both dental providers and otolaryngologists treat these patients, and as such they may present in either setting.

SYMPTOMS AND DIAGNOSIS

A patient presenting with unilateral sinus disease should pique the provider's interest and raise the clinical suspicion of OS. However, there remain several other important causes of unilateral sinus disease on the differential: antrochoanal polyp, inverted papilloma, squamous cell carcinoma, and allergic fungal sinusitis, to name a few. Nevertheless, there are important findings to help the clinician yield a diagnosis of OS. Most studies agree that a distinguishing symptom of OS from other causes of acute or chronic sinusitis is foul smelling/tasting rhinorrhea.[5,19,25] A study by Workman and colleagues[7] and the more recent findings of Simuntis and colleagues[24] emphatically conclude that malodorous secretions are the hallmark of OS, and the significance of a thorough history taking should not be understated. Other less unique symptoms include facial pain and pressure, and nasal congestion. Surprising is the consistency at which less than half of patients report dental pain.[21,25] Symptoms can be present from a few weeks in acute cases to several years in chronic OD.[14,25,27] Patients may report a preceding history of dental procedure such as recent dental implant or extraction or may have not seen a dental provider in many years.

On clinical examination, even by a dental professional, the identification of the offending tooth may not be obvious, owing in part to the varied inciting dental pathologies. This also makes sense considering the relatively low reporting rate of associated tooth pain. This step, however, should not be skipped, as sometimes carious teeth or extraction-site oroantral fistulas are readily apparent. Interestingly, a 2019 retrospective chart review on acute sinusitis patients from an otorhinolaryngology clinic found that only 8.1% of provider notes mentioned examination of the teeth: a clear opportunity for improvement in the diagnostic value of the physical examination.[27] Similarly to other presentations of sinusitis, endoscopic examination of OS may yield findings of purulent secretions in the middle meatus, and if the patient has already undergone surgical antrostomy, findings of foreign bodies or projecting tooth roots/implants into the maxillary sinus floor may be demonstrated. Given the subtle findings on clinical examination, a provider must have a high index of suspicion before ordering imaging studies or the diagnosis of the OS may be missed.

IMAGING

With the advent of improved accessibility of in-office imaging techniques, there has been increasing awareness of the radiologic features of OS. Two-dimensional (2D) imaging studies that can be used—albeit with limited efficacy—include periapical, panoramic, and Waters radiographs.[28] All 2D studies have the same limitation in that they try to portray a three-dimensional (3D) space in a flat image that often compromises anatomic relationships because of its superimposition, making it difficult to identify periodontal disease (**Fig. 4**). In addition, the posterior maxillary teeth are poorly visualized on these studies.[29] By far the most common imaging study currently used for rhinologic evaluation is a noncontrast CT scan of the sinuses, and several published

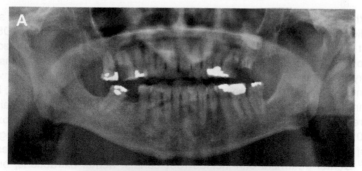

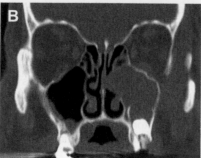

Fig. 4. (*A*) Panoramic radiograph and (*B*) computed tomography scan of the same patient with left unilateral maxillary odontogenic sinusitis caused by dental implant. Radiograph utility is limited by overlapping anatomic structures.

works have been dedicated to increasing awareness of the relevant clinical findings that suggest OS.[8,10,29,30]

Conventional CT and CBCT are 3D studies that eliminate the superimposition of anatomic structures and are superior at identifying changing densities in bony structures. In addition, they provide the potential to image all of the paranasal sinuses rather than just the maxillaries. Nevertheless, the odontogenic causes of maxillary sinusitis may be missed by radiologists up to 60% of the time.[8,23] For this reason, it is imperative for both dental providers and otolaryngologists to review images themselves and to supplement with a physical examination. Bomeli and colleagues[12] identified 3 key radiographic findings suggestive of dental etiology in their retrospective review of 101 CT scans of unilateral and bilateral maxillary sinus fluid: (1) oroantral fistula, (2) periodontal disease with periapical abscess, and (3) a projection molar/premolar tooth root with periodontal disease. Additionally, they found an increasing likelihood of a dental source with increasing levels of maxillary fluid (mucosal thickening also showed a similar trend). This finding was supported by a more recent Swedish study with similar results: patients with unilateral OS had significantly more swelling and congestion of the maxillary sinuses than patients with nonodontogenic cause.[3] Another key point of radiologic studies is that 75% of cases of unilateral maxillary sinusitis (or more extensive) with a patent ethmoid infundibulum can be attributed to an oral cavity source.[8] Otolaryngologists should thus keep this in mind when considering cases of failed functional ESS. Although the likelihood of OS increases when radiographic findings are unilateral, Saibene and colleagues[9] found that almost 20% of 315 surgically treated cases of OS were bilateral.

TREATMENT AND MANAGEMENT

Although there is a large role for medical therapy in cases of classic chronic sinusitis, most studies focus on a combination of medical and surgical treatment for OS. There does exist controversy, however, on timing and sequence of surgical procedures to treat the oral cavity source and the paranasal sinus disease. Surgical management of maxillary sinus disease classically included the Caldwell-Luc procedure, which involves completely stripping the respiratory epithelium of the maxillary sinus, but now more commonly includes ESS as the gold standard.[31] Antibiotics are the mainstay of medical treatment. Multiple small-sized studies have found that only approximately 15% to 20% of OS cases resolved with antibiotics alone and that an average of 2.6 courses of antibiotics has been trialed before proceeding to surgery in cases of failure.[14,18,19] Dental treatment can include root canals, dental extractions, or buccal flaps for oroantral fistulas, depending on the pathologic profile. However, if surgical treatment is necessary, should the tooth or sinus be treated first?

It is not uncommon for OS patients to present to the otolaryngologist's office only to be referred for dental evaluation once OS has been suspected.[2] In fact, the American Association of Endodontists recommends treating the primary endodontic infection before undertaking ESS.[32] Tomomatsu and coworkeres[33] studied 39 patients with OS and found that 20 patients improved after dental treatment and a course of antibiotics (length of antibiotic treatment depended on chronicity of symptoms). The other 19 patients required ESS for symptom and radiographic resolution. This suggests that although treatment of the primary source of infection may prevent more extensive surgery, ESS will be necessary in some cases.

In a study of 43 OS patients (22 improved with medical and dental therapy alone), Mattos and colleagues[21] identified involvement of the osteomeatal complex and a dental procedure before developing OS symptoms as predictive factors for needing

ESS. Other studies have seconded osteomeatal complex involvement as a critical factor toward requiring surgical management; less commonly, osteomeatal complex aperture width, increased Lund-Makay score, symptom duration, and condition of the maxillary sinus floor have been found to be predictive.[14,33] In one prospective study of implant-related sinusitis, 80% of patients failed to improve after a trial of antibiotics and required functional ESS.[19] All of the studied patients eventually improved despite implants protruding into the maxillary sinus, which remained *in situ*. This is a reassuring finding for those patients who are reluctant to have costly implants removed. Moreover, Craig and colleagues[18] published a series of 37 patients with symptomatic OS and allowed patients to choose primary dental treatment (n = 11) or ESS (n = 26). The group undergoing ESS had faster resolution of symptoms based on the SNOT-22 and endoscopic findings, and the investigators promoted ESS as first-line treatment in OS. However, that is also not to say that a patient cannot undergo both an intraoral approach for source control and ESS simultaneously, as was proved feasible by Kende and colleagues.[31] Clearly, based on the current state of the literature, more prospective studies are needed to clarify the optimal surgical treatment of this disease.

MICROBIOLOGY

Because of the contamination of the maxillary sinus with oral cavity pathogens, OS requires thoughtfulness in its antibiotic treatments. One study on microbiological samples from chronic sinusitis and odontogenic sinusitis found that only 60% of chronic sinusitis samples grew microbes, whereas all of the OS samples had a large microbial burden and led to bacterial growth.[22] Instead of the usual *Streptococcus pneumoniae*, *Moraxella catarrhalis*, and *Haemophilus influenzae* that regularly cause most cases of nonodontogenic sinusitis, cultures from multiple studies of OS have shown an increased incidence of polymicrobial infections. Isolates have grown oral anaerobes such as *Peptostreptococcus* and *Prevotella* spp. as well as aerobic bacteria such as *Staphylococcus aureus*.[2,5,14,34] As such, respiratory fluroquinolones are frequently used to treat OS.[14,22] In addition, fungal isolates, namely *Aspergillus* and *Candida*, have been found in rare cases of OS. Duration of antibiotic therapy seems to vary anywhere from to 1 week to 3 months and usually correlates with symptom duration.

SUMMARY

OS is a unique cause of sinus disease that deserves special consideration. An astute clinician can elicit historical findings such as recent dental work and symptoms such as unilateral facial pain and foul drainage, despite a relatively benign oral cavity examination. Otolaryngologists and dental professionals who work together to care for these patients must be able to interpret imaging studies for dental disorder, such as periapical abscesses and periodontal disease, because radiology reports may fail to comment on these common findings. Treatment is frequently some combination of antibiotic therapy, dental procedures, and ESS. More prospective studies on this topic are needed to determine the best direction of care for this patient population.

DISCLOSURE

The authors have nothing to disclose.

REFERENCES

1. Smith KA, Orlandi RR, Rudmik L. Cost of adult chronic rhinosinusitis: a systematic review. Laryngoscope 2015;125(7):1547–56.
2. Longhini AB, Branstetter BF, Ferguson BJ. Unrecognized odontogenic maxillary sinusitis: a cause of endoscopic sinus surgery failure. Am J Rhinol Allergy 2010;24(4):296–300.
3. Vestin Fredriksson M, Ohman A, Flygare L, et al. When maxillary sinusitis does not heal: findings on CBCT scans of the sinuses with a particular focus on the occurrence of odontogenic causes of maxillary sinusitis. Laryngoscope Investig Otolaryngol 2017;2(6):442–6.
4. Bauer WH. Maxillary sinusitis of dental origin. Am J Orthod Oral Surg 1943;29(3): B133–51.
5. Kim SM. Definition and management of odontogenic maxillary sinusitis. Maxillofac Plast Reconstr Surg 2019;41(1):13.
6. Maillet M, Bowles WR, McClanahan SL, et al. Cone-beam computed tomography evaluation of maxillary sinusitis. J Endod 2011;37(6):753–7.
7. Workman AD, Granquist EJ, Adappa ND. Odontogenic sinusitis: developments in diagnosis, microbiology, and treatment. Curr Opin Otolaryngol Head Neck Surg 2018;26(1):27–33.
8. Pokorny A, Tataryn R. Clinical and radiologic findings in a case series of maxillary sinusitis of dental origin. Int Forum Allergy Rhinol 2013;3(12):973–9.
9. Saibene AM, Pipolo GC, Lozza P, et al. Redefining boundaries in odontogenic sinusitis: a retrospective evaluation of extramaxillary involvement in 315 patients. Int Forum Allergy Rhinol 2014;4(12):1020–3.
10. Whyte A, Boeddinghaus R. Imaging of odontogenic sinusitis. Clin Radiol 2019; 74(7):503–16.
11. Lechien JR, Filleul O, Costa de Araujo P, et al. Chronic maxillary rhinosinusitis of dental origin: a systematic review of 674 patient cases. Int J Otolaryngol 2014; 2014:465173.
12. Bomeli SR, Branstetter BF, Ferguson BJ. Frequency of a dental source for acute maxillary sinusitis. Laryngoscope 2009;119(3):580–4.
13. Troeltzsch M, Pache C, Troeltzsch M, et al. Etiology and clinical characteristics of symptomatic unilateral maxillary sinusitis: a review of 174 cases. J Craniomaxillofac Surg 2015;43(8):1522–9.
14. Lee KC, Lee SJ. Clinical features and treatments of odontogenic sinusitis. Yonsei Med J 2010;51(6):932–7.
15. Selden HS. The endo-antral syndrome: an endodontic complication. J Am Dent Assoc 1989;119(3):397–8.
16. Selden HS. Endo-antral syndrome and various endodontic complications. J Endod 1999;25(5):389–93.
17. Maloney PL, Doku HC. Maxillary sinusitis of odontogenic origin. J Can Dent Assoc (Tor) 1968;34(11):591–603.
18. Craig JR, McHugh CI, Griggs ZH, et al. Optimal timing of endoscopic sinus surgery for odontogenic sinusitis. Laryngoscope 2019;129(9):1976–83.
19. Kim SJ, Park JS, Kim HT, et al. Clinical features and treatment outcomes of dental implant-related paranasal sinusitis: a 2-year prospective observational study. Clin Oral Implants Res 2016;27(11):e100–4.
20. Matsumoto Y, Ikeda T, Yokoi H, et al. Association between odontogenic infections and unilateral sinus opacification. Auris Nasus Larynx 2015;42(4):288–93.

21. Mattos JL, Ferguson BJ, Lee S. Predictive factors in patients undergoing endoscopic sinus surgery for odontogenic sinusitis. Int Forum Allergy Rhinol 2016; 6(7):697–700.

22. Saibene AM, Vassena C, Pipolo C, et al. Odontogenic and rhinogenic chronic sinusitis: a modern microbiological comparison. Int Forum Allergy Rhinol 2016; 6(1):41–5.

23. Wang KL, Nichols BG, Poetker DM, et al. Odontogenic sinusitis: a case series studying diagnosis and management. Int Forum Allergy Rhinol 2015;5(7): 597–601.

24. Simuntis R, Vaitkus J, Kubilius R, et al. Comparison of sino-nasal outcome test 22 symptom scores in rhinogenic and odontogenic sinusitis. Am J Rhinol Allergy 2019;33(1):44–50.

25. Longhini AB, Ferguson BJ. Clinical aspects of odontogenic maxillary sinusitis: a case series. Int Forum Allergy Rhinol 2011;1(5):409–15.

26. Melan I, Lindahl L, Andresson L, et al. Chronic maxillary sinusitis definition, diagnosis and relation to dental infections and nasal polyposis. Acta Otolaryngol 1986;101:320–7.

27. Wuokko-Landen A, Blomgren K, Valimaa H. Acute rhinosinusitis—are we forgetting the possibility of a dental origin? A retrospective study of 385 patients. Acta Otolaryngol 2019;139(9):783–7.

28. Shahbazian M, Jacobs R. Diagnostic value of 2D and 3D imaging in odontogenic maxillary sinusitis: a review of literature. J Oral Rehabil 2012;39(4):294–300.

29. de Lima CO, Devito KL, Baraky Vasconcelos LR, et al. Correlation between endodontic infection and periodontal disease and their association with chronic sinusitis: a clinical-tomographic study. J Endod 2017;43(12):1978–83.

30. Khorramdel A, Shirmohammadi A, Sadighi A, et al. Association between demographic and radiographic characteristics of the Schneiderian membrane and periapical and periodontal diseases using cone-beam computed tomography scanning: a retrospective study. J Dent Res Dent Clin Dent Prospects 2017; 11(3):170–6.

31. Kende P, Mathai PC, Landge J, et al. Combined endoscopic and intra-oral approach for chronic maxillary sinusitis of dental origin—a prospective clinical study. Oral Maxillofac Surg 2019;23(4):429–37.

32. Tataryn R, Lewis M, Horalek AL, et al. Maxillary sinusitis of endodontic origin: AAE position statement. Chicago (IL): American Association of Endodontists; 2018. Available at: https://www.aae.org/specialty/wp-content/uploads/sites/2/2018/04/AAE_PositionStatement_MaxillarySinusitis.pdf.

33. Tomomatsu N, Uzawa N, Aragaki T, et al. Aperture width of the osteomeatal complex as a predictor of successful treatment of odontogenic maxillary sinusitis. Int J Oral Maxillofac Surg 2014;43(11):1386–90.

34. Zirk M, Dreiseidler T, Pohl M, et al. Odontogenic sinusitis maxillaris: a retrospective study of 121 cases with surgical intervention. J Craniomaxillofac Surg 2017; 45(4):520–5.

Management of Sinusitis in the Cystic Fibrosis Patient

Somtochi Okafor, BA, Kathleen M. Kelly, MD, Ashleigh A. Halderman, MD*

KEYWORDS

- Cystic fibrosis • Sinusitis • Chronic rhinosinusitis • Endoscopic sinus surgery
- Medical management

KEY POINTS

- Cystic fibrosis (CF) associated chronic rhinosinusitis (CRS) is a particularly recalcitrant form of CRS managed both medically and surgically.
- Medical management includes nasal saline rinses, corticosteroids, antibiotics, and mucolytics/surfactants, but the optimal approach to treating CF-associated CRS is not well defined and guidelines are lacking.
- Surgical management of CF-associated CRS differs from that of non-CF CRS in several respects, particularly with management of the maxillary sinus.

INTRODUCTION

Cystic fibrosis (CF) is the most common lethal genetic disease in Caucasians.[1] It is a result of mutations in the cystic fibrosis transmembrane conductance regulator (CFTR) gene causing defective anion (chloride and bicarbonate) transport across secretory epithelium. The consequence of this altered anion transport is abnormally viscous secretions in the airways and other organ systems up to 30 to 60 times more viscous than normal.[2] In the paranasal sinuses, these secretions obstruct sinus ostia, creating hypoxic conditions that lead to increased edema and secondary ciliary dyskinesia.[3,4] These factors, coupled with the marked disruption of normal mucociliary clearance (MCC), result in chronic bacterial infection.[3,4] The host inflammatory response elicited from chronic bacterial infection further damages the mucosa leading to goblet cell hyperplasia, squamous metaplasia, and loss of ciliated cells.[3] These pathologic changes account for the prevalence of chronic rhinosinusitis (CRS) in CF approaching 100%.[4]

CF-associated CRS (CF-CRS) is different from non–CF-associated CRS (non-CF CRS) in numerous ways. There is a high incidence of nasal polyps in CF-CRS ranging from 7% to 66% of patients, and these polyps can present in early childhood.[5]

Department of Otolaryngology–Head and Neck Surgery, University of Texas Southwestern Medical Center, 2001 Inwood Road, Dallas, TX 75390, USA
* Corresponding author.
E-mail address: ashleigh.halderman@utsouthwestern.edu

Immunol Allergy Clin N Am 40 (2020) 371–383
https://doi.org/10.1016/j.iac.2019.12.008   immunology.theclinics.com
0889-8561/20/© 2019 Elsevier Inc. All rights reserved.

Compared with non-CF CRS, the diseased sinonasal mucosa in CF typically demonstrates higher numbers of neutrophils, macrophages, and levels of interferon-γ and interleukin (IL)-8 consistent with helper T cell type 1 (Th-1) skewed inflammation.[6] By contrast, non-CF CRS with polyps exhibits a Th-2 type of inflammation hallmarked by elevated levels of eosinophils, IL-4, IL-5, and IL-10.[6] Significant differences also exist in the development of the paranasal sinuses. Radiographic findings common in CF-CRS include higher rates of hypoplastic maxillary sinuses, hypoplastic or aplastic frontal and sphenoid sinuses, and increased incidence of osteitis/bone sclerosis.[7,8] Mucocele formation is also more common in CF-CRS.[7]

Despite the prevalence of sinonasal involvement on radiographic imaging nearing 100% and the fact that most patients with CF fulfill criteria for CRS, only 10% to 15% of patients complain of sinonasal symptoms.[9–11] The reasons for this disconnect between prevalence and portion of CF patients presenting with complaints are unclear. CF patients with polyps tend to present with complaints of nasal obstruction compared with those without polyps who most commonly present with headaches.[4] Other symptoms of CRS include nasal obstruction, rhinorrhea, hyposmia/anosmia, and facial pain.[12]

Pulmonary decline is the most common cause of death in CF; therefore, treatment and interventions for pulmonary disease in these patients has been a major focal point in the literature. As the life expectancy of CF patients has steadily improved over time, largely attributable to advancements made in the treatment of CF lung disease, interest in nonlethal aspects of the disease including CRS has increased.[13] The management of CF-CRS is important for 2 particular reasons. The first is explained under the unified airway model, which views the entire respiratory system as a single functional unit, meaning the paranasal sinuses and lungs are uniformly affected by infectious and inflammatory insults.[14] In other words, diseases of the upper and lower airways affect one another. Support for this theory comes from numerous studies demonstrating high concordance rates between cultures from the sinonasal passages and from bronchoalveolar lavage both before and after lung transplant.[15–18] Also, there is evidence to suggest that CF-CRS may contribute to bacterial seeding of the lower airways, pulmonary decline, and allograft rejection in post-transplant patients.[11,15,19] Second, CF-CRS contributes to reductions in the quality of life (QoL) reported by CF patients. Although this pales in comparison to treatment and maintenance of pulmonary function, as survival of CF patients has steadily improved the focus in research and clinical care has begun to shift to include consideration of how aspects of CF affect QoL. Given that this has been a more recent change, the literature on management of CF-CRS is somewhat limited and specific guidelines are lacking. This review examines the current literature to provide an outline of the medical and surgical management of CF-CRS.

MEDICAL MANAGEMENT

Medical therapy represents the mainstay of management of CRS in patients with CF. Broadly speaking, medical management consists of nasal toilet accomplished through high-volume saline rinses and in-office debridements, topical and systemic anti-inflammatory medications and antimicrobials, surfactants, and mucolytics, and possibly the new class of medications known collectively as CF-targeted therapies. A review of each of these medical options follows.

Saline Irrigation

Intranasal saline irrigations serve as one of the mainstays of maintenance therapy. Irrigating with isotonic saline mechanically debrides the inspissated secretions and crusting common in CF.[2,20,21] Large-volume isotonic saline irrigation has been established as an effective therapy for improving symptoms and disease-specific QoL outcomes in patients with non-CF CRS.[22,23] Although various delivery mechanisms exist, the squeeze bottle and neti pot seem to provide the best delivery to the paranasal sinuses.[21] The delivery of topical saline into the sinuses is further improved with endoscopic sinus surgery (ESS).[24] Aside from the established efficacy of saline rinses, this has the additional benefits of low cost and a favorable side-effect profile. Saline rinses can further function as a vehicle by which higher concentrations of antibiotics and corticosteroids can be delivered topically to the sinuses.

Because hypertonic saline has been beneficial in the management of CF pulmonary disease, its use has been explored for the treatment of CF-CRS. In a randomized, double-blind controlled trial, Mainz and colleagues[25] investigated inhalation of hypertonic saline (6.0%) versus isotonic saline and found no significant differences between the 2 concentrations. Of importance is that hypertonic saline can be irritating to the sinonasal mucosa and is associated with a higher rate of adverse reactions that may affect compliance.[26,27] Given the lack of added benefit with an increased rate of adverse events, nasal saline irrigations with hypertonic saline are not recommended over isotonic saline.

CORTICOSTEROIDS

Systemic and/or topical steroids are popular adjunct treatments used in the management of non-CF CRS. Importantly, as already detailed, CF-CRS differs from non-CF CRS in that it demonstrates a neutrophil-predominated inflammatory response. Neutrophils are generally less responsive to steroids than are eosinophils.[20] Therefore, research on steroids in non-CF CRS serves as a poor proxy. To the authors' knowledge, there are no studies investigating the use of systemic steroids for treatment of CF-CRS. Given the potential for severe adverse events associated with systemic steroids, particularly in the CF population where pancreatic function is often compromised and diabetes is present, great care must be exercised in the use of this treatment approach for CF-CRS, particularly when no efficacy has been established.

Topical steroids provide effective treatment of allergic rhinitis and non-CF CRS.[28,29] Unlike systemic steroids, the use of topical steroids in CF-CRS has been studied. Several studies have demonstrated improvement in either nasal endoscopic or nasal polyp scores in CF-CRS with the use of topical intranasal steroids.[30–33] Interestingly, however, most of these studies failed to show a corresponding improvement in sinonasal symptoms.[30,31,33] Given the insignificant level of systemic absorption, favorable side-effect profile, and likely efficacy in improving endoscopic appearance and polyp size, topical intranasal steroids can be used in the treatment of CF-CRS, particularly when concomitant allergic rhinitis is present.

Mucolytics and Surfactants

Dornase alfa, a recombinant human deoxyribonuclease, hydrolyzes DNA fragments produced by neutrophil degradation in mucus of CF patients, thus resulting in decreased mucus viscosity and improvement in MCC.[34] Mainz and colleagues[35] performed a double-blind crossover study investigating the use of intranasal dornase alfa versus isotonic saline, which revealed that dornase alfa improved clinical symptoms and QoL as measured by the Sino-Nasal Outcome (SNOT-20) questionnaire to a significantly greater degree than saline. Shah and colleagues[34] conducted a systematic review of the use of intranasal dornase alfa for CF-CRS and concluded that intranasal dornase alfa seems to improve sinonasal symptoms to a greater degree than saline alone. Whereas the findings on symptoms were consistent throughout the systematic review, the impact of intranasal dornase alfa on pulmonary function, computed tomography (CT) scores, and endoscopy scores was variable, leading the investigators to conclude that a further study is necessary to further elucidate the true efficacy of intranasal dornase alfa in CF-CRS.[34] Unfortunately, the cost of this medication represents a significant barrier to widespread use.

Baby shampoo used in combination with isotonic saline irrigation has been suggested as a possible low-risk and inexpensive mucolytic.[9] Previous studies have observed symptomatic improvement in non-CF patients with CRS as well as in post-ESS patients using the combination of normal saline and baby shampoo in comparison with normal saline alone.[36,37] In the authors' experience, anecdotally the addition of baby shampoo to saline rinses seems to provide some benefit in CF-CRS patients with sinonasal crusting, particularly in the postoperative period after ESS. Ultimately, more studies are necessary to better define the effectiveness of baby shampoo in the CF population.

Antimicrobials

Systemic antibiotics are the standard treatment of both sinonasal and pulmonary exacerbations in CF. Depending on the severity of the exacerbation, this can be in either oral or intravenous (IV) form. In general, antibiotic treatment should cover common pathogens afflicting CF patients such as *Pseudomonas aeruginosa* and *Staphylococcus aureus*, and preferably the choice of antibiotic should be directed by culture when possible.[20] Of note, prophylactic antibiotic treatment is not commonly used in CF patients.[9]

Macrolide antibiotics, most notably azithromycin and clarithromycin, have garnered interest for use in CF given their ability to incite neutrophil chemotaxis, decrease mucus production, and inhibit cytokine release, thereby modulating the inflammatory response.[38] Azithromycin is a common maintenance drug in CF patients given its ability to reduce airway inflammation and decrease pulmonary deterioration.[20,39] In light of the pathophysiology behind CF-CRS, macrolides are an intriguing option for managing acute sinonasal exacerbations. However, specific studies analyzing the effects of macrolides on acute and CRS in CF patients must be conducted before strong recommendations can be made.

Topical antibiotics are another intriguing option for the management of CF-CRS given the low rate of systemic effects and ability to deliver higher concentrations directly to the infected sinuses.[40] Furthermore, several studies have established topical antibiotics to be efficacious in this patient population. A systematic review by Lim and colleagues[40] found level IIb evidence supporting the use of topical antibiotics in CF-CRS. Intranasal tobramycin has perhaps been the most well-studied antibiotic and has been associated with significant improvements in QoL, reduced *P aeruginosa* colonization of the sinuses, and improvement in sinus inflammation on serial MRI.[41,42] It is important that many of these studies investigated the use of topical antibiotics in patients who had undergone prior ESS given the significant improvement in delivery of topical medications to the sinuses after surgery. Topical antibiotics have also shown efficacy in the immediate postoperative period (see later discussion). Given the aforementioned, topical antibiotics represent an option in the treatment of CF-CRS, particularly in patients with prior ESS.

Cystic Fibrosis Transmembrane Conductance Regulator Modulator Therapies

With the advent of more advanced molecular genetic research, new therapies such as ivacaftor, resveratrol, and Orkambi (a combination of ivacaftor and lumacaftor) represent innovative treatments for CF. Ivacaftor is a CFTR potentiator used in patients with at least one copy of G551D or other mutations affecting channel gating.[43] Most studies surrounding ivacaftor have illustrated its positive effects on CF pulmonary lung disease with limited mention of its effects on CF-CRS.[2] However, in a multicenter prospective cohort study, McCormick and colleagues[44] revealed significant improvements in CF-related sinonasal QoL following treatment with ivacaftor.

The combination drug Orkambi, consisting of ivacaftor and lumacaftor, represents another CFTR-targeted therapy. Lumacaftor is a "corrector" and functions to correct folding defects that prevent transport of CFTR proteins to the apical cell surface.[9] The combination of ivacaftor and lumacaftor has shown improvement in forced expiratory volume in 1 second and reduction of pulmonary exacerbation, but the impact on CF-CRS has not yet been delineated.[38]

CFTR modulator therapies have shown tremendous promise in the treatment of the lower airways thus far. Under the unified airway model, one could theorize that the upper airways would benefit as well, but this remains to be established through clinical research.

SURGICAL MANAGEMENT
Patient Selection

In the absence of current consensus regarding indications for surgery in CF-CRS, ESS is often offered to those patients with persistent symptoms despite maximal medical therapy.[45–48] The term "maximal medical therapy" is further poorly defined and varies significantly in practice. In the current literature, most studies do not use set criteria for operative candidates, instead leaving decision-making up to the primary surgeon. In fact, most studies do not report individual selection criteria, instead citing failure of medical management, which as stated previously is poorly defined for this patient population.

Keck and Rozsasi[49] offered surgery to patients if they had persistent symptoms despite 6 weeks of local steroids. By contrast, Virgin and colleagues[50] required patients to have persistent symptoms despite a minimum of antibiotics for 2 weeks coupled with panmucosal sinus disease on CT scan. In other studies, sinonasal symptoms and pulmonary status were considered rather than endoscopic or CT findings.[51] As discussed next, ESS seems to improve sinonasal symptoms and QoL. Therefore, it is reasonable to offer surgery to patients with persistent sinonasal symptoms despite adequate medical care. The impact of surgery on pulmonary function tests (PFTs) and number of exacerbations is less clear; therefore, recommending surgery on declining lung function and increasing exacerbations is less well supported. Similar to non-CF CRS, surgery is indicated for disease recalcitrant to maximal medical therapy, mucocele(s), impending complications from acute sinusitis, and fungal sinusitis.

Surgical Approach

The goal of ESS in CF patients is to provide large cavities to facilitate nasal hygiene, drug delivery, and endoscopic debridement in the clinic given CF-associated impaired MCC and tenacious secretions. In general, more aggressive surgical procedures are used in the CF population in an effort to improve effectiveness of nasal irrigations (and thus the delivery of topical medications), allow for better debridements in the office, achieve better control of sinonasal bacteria, and decrease the rate of revision surgery.[15,50,52,53]

Management of the maxillary sinus is of particular interest in CF patients. Owing to the position of the natural os, drainage of this sinus is against gravity and is therefore significantly affected in CF. In this patient population, the maxillary sinus serves as a reservoir for chronic infections of the sinuses and possibly the lungs.[54] Given these factors, many advocate for the creation of gravity-dependent drainage pathways via more extensive maxillary antrostomies. Two extended procedures frequently used in CF patients to achieve gravity-dependent drainage are the endoscopic megamaxillary antrostomy (EMMA) and the modified endoscopic medial maxillectomy (MEMM).

EMMA involves removing the posterior half of the inferior turbinate and extending the antrostomy to the floor of the nose. This technique is thought to facilitate gravity-dependent drainage and maximum delivery of saline and topical medications as well as providing access for clinic-based debridements.[23,55] EMMA has been established as a safe and effective method for managing recalcitrant maxillary sinusitis in CF patients, with improvement in QoL and sinonasal symptoms, and reduction in the frequency of hospitalizations and the need for IV antibiotics.[53]

By contrast, MEMM consists of removing the medial maxillary wall down to or beyond the nasal floor with removal of the posterior two-thirds of the inferior turbinate, thus marsupializing the maxillary sinus into the nasal cavity. MEMM has been shown to improve effectiveness of nasal irrigations and thus the delivery of topical medications, increase accessibility for debridement in clinic, improve sinonasal symptom scores, and reduce the frequency of hospital admissions and the need for IV antibiotics.[50,53,56]

The ethmoid sinuses are also frequently addressed along with the maxillary, especially if polyps are present. CF patients show a high rate of osteitis throughout the sinuses as well as aplasia or hypoplasia of the frontal and sphenoid sinuses.[7,57] Therefore, review of preoperative CT scans is of great importance for surgical planning. If the sphenoid sinuses have significant disease, methods such as posterior septectomy and removal of the intrasinus septum or nasalization of the sinus may be considered to create the largest sphenoidotomy possible. For the frontal sinuses, if the patient's anatomy is amenable, a modified endoscopic Lothrop procedure may be considered for particularly recalcitrant frontal sinus disease or when complete stenosis of the frontal outflow tract has occurred.[58]

Perioperative Antibiotics

CF patients undergoing ESS often receive additional preoperative or postoperative antibiotic therapy beyond their typical maintenance regimens. Preoperative antibiotic regimens vary greatly between institutions, with some advocating preoperative treatment either as prophylaxis or directed by sputum culture.[59,60] Others have used antibiotics only postoperatively, based on cultures taken at the time of surgery.[50,51]

The use of antibiotics postoperatively is perhaps the most well studied, and the literature has shown benefits of antibiotics in this setting. Aanaes and colleagues[61] treated post-ESS patients with 2 weeks of IV antibiotics directed at colonizing bacteria in addition to 6 months of colistin nasal irrigations and 12 months of topical nasal steroids. Following this regimen, the investigators demonstrated eradication of pathogenic bacteria in 67% of study patients at 6 months postoperatively.[61] In a study by Virgin and colleagues,[50] a postoperative regimen of 3 weeks of culture-directed antibiotics, 3 to 8 weeks of oral prednisone, and saline rinses twice daily with the addition of both a topical steroid and antibiotic after the cavities were healed for the remainder of the study resulted in significant improvements in SNOT-22 scores and Lund-Kennedy endoscopic scores, and a decreased number of admissions for pulmonary exacerbations for 12 months after surgery. Both of these studies are examples of intensive medical management following surgery with impressive results.

Adding a significant number of components to an already exhaustive medical regimen that may take several hours each day can affect the QoL and compliance of CF patients. Therefore, it is interesting that Vital and colleagues[15] showed that a regimen consisting only of twice-daily isotonic nasal saline douches after ESS in patients after lung transplantation resulted in eradication of *Pseudomonas* in the sinuses and lungs in 35%, and eradication from the lungs in 62%.

At present there are no guidelines, recommendations, or "gold standards" for perioperative antibiotics in CF patients undergoing sinus surgery. Given the limited number of studies and significant variation of preoperative and postoperative regimens described, further research is needed to better elucidate the most optimal approach.

Postoperative Irrigation

Nasal saline irrigations following sinus surgery have been associated with better healing and decreased rates of scarring/synechiae and ostial stenosis.[62] Most studies in the current literature used saline irrigations as standard postoperative management starting 24 to 48 hours after surgery.[19,50,60,61,63] Addition of antibiotics and/or steroids to saline irrigations is another popular adjunctive therapy for patients with CF after ESS.[50,61,64] As stated earlier, studies using topical antibiotic and steroid rinses as part of a post-ESS regimen have shown high rates of eradication of pathogenic bacteria in the sinuses and lungs, significant improvements in symptoms and endoscopy scores, reduced number of hospitalizations from pulmonary exacerbations, and even a reduction in revision or salvage surgeries.[50,61,64]

Postoperative Debridements

It is well established that post-ESS debridements reduce the incidence of scarring/synechiae and ostial stenosis, and in general promote better healing, and most studies advocate for in-office debridements as an important element of disease maintenance.[49,50,61,62] Similar to perioperative antibiotics, no guidelines or recommendations for the timeline or number of postoperative debridements following ESS exist, and there is considerable variability in the current literature. It is the authors' experience that because of chronic inflammation, infection, and mucostasis, patients with CF demonstrate a propensity for scarring and crusting; hence, regular in-office debridements are performed on a weekly or every-other-week basis for a variable amount of time after ESS. Close follow-up is often necessary in these patients for a month or more after ESS to ensure that ostial stenosis is not occurring and to remove crusts that could lead to scarring or postobstructive disease and infection.

Impact of Surgery

Often, otolaryngologists are encouraged by pulmonary and transplant teams to perform ESS on patients who are experiencing an increased number of pulmonary exacerbations or declining pulmonary function. Following lung transplant, otolaryngologists are often consulted to perform sinus surgery out of concerns the sinuses will "seed" the lower airways. However, the impact of ESS on factors including the number of pulmonary exacerbations/hospitalizations/need for IV antibiotics, PFTs, and bacterial colonization of the lower airways is poorly understood and the literature has shown conflicting results. Studies have, however, consistently shown that ESS for CF patients improves QoL and decreases sinonasal symptoms while also often improving endoscopic scores.[65–67] Therefore, it is reasonable to counsel patients that they can anticipate improvements in these parameters after surgery.

Based on the current literature, no conclusions can be drawn on the impact of ESS on number of and/or length of hospitalizations or the need for antibiotics, as the studies have shown mixed results.[59,66–69] The same can be said for the impact of ESS on the need for antibiotics.[59,68,69] Regarding PFTs, a meta-analysis and a separate systematic review both failed to show significant improvements in lung function after ESS.[66,67] Additional studies not included in either the meta-analysis or systematic review also failed to show improvement in PFTs.[65,68,70] The lack of clear improvement in lung function after ESS is intriguing, especially in light of the finding of Ayoub and colleagues[65] that decline in pulmonary function may disproportionally contribute to the decision to perform ESS.

One reason why the literature has shown such conflicting results is that the severity and impact of the disease can differ significantly between CF patients. Advancements in understanding the molecular and functional impact of various mutations to the CFTR protein has led to the classification of CF patients as high-risk and low-risk based on genotype. A patient's genotype has been shown to correlate with age at diagnosis, mortality, pancreatic function, and burden of radiographic sinus disease.[57,71–75] Furthermore, there is emerging evidence that patients may respond differently to interventions depending on the severity of their disease.[59,76] Clearly this remains an area for which ongoing research is necessary.

Another aspect for which the literature has demonstrated inconsistent results is in the ability of ESS to alter the microbiome or bacterial burden in the lungs. One particular area where this is of significant interest is the lung transplant population. Chronic sinonasal bacterial colonization has been proposed as a contributing factor to the development of bronchiolitis obliterans or allograft rejection.[61] It has therefore been postulated that ESS in combination with routine nasal medical management may reduce the risk of bacterial colonization of transplanted lungs.[19,77] However, some studies have shown no difference in recolonization rates after ESS in patients after lung transplantation, and the efficacy of prophylactic ESS in post-transplant patients is a matter of debate.[78]

Even after surgical intervention, relapse rates in this patient population are quoted as high as 50% in the first 1.5 to 2 years, and 46% to 100% after 2 to 4 years.[41,79] Similar to non-CF CRS, factors such a severity of polyps on initial presentation are significantly more likely to require revision ESS.[51] Other risk factors for relapse or recurrence include incomplete surgery and suboptimal adjunctive antibiotic therapy.[35,80]

SUMMARY

CF-CRS represents one of the more recalcitrant forms of CRS. The potential impact of CF-CRS on the lower airways and overall well-being of CF patients could be significant, but to date is not well defined. Both medical and surgical management play critical roles in the management of CF-CRS, but guidelines defining best practice are lacking. With the advent of CFTR modulator therapies, the understanding, management, and possibly even the epidemiology of CF-CRS will continue to evolve. Therefore, now more than ever, high-level research focusing on the treatment of CRS in this patient population is critical.

DISCLOSURE

The authors have nothing to disclose.

REFERENCES

1. Grosse SD, Boyle CA, Botkin JR, et al. Newborn screening for cystic fibrosis: evaluation of benefits and risks and recommendations for state newborn screening programs. MMWR Recomm Rep 2004;53(RR-13):1–36.
2. Chaaban MR, Kejner A, Rowe SM, et al. Cystic fibrosis chronic rhinosinusitis: a comprehensive review. Am J Rhinol Allergy 2013;27(5):387–95.
3. Gysin C, Alothman GA, Papsin BC. Sinonasal disease in cystic fibrosis: clinical characteristics, diagnosis, and management. Pediatr Pulmonol 2000;30(6):481–9.

4. Gentile VG, Isaacson G. Patterns of sinusitis in cystic fibrosis. Laryngoscope 1996;106(8):1005–9.

5. Farrell PM, Rosenstein BJ, White TB, et al. Guidelines for diagnosis of cystic fibrosis in newborns through older adults: cystic fibrosis foundation consensus report. J Pediatr 2008;153(2):S4–14.

6. Sobol SE, Christodoulopoulos P, Manoukian JJ, et al. Cytokine profile of chronic sinusitis in patients with cystic fibrosis. Arch Otolaryngol Head Neck Surg 2002; 128(11):1295–8.

7. Orlandi RR, Wiggins RH 3rd. Radiological sinonasal findings in adults with cystic fibrosis. Am J Rhinol Allergy 2009;23(3):307–11.

8. Kang SH, Piltcher OB, de Tarso Roth Dalcin P. Sinonasal alterations in computed tomography scans in cystic fibrosis: a literature review of observational studies. Int Forum Allergy Rhinol 2014;4(3):223–31.

9. Hamilos DL. Chronic rhinosinusitis in patients with cystic fibrosis. J Allergy Clin Immunol Pract 2016;4(4):605–12.

10. Fokkens WJ, Lund VJ, Mullol J, et al. European position paper on rhinosinusitis and nasal polyps 2012. Rhinol Suppl 2012;23. 3 p preceding table of contents, 1-298.

11. Aanaes K. Bacterial sinusitis can be a focus for initial lung colonisation and chronic lung infection in patients with cystic fibrosis. J Cyst Fibros 2013; 12(Suppl 2):S1–20.

12. Rosenfeld RM, Piccirillo JF, Chandrasekhar SS, et al. Clinical practice guideline (update): adult sinusitis executive summary. Otolaryngol Head Neck Surg 2015;152(4):598–609.

13. Hurley MN, McKeever TM, Prayle AP, et al. Rate of improvement of CF life expectancy exceeds that of general population—observational death registration study. J Cyst Fibros 2014;13(4):410–5.

14. Krouse JH, Brown RW, Fineman SM, et al. Asthma and the unified airway. Otolaryngol Head Neck Surg 2007;136(5 Suppl):S75–106.

15. Vital D, Hofer M, Boehler A, et al. Posttransplant sinus surgery in lung transplant recipients with cystic fibrosis: a single institutional experience. Eur Arch Otorhinolaryngol 2013;270(1):135–9.

16. Roby BB, McNamara J, Finkelstein M, et al. Sinus surgery in cystic fibrosis patients: comparison of sinus and lower airway cultures. Int J Pediatr Otorhinolaryngol 2008;72(9):1365–9.

17. Mainz JG, Naehrlich L, Schien M, et al. Concordant genotype of upper and lower airways P aeruginosa and S aureus isolates in cystic fibrosis. Thorax 2009;64(6): 535–40.

18. Ciofu O, Johansen HK, Aanaes K, et al. P. aeruginosa in the paranasal sinuses and transplanted lungs have similar adaptive mutations as isolates from chronically infected CF lungs. J Cyst Fibros 2013;12(6):729–36.

19. Holzmann D, Speich R, Kaufmann T, et al. Effects of sinus surgery in patients with cystic fibrosis after lung transplantation: a 10-year experience. Transplantation 2004;77(1):134–6.

20. Mainz JG, Koitschev A. Management of chronic rhinosinusitis in CF. J Cyst Fibros 2009;8(Suppl 1):S10–4.

21. Illing EA, Woodworth BA. Management of the upper airway in cystic fibrosis. Curr Opin Pulm Med 2014;20(6):623–31.

22. Chong LY, Head K, Hopkins C, et al. Saline irrigation for chronic rhinosinusitis. Cochrane Database Syst Rev 2016;(4):CD011995.

23. Rudmik L, Hoy M, Schlosser RJ, et al. Topical therapies in the management of chronic rhinosinusitis: an evidence-based review with recommendations. Int Forum Allergy Rhinol 2013;3(4):281–98.
24. Harvey RJ, Goddard JC, Wise SK, et al. Effects of endoscopic sinus surgery and delivery device on cadaver sinus irrigation. Otolaryngol Head Neck Surg 2008; 139(1):137–42.
25. Mainz JG, Schumacher U, Schädlich K, et al. Sino nasal inhalation of isotonic versus hypertonic saline (6.0%) in CF patients with chronic rhinosinusitis—results of a multicenter, prospective, randomized, double-blind, controlled trial. J Cyst Fibros 2016;15(6):e57–66.
26. Elkins MR, Robinson M, Rose BR, et al. A controlled trial of long-term inhaled hypertonic saline in patients with cystic fibrosis. N Engl J Med 2006;354(3):229–40.
27. Donaldson SH, Bennett WD, Zeman KL, et al. Mucus clearance and lung function in cystic fibrosis with hypertonic saline. N Engl J Med 2006;354(3):241–50.
28. Wise SK, Lin SY, Toskala E, et al. International consensus statement on allergy and rhinology: allergic rhinitis. Int Forum Allergy Rhinol 2018;8(2):108–352.
29. Orlandi RR, Kingdom TT, Hwang PH. International consensus statement on allergy and rhinology: rhinosinusitis. Int Forum Allergy Rhinol 2016;6(Suppl 1): S22–209.
30. Zemke AC, Nouraie SM, Moore J, et al. Clinical predictors of cystic fibrosis chronic rhinosinusitis severity. Int Forum Allergy Rhinol 2019;9(7):759–65.
31. Hadfield PJ, Rowe-Jones JM, Mackay IS. A prospective treatment trial of nasal polyps in adults with cystic fibrosis. Rhinology 2000;38(2):63–5.
32. Donaldson JD, Gillespie CT. Observations on the efficacy of intranasal beclomethasone dipropionate in cystic fibrosis patients. J Otolaryngol 1988;17(1):43–5.
33. Costantini D, Di Cicco M, Giunta A, et al. Nasal polyposis in cystic fibrosis treated by beclomethasone dipropionate. Acta Univ Carol Med (Praha) 1990;36(1–4): 220–1.
34. Shah GB, De Keyzer L, Russell JA, et al. Treatment of chronic rhinosinusitis with dornase alfa in patients with cystic fibrosis: a systematic review. Int Forum Allergy Rhinol 2018;8(6):729–36.
35. Mainz JG, Schien C, Schiller I, et al. Sinonasal inhalation of dornase alfa administered by vibrating aerosol to cystic fibrosis patients: a double-blind placebo-controlled cross-over trial. J Cyst Fibros 2014;13(4):461–70.
36. Chiu AG, Palmer JN, Woodworth BA, et al. Baby shampoo nasal irrigations for the symptomatic post-functional endoscopic sinus surgery patient. Am J Rhinol 2008;22(1):34–7.
37. Isaacs S, Fakhri S, Luong A, et al. The effect of dilute baby shampoo on nasal mucociliary clearance in healthy subjects. Am J Rhinol Allergy 2011;25(1):e27–9.
38. Tipirneni KE, Woodworth BA. Medical and surgical advancements in the management of cystic fibrosis chronic rhinosinusitis. Curr Otorhinolaryngol Rep 2017;5(1):24–34.
39. Jaffe A, Francis J, Rosenthal M, et al. Long-term azithromycin may improve lung function in children with cystic fibrosis. Lancet 1998;351(9100):420.
40. Lim M, Citardi MJ, Leong JL. Topical antimicrobials in the management of chronic rhinosinusitis: a systematic review. Am J Rhinol 2008;22(4):381–9.
41. Mainz JG, Schaedlich K, Schien C, et al. Sinonasal inhalation of tobramycin vibrating aerosol in cystic fibrosis patients with upper airway *Pseudomonas aeruginosa* colonization: results of a randomized, double-blind, placebo-controlled pilot study. Drug Des Devel Ther 2014;8:209–17.

42. Graham SM, Launspach JL, Welsh MJ, et al. Sequential magnetic resonance imaging analysis of the maxillary sinuses: implications for a model of gene therapy in cystic fibrosis. J Laryngol Otol 1999;113(4):329–35.
43. Cho DY, Zhang S, Lazrak A, et al. Resveratrol and ivacaftor are additive G551D CFTR-channel potentiators: therapeutic implications for cystic fibrosis sinus disease. Int Forum Allergy Rhinol 2019;9(1):100–5.
44. McCormick J, Cho DY, Lampkin B, et al. Ivacaftor improves rhinologic, psychologic, and sleep-related quality of life in G551D cystic fibrosis patients. Int Forum Allergy Rhinol 2019;9(3):292–7.
45. Bhattacharyya N. Clinical outcomes after endoscopic sinus surgery. Curr Opin Allergy Clin Immunol 2006;6(3):167–71.
46. Ikeda K, Oshima T, Furukawa M, et al. Restoration of the mucociliary clearance of the maxillary sinus after endoscopic sinus surgery. J Allergy Clin Immunol 1997; 99(1 Pt 1):48–52.
47. Ikeda K, Tamura G, Shimomura A, et al. Endoscopic sinus surgery improves pulmonary function in patients with asthma associated with chronic sinusitis. Ann Otol Rhinol Laryngol 1999;108(4):355–9.
48. Poetker DM, Smith TL. Adult chronic rhinosinusitis: surgical outcomes and the role of endoscopic sinus surgery. Curr Opin Otolaryngol Head Neck Surg 2007;15(1):6–9.
49. Keck T, Rozsasi A. Medium-term symptom outcomes after paranasal sinus surgery in children and young adults with cystic fibrosis. Laryngoscope 2007; 117(3):475–9.
50. Virgin FW, Rowe SM, Wade MB, et al. Extensive surgical and comprehensive postoperative medical management for cystic fibrosis chronic rhinosinusitis. Am J Rhinol Allergy 2012;26(1):70–5.
51. Rickert S, Banuchi VE, Germana JD, et al. Cystic fibrosis and endoscopic sinus surgery: relationship between nasal polyposis and likelihood of revision endoscopic sinus surgery in patients with cystic fibrosis. Arch Otolaryngol Head Neck Surg 2010;136(10):988–92.
52. Batra PS, Kern RC, Tripathi A, et al. Outcome analysis of endoscopic sinus surgery in patients with nasal polyps and asthma. Laryngoscope 2003;113(10): 1703–6.
53. Crockett DJ, Wilson KF, Meier JD. Perioperative strategies to improve sinus surgery outcomes in patients with cystic fibrosis: a systematic review. Otolaryngol Head Neck Surg 2013;149(1):30–9.
54. Woodworth BA, Ahn C, Flume PA, et al. The delta F508 mutation in cystic fibrosis and impact on sinus development. Am J Rhinol 2007;21(1):122–7.
55. Thomas WW 3rd, Harvey RJ, Rudmik L, et al. Distribution of topical agents to the paranasal sinuses: an evidence-based review with recommendations. Int Forum Allergy Rhinol 2013;3(9):691–703.
56. Zheng Z, Safi C, Gudis DA. Surgical management of chronic rhinosinusitis in cystic fibrosis. Med Sci (Basel) 2019;7(4) [pii:E57].
57. Halderman AA, Lee S, London NR, et al. Impact of high- versus low-risk genotype on sinonasal radiographic disease in cystic fibrosis. Laryngoscope 2019;129(4): 788–93.
58. Jaberoo MC, Pulido MA, Saleh HA. Modified Lothrop procedure in cystic fibrosis patients: does it have a role? J Laryngol Otol 2013;127(7):666–9.
59. Khalfoun S, Tumin D, Ghossein M, et al. Improved lung function after sinus surgery in cystic fibrosis patients with moderate obstruction. Otolaryngol Head Neck Surg 2018;158(2):381–5.

60. Luparello P, Lazio MS, Voltolini L, et al. Outcomes of endoscopic sinus surgery in adult lung transplant patients with cystic fibrosis. Eur Arch Otorhinolaryngol 2019; 276(5):1341–7.
61. Aanaes K, von Buchwald C, Hjuler T, et al. The effect of sinus surgery with intensive follow-up on pathogenic sinus bacteria in patients with cystic fibrosis. Am J Rhinol Allergy 2013;27(1):e1–4.
62. Rudmik L, Soler ZM, Orlandi RR, et al. Early postoperative care following endoscopic sinus surgery: an evidence-based review with recommendations. Int Forum Allergy Rhinol 2011;1(6):417–30.
63. Fuchsmann C, Ayari S, Reix P, et al. Contribution of CT-assisted navigation and microdebriders to endoscopic sinus surgery in cystic fibrosis. Int J Pediatr Otorhinolaryngol 2008;72(3):343–9.
64. Moss RB, King VV. Management of sinusitis in cystic fibrosis by endoscopic surgery and serial antimicrobial lavage. Reduction in recurrence requiring surgery. Arch Otolaryngol Head Neck Surg 1995;121(5):566–72.
65. Ayoub N, Thamboo A, Habib A-R, et al. Determinants and outcomes of upfront surgery versus medical therapy for chronic rhinosinusitis in cystic fibrosis. Int Forum Allergy Rhinol 2017;7(5):450–8.
66. Liang J, Higgins TS, Ishman SL, et al. Surgical management of chronic rhinosinusitis in cystic fibrosis: a systematic review. Int Forum Allergy Rhinol 2013;3(10): 814–22.
67. Macdonald KI, Gipsman A, Magit A, et al. Endoscopic sinus surgery in patients with cystic fibrosis: a systematic review and meta-analysis of pulmonary function. Rhinology 2012;50(4):360–9.
68. Henriquez OA, Wolfenden LL, Stecenko A, et al. Endoscopic sinus surgery in adults with cystic fibrosis: effect on lung function, intravenous antibiotic use, and hospitalization. Arch Otolaryngol Head Neck Surg 2012;138(12):1167–70.
69. Kempainen RR, Sajan JA, Pylkas AM, et al. Effect of endoscopic sinus surgery on pulmonary status of adults with cystic fibrosis. Otolaryngol Head Neck Surg 2012;147(3):557–62.
70. Abuzeid WM, Song C, Fastenberg JH, et al. Correlations between cystic fibrosis genotype and sinus disease severity in chronic rhinosinusitis. Laryngoscope 2018;128(8):1752–8.
71. McKone EF, Goss CH, Aitken ML. CFTR genotype as a predictor of prognosis in cystic fibrosis. Chest 2006;130(5):1441–7.
72. McKone EF, Emerson SS, Edwards KL, et al. Effect of genotype on phenotype and mortality in cystic fibrosis: a retrospective cohort study. Lancet 2003; 361(9370):1671–6.
73. Ferril GR, Nick JA, Getz AE, et al. Comparison of radiographic and clinical characteristics of low-risk and high-risk cystic fibrosis genotypes. Int Forum Allergy Rhinol 2014;4(11):915–20.
74. Castellani C, Cuppens H, Macek M, et al. Consensus on the use and interpretation of cystic fibrosis mutation analysis in clinical practice. J Cyst Fibros 2008; 7(3):179–96.
75. Berkhout MC, van Rooden CJ, Rijntjes E, et al. Sinonasal manifestations of cystic fibrosis: a correlation between genotype and phenotype? J Cyst Fibros 2014; 13(4):442–8.
76. Halderman AA, West N, Benke J, et al. F508del genotype in endoscopic sinus surgery: do differences in outcomes exist between genotypic subgroups? Int Forum Allergy Rhinol 2017;7(5):459–66.

77. Hofer M, Benden C, Inci I, et al. True survival benefit of lung transplantation for cystic fibrosis patients: the Zurich experience. J Heart Lung Transplant 2009; 28(4):334–9.
78. Leung MK, Rachakonda L, Weill D, et al. Effects of sinus surgery on lung transplantation outcomes in cystic fibrosis. Am J Rhinol 2008;22(2):192–6.
79. Rowe-Jones JM, Mackay IS. Endoscopic sinus surgery in the treatment of cystic fibrosis with nasal polyposis. Laryngoscope 1996;106(12 Pt 1):1540–4.
80. Davidson TM, Murphy C, Mitchell M, et al. Management of chronic sinusitis in cystic fibrosis. Laryngoscope 1995;105(4 Pt 1):354–8.

Moving?

Make sure your subscription moves with you!

To notify us of your new address, find your **Clinics Account Number** (located on your mailing label above your name), and contact customer service at:

Email: journalscustomerservice-usa@elsevier.com

800-654-2452 (subscribers in the U.S. & Canada)
314-447-8871 (subscribers outside of the U.S. & Canada)

Fax number: 314-447-8029

Elsevier Health Sciences Division
Subscription Customer Service
3251 Riverport Lane
Maryland Heights, MO 63043

*To ensure uninterrupted delivery of your subscription, please notify us at least 4 weeks in advance of move.

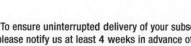
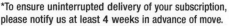

ELSEVIER

Moving?

Make sure your subscription moves with you!

To notify us of your new address, find your Clinics Account Number (located on your mailing label above your name) and contact customer service at:

Email: journalscustomerservice-usa@elsevier.com

800-654-2452 (subscribers in the U.S. & Canada)
314-447-8871 (subscribers outside of the U.S. & Canada)

Fax number: 314-447-8029

Elsevier Health Sciences Division
Subscription Customer Service
3251 Riverport Lane
Maryland Heights, MO 63043

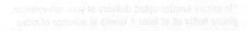

Printed and bound by CPI Group (UK) Ltd, Croydon, CR0 4YY

21/10/2024

01777184-0001